PRINCIPLES AND PRACTICE OF

High Dependency Nursing

For Baillière Tindall:

Commissioning Editor: Alex Mathieson, Ninette Premdas
Project Development Manager: Mairi McCubbin
Project Manager: Derek Robertson
Designer: Judith Wright, George Ajayi

PRINCIPLES AND PRACTICE OF
High Dependency Nursing

Edited by

Mandy Sheppard

RN ENB100
Training and Development Consultant, Kent, UK

Mike Wright

MBA RN DMS CHSM ENB100
Directorate Manager and Head of Nursing - Anaesthesia and Theatre Services,
Guy's and St Thomas' Hospital Trust, London, UK

Foreword by

Ruth Endacott

MA PhD RGN DipN(Lond) RNT
Independent Adviser and Researcher in Critical Care Nursing,
Crediton, UK

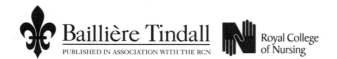

Baillière Tindall
PUBLISHED IN ASSOCIATION WITH THE RCN

Royal College
of Nursing

EDINBURGH LONDON NEW YORK PHILADELPHIA ST LOUIS SYDNEY TORONTO 2000

BAILLIÈRE TINDALL
An imprint of Harcourt Publishers Limited

First published 2000

ISBN 0 7020 2117 2

British Library Cataloguing in Publication Data
A catalogue record for this book is available from the British Library

Library of Congress Cataloging in Publication Data
A catalog record for this book is available from the Library of Congress

Note
Medical knowledge is constantly changing. As new information becomes
available, changes in treatment, procedures, equipment and the use of drugs
become necessary. The editors and contributors and the publishers have, as
far as it is possible, taken care to ensure that the information given in this
text is accurate and up-to-date. However, readers are strongly advised to
confirm that the information, especially with regard to drug usage, complies
with the latest legislation and standards of practice.

The
publisher's
policy is to use
**paper manufactured
from sustainable forests**

Printed in China
EPC/01

Contents

Contributors

Helena Baxter BSc(Hons) MSc RGN
Clinical Nurse Specialist, Tissue Viability, Guy's and St Thomas' Hospital Trust, London

11   Pain management

Heather Carroll BA(Hons) MSc CertEd RGN RNT ENB136
Freelance Lecturer, Bristol, UK

10   Fluid and electrolytes

Andrew Cook BSc(Hons) RGN ENB199, 998
A & E Senior Nurse Manager, East Surrey Hospital – Surrey and Sussex Healthcare NHS Trust, Redhill, UK

9   Medical emergencies

Nigel Davies BSc MSc CertEd RGN ENB254
Senior Lecturer/Clinical Practitioner, Faculty of Health, South Bank University, London, UK

6   Cardiac care

Deborah Dawson BSc(Hons) RGN ENB100
Directorate Nurse Manager, Critical Care and Support Services, Royal Sussex County Hospital, Brighton, UK

7   Neurological care

Debbie Field BSc(Hons) MSc DipNurs ENB249 RGN
Clinical Research Fellow, Academic Anaesthetic Department, Division of Anaesthesia, Middlesex and University College Hospitals, London, UK

5   Respiratory care

Paul Mulligan BSc RGN DipNurs(Lond)
Senior Resuscitation Officer, Resuscitation Training Department, Guy's and St Thomas' Hospital Trust, London, UK

4   Social issues in high dependency care

Jo Norman RN
Formerly Senior Nurse, Accident and Emergency Department, Bromley Hospital NHS Trust, Bromley, UK

9   Medical emergencies

Mandy Sheppard RN ENB100
Training and Development Consultant, Kent, UK

1   *The development, role and function of high dependency care*

John Allen Wilkinson BSc(Hons) MSc RGN RMN DipN DipEd ENB100
Head of Continuing Professional Development, School of Health Studies,
Homerton College Cambridge, Addenbrooke's Hospital, Cambridge, UK

3   *Interpersonal issues in high dependency care*

Mike Wright MBA RN DMS CHSM ENB100
Directorate Manager and Head of Nursing - Anaesthesia and Theatre Services,
Guy's and St Thomas' Hospital Trust, London, UK

2   *The management of high dependency care*

Guy Young RN ENB100
Senior Nurse, Clinical Development, Anaesthesia and Theatre Services, Guy's and
St Thomas' Hospital Trust, London, UK

8   *Post-anaesthetic and post-operative care*

Foreword

The health service has seen many changes during the past decade, not just in the configuration of services and the roles of clinicians, but also in the expectations of the public. This is particularly evident in the provision of care for patients who are, or are at risk of becoming, seriously ill. These changes take various forms: the development of 'patient at risk' or 'medical emergency' teams, the increase in high dependency facilities and the media interest in problems with bed availability.

At the time of writing this foreword, high dependency care is high on the agenda of policy makers and clinicians. Intensive care is beset with problems of closed beds, nurse recruitment and debates about the appropriateness of intensive care for certain patients (for example, those who are too sick or too well to benefit). At the same time studies are highlighting delays in identifying ward patients who would benefit from intensive care. It is suggested that one possible solution to these problems is the establishment of more high dependency facilities. However, whilst the number of high dependency facilities is increasing, there is also a call for more evidence regarding the benefits they bring.

Aside from these debates, the number of highly dependent patients is increasing in both hospital and community settings. Hence many of the nurses (and midwives) who will be managing these patients will not be working in formal high dependency units, but will be caring for these patients in more general ward and other settings. This broadening of the scope of high dependency care is reflected in the Department of Health 1996 *Guidelines for Admission to and Discharge from Intensive Care and High Dependency Units* where high dependency is defined as a level of care, not a location. Developing a text that addresses the diversity of the high dependency patient population is a considerable challenge. Sheppard and Wright and their co-authors have met this challenge admirably and provide us with a text which more than meets those requirements.

Definitions of high dependency care emphasise the intensity of nursing required. High dependency nursing care is often provided without the back-up of technology-intensive units, and the sophisticated monitoring equipment that goes with them. In this situation, the patient is even more reliant on the eyes, ears and touch of the nurse to detect changes in his condition. Perhaps more crucially, the high dependency patient is looking to the nurse to provide the level of confidence that comes with skilled practice, combined with an understanding of the patient's many anxieties about what may be happening to him. Providing this level of nursing intensity can have an impact on the practitioner. The complex fluid and drug management, constant observation, assessment and reassurance required by a patient who is 'on the brink', place an enormous responsibility on the nurse. Where high dependency care is provided outside designated areas, this responsibility is often enhanced by difficulties in accessing medical expertise at the appropriate time. This text provides the reader with a wealth of insight into both clinical and professional dimensions of high dependency care, incorporating central issues such as stress and communication.

In many settings, high dependency nursing encompasses the use of varying degrees of technology to provide an on-going picture of the patient's physiological status and enable timely interventions to prevent further deterioration. The use of such technology is addressed within the scope of this text and should provide a bedrock for nursing knowledge in this field. However, the authors rightly place firm emphasis on the non-invasive assessment skills used by nurses.

It is important to balance the emphasis on nursing skills and responsibilities with an appreciation of the wider context of high dependency care. Establishing a high dependency service (not necessarily in a high dependency area) requires more than just the right number of nurses; it requires the appropriate equipment, education, support services and medical expertise in order to anticipate and respond to the patient's changing needs. Similarly, the nursing role in high dependency care involves more than direct care giving. The nurse is usually the central point of contact and will co-ordinate the activities of, for example, the doctors. This role is of particular importance with high dependency patients who may have more than one team of doctors involved in their care.

Given this complex situation in which high dependency care is provided, the need for a text such as this is evident. Moreover, Sheppard and Wright have achieved a balance between the organisational and clinical aspects of high dependency care, with each chapter providing working examples from practice. The breadth and depth of topics addressed in the book reflect the scope of high dependency nursing and should also enable a greater understanding of the political aspects of high dependency care. It is increasingly important for nurses to understand this political context in order to influence policy decisions at local, regional and national level.

This text will be invaluable for qualified nurses and midwives working in a variety of settings and for students of nursing and midwifery.

Ruth Endacott

Preface

Most nurses, either during training or subsequently in their careers, will be involved in the care of patients who require that little bit extra: patients whose condition sets them apart from the general ward population, yet does not warrant admission to an intensive care unit; patients who need closer observation, monitoring and, if necessary, rapid and coordinated intervention.

Most nurses will care for a highly dependent patient at some stage. High dependency care is by no means a new phenomenon but what has changed in recent times is the professional and political recognition that high dependency care is an increasingly vital element of acute hospital services. This has, in part, been prompted by a shift in the dynamics of inpatient care: advances in technology, reduced lengths of stay, improved treatments for chronic illnesses, and access to day surgery are some of the key factors that have combined to produce a concentration of potentially sicker inpatients.

It is essential that patients who require high dependency care are placed in an appropriate setting, where resources, skills and expertise are available and focused to achieve optimum effect. This is an ongoing process which has already seen the development of high dependency units in many hospitals, and also designated areas within wards where planned high dependency work can be undertaken. High dependency care also occurs as routine activity in a variety of hospital settings, including post-operative recovery rooms or accident and emergency departments. Equally, though, there are patients who suddenly and unexpectedly require an enhanced level of care. It is inevitable that the immediate intervention has to be undertaken at that point but all efforts should then be made to transfer the patient to a designated high dependency area as soon as is reasonably practicable. It is at this point that more competent nursing assessment, care and evaluation becomes crucial, both to provide appropriate high-quality patient care and, where possible, to prevent further deterioration.

It is an opportune time, then, to capture in one book the expertise of academics, managers and practitioners who have been involved in the development of the high dependency concept. The authors have been committed to:

- reflect the diversity of high dependency and its many care settings
- provide a foundation of clinical application
- focus on high dependency care as an entity in its own right.

Some chapters are devoted to specific body systems, which will assist nurses in the clinical areas when assessing their patients and planning care interventions. Other chapters address broader issues, such as pain control, or social issues, which are applicable to a wide range of patients.

The Editors would like to thank the authors for the hard work and attention to detail involved in writing the book. They hope it will be a valuable resource to all nurses working in the high dependency areas, and for managers who may have to develop a high dependency facility, assess staffing requirements or the financial implications of high dependency care.

Kent and London 1999   Mandy Sheppard
                                                             Mike Wright

General issues in high dependency care

The development, role and function of high dependency care

Mandy Sheppard

Key learning objectives

- To appreciate how the historical development of high dependency care has led to the current status of the service in the UK.
- To understand the complex and variable nature of high dependency care with specific reference to:
  - what constitutes high dependency care
  - which patients need high dependency care
  - where high dependency care is undertaken.
- To utilise the background information in the ongoing development of high dependency care.

INTRODUCTION

High dependency care is not a new concept. It is inherent within human nature to recognise that as individuals become sicker and more dependent, an increased level of care and attention is required.

In healthcare, high dependency care has been recognised, albeit informally, for many years. In more recent times, there have been attempts to clarify what high dependency care is and what constitutes a high dependency care unit (HDU) (Department of Health 1996).

The HDU is not, however, necessarily synonymous with high dependency care. Patients may require high dependency care (anticipated or otherwise) at various stages of a hospital stay. For example, after a general anaesthetic, it is expected that a patient will require close monitoring and observation, usually in a recovery ward. For this period of time the patient is undoubtedly highly dependent, and the level of nursing resource and monitoring equipment is greater than on a general ward. Although recovery wards are not generally labelled as HDUs, the nurses are, however, routinely practising high dependency care.

Theoretically, any patient in an acute hospital setting could unexpectedly deteriorate and become highly dependent, possibly requiring transfer to a critical care environment. With this possibility in mind, while it would be unreasonable to expect all nurses working in general areas to be competent in all aspects of high dependency nursing, it would be sensible for those nurses to have an appreciation of the fundamental principles of high dependency care. This may help to prevent further deterioration in a patient's condition and could possibly avert the need for the patient to be transferred for high dependency care. If such a transfer were inevitable, it would place the nurse in a position to provide appropriate and timely care until and during the transfer. Equally, there are many clinical areas where a significant proportion of patients require high dependency care, but perhaps only for short periods of time. This would include the accident and emergency department, the acute admissions ward or the medical assessment

> The concept of a designated high dependency unit may be new, but the quality of care implied is not. Patients have always needed varying levels of care at varying stages of their illness.

ward/unit. Nurses working in these areas are not working in formal HDUs but it is nonetheless imperative that they are competent in many aspects of high dependency care nursing.

THE DEVELOPMENT OF HIGH DEPENDENCY CARE

The first reference to high dependency care was probably in 1852 when Florence Nightingale wrote: 'It is valuable to have one place where post operative and other patients requiring close attention can be watched' (Jennett 1990).

During the 1940s, post-operative recovery rooms were introduced, significantly reducing the morbidity and mortality of post-operative patients (Oh 1996). This development allowed the close observation of patients and was in fact high dependency care. The use of intermittent positive pressure ventilation (IPPV) during the poliomyelitis epidemic of the 1950s prompted the development of intensive care.

In 1967, a report from the British Medical Association asserted that the presence of an intensive care unit (ICU) in a hospital would improve the care and outcome of seriously ill patients. The report also stated that at that time many hospitals were considering the setting up of ICUs (Hopkinson 1996). The 1960s also saw the use of continuous electrocardiogram (ECG) monitoring for patients with myocardial infarction and subsequently the development of specialised high dependency areas: coronary care units (CCUs).

In many ways, the subsequent and rapid growth of intensive care overshadowed the formal and documented development of high dependency care, which still occurred in specialised areas such as post-operative recovery rooms and CCUs. Other specialised forms of high dependency care were also introduced such as renal and bone marrow transplant units.

Patients in the general hospital environment requiring high dependency care were (and in some cases still are) cared for in general wards, often situated in an area of the ward that enabled close observation, i.e. at the entrance to the ward, or in close proximity to the 'nurses' station'. Sometimes these patients were 'specialled', whereby the nurse : patient ratio increased from the normal ratio for general ward patients. Although the distinction between a general ward patient and a patient of higher dependency was blurred, there was, however, a clear recognition that certain patients required more nursing resource and closer observation – two essential elements of high dependency care.

Some of these patients would deteriorate further and would require, if available, intensive care facilities. The requirement of IPPV was a common indication for admission to intensive care but generally the distinction between high dependency care and intensive care was unclear.

During the 1970s and 1980s specialised high dependency care, as previously discussed, became established and although a few hospitals developed designated general clinical areas for highly dependent patients, the majority of such patients remained scattered throughout the hospital, cared for in general wards. Intensive care continued its rapid development, aided by advances in technology and in response to healthcare needs.

In 1986, the government of the time proposed the Resource Management Initiative which was introduced in six pilot hospitals and, in 1989, the introduction of the NHS internal market (Mohan 1995) placed increased pressure on all providers of healthcare to demonstrate cost effectiveness. Intensive care was no exception and the requirement to justify the high costs associated with the service was increased. Cost and the rising demand for intensive care prompted closer scrutiny into the types of patient being admitted. Two categories of patient caused concern: firstly, the patients who were 'too sick' – that is, intensive care was unlikely to benefit them; secondly, the patients who were 'too well' – that is, intensive care was being used inappropriately and this could possibly prevent the timely admission of patients genuinely requiring the service. There was a growing awareness of the latter category, the high dependency patient, too sick for a general ward yet not sick enough for intensive care. This was a predicament and remains so for many hospitals – where should this category of patient be cared for?

In 1988 the report 'Intensive Care Services – provision for the future' (Association of Anaesthetists 1988) highlighted the need for effective use of intensive care and made recommendations about the size, location, workload and staffing of ICUs. Within that report a definition of a high dependency care unit was given as 'An area for patients who require more intensive observation and/or nursing care than would be expected on a general ward. It would not normally include patients requiring mechanical ventilation or invasive monitoring'.

Also in 1988, an article was published showing that within 1 year of setting up an HDU, ward mortality in the hospital fell by 13.3% (Franklin et al 1988). A King's Fund Panel was then set up which questioned (among other things) the lack of evidence that could justify which patients were most likely to benefit from intensive care (King's Fund Panel 1989). Both the Intensive Care Society in the report 'The Intensive Care Service in the UK' (Intensive Care Society 1990) and the Association of Anaesthetists in their report 'The High Dependency Unit – Acute care for the future' (Association of Anaesthetists 1991), highlighted the problem over this 'middle band' of patient – the highly dependent patient.

In the Association of Anaesthetists' report, a survey was published of 339 acute hospitals and a further 96 hospitals which performed only elective surgery. Only 55 of these hospitals had a designated HDU and of these 48 also had an ICU. The survey also revealed that many of the patients located on the ICU in fact required high dependency care and that many of the patients on the general wards should have been cared for in an HDU.

This report went on to describe the concept of 'Progressive Patient Care'. It noted how patients require varying levels of care during a hospital stay, and that traditional methods of providing high dependency care by 'specialling' individual patients in general wards diluted expertise and were both inefficient and uneconomic. The report went on to define Progressive Patient Care as 'a system of organising patient care in which patients are grouped together in units depending on their need for care as determined by their degree of illness rather than by traditional factors such as medical or surgical specialty. The three usual levels of care are intensive, intermediate and minimal or self care.' In 1993 a study was undertaken on behalf of the Department of Health to investigate the provision of intensive care in England (Metcalfe & McPherson 1995). Although it primarily concentrated on intensive care, it also highlighted aspects of high dependency care. The report revealed a significant variation in the provision of high dependency care. Only 34 of the acute hospitals in England with an ICU also had an HDU. In many hospitals there was a complete absence of high dependency beds, while in others there would be an HDU but not an ICU. Consultants who participated in the study indicated that 65% of the inappropriate admissions to the ICU would have been more appropriately admitted to an HDU. The report suggested that there may well be a requirement for more high dependency beds.

In 1994 Kilpatrick and colleagues published an article which mirrored parts of the 1991 Association of Anaesthetists' report. Specifically, the article said that it made both clinical and economic sense to have ill patients confined to specialised areas and not scattered throughout the hospital. In this way, problems could be anticipated early and intervention could be timely (Kilpatrick et al 1994). Several other articles were published in relation to the demand for intensive care and how the effective use of high dependency may also enable the effective use of intensive care services (Bion 1994, Peacock & Edbrooke 1995, Ryan 1995).

In December 1995, a 10-year-old boy was transferred a total of four times in 12 hours by ambulance because of a shortage of intensive care beds. Following this, health authorities were asked to review their emergency services and to consider a national database of intensive care beds. Notably, the then Health Secretary Stephen Dorrell asked health authorities to make more use of 'intermediate, high dependency beds' (Carnall 1996). Although there had been numerous reports and medical papers, all supporting the need for high dependency care, this political statement was highly significant in the recognition of high dependency care. It prompted healthcare providers (Trusts) to examine how they proposed to care for this group of patients.

In 1995, Rennie wrote that 'at present less than 10% of UK hospitals have HDUs' (Rennie 1995). This article also highlighted the need to make better use of intensive care facilities and argued some cost implications. 1996 was one of the most significant years in terms of high dependency care. The beginning of the year saw the publication of 'The Report of the Joint Working Party on Graduated Care' (Royal College of Anaesthetists & Royal College of Surgeons 1996). In many ways, the report reiterated but also expanded on the Association of Anaesthetists' report, Graduated Care being conceptually akin to Progressive Patient Care. This new report had far-reaching consequences for not only the design of modern hospitals but also the traditional method of care organisation and delivery in the UK. It quoted the Report of the National Confidential Enquiry into Peri-operative Deaths 1992–3 which had found that: 'Overall there is an inadequate provision of high dependency units across the country and this is something that should be addressed very urgently by both clinicians and managers. It is pointless to perform major surgery on patients who are physiologically compromised unless there are facilities for these patients to recover post-operatively.'

So by 1996 there was a significant and growing body of evidence that justified the need for high dependency care. It was accepted that high dependency care was a category between the general ward and intensive care, but although this category was recognised and accepted, ambiguity remained: what *defined* a highly dependent patient and what exactly was high dependency care? In March of that year, the Department of Health published 'Guidelines on Admission to and Discharge from Intensive Care and High Dependency Units' (Department of Health 1996). These guidelines were produced by a working party which comprised clinicians (nursing and medical), health service managers and members of the NHS Executive. Their terms of reference had been: 'To produce national guidelines which are evidence-based (or based on clear professional consensus) and which set out specific indications for admission to and discharge from intensive care; to produce clear and practical definitions of intensive care and high dependency units and other levels of care above that expected on a general hospital ward; and to cover in the guidelines the nature of the relationship which should exist between the different levels of such care'. The guidelines defined not only what high dependency care should provide but also for whom it is appropriate.

In March 1997 a new method of data collection was described, the so-called Augmented Care Period (ACP) Dataset (Department of Health 1997). The ACP Dataset, the use of which became mandatory later that year, was designed to capture information regarding the level and location of intensive and high dependency care being practised in acute hospitals.

The first high dependency care areas to be formally recognised were post-operative recovery rooms in the 1940s. At the end of the 1990s high dependency has undoubtedly progressed and its profile has been raised in the acute care setting.

THE ROLE AND FUNCTION OF HIGH DEPENDENCY CARE

It is generally accepted and agreed that high dependency is a level of care between a general ward and the ICU. It is implicit in this statement then, that high dependency will not be uniform throughout the UK; wards and ICUs differ from hospital to hospital.

It is right that there are national definitions of what high dependency care is and for whom it is appropriate; it would be wrong, however, to be overly restrictive or prescriptive. It is vital that there are national guidelines and standards to develop, safeguard and improve the service, but within these there has to be capacity for local high dependency services to be fully integrated into the local hospital service.

> National standards and safeguards are vital. But on a local basis, high dependency care has to be fully integrated with the culture of your own hospital.

The high dependency patient

The UK Department of Health document 'Guidelines on admission to and discharge from Intensive Care and High Dependency Units' (Department of Health 1996) describes four main categories of patient for whom high dependency care is appropriate (Box 1.1).

Within the same guidelines the categories of organ system monitoring and support are also detailed (Box 1.2).

■ **BOX 1.1** Categories of high dependency patient (DOH 1996)

1 Patients requiring single organ support (excluding advanced respiratory support)
2 Patients requiring more detailed observation/monitoring than can safely be provided on a general ward
3 Patients who no longer need intensive care but are not well enough for a general ward
4 Post-operative patients who need close monitoring for more than a few hours

---

Patients requiring single organ support

It usually fairly clear which patients fall into category 1; most of the criteria for single organ support are tangible and objective. One of the difficulties associated with this category, however, is that the patients requiring advanced respiratory support (i.e. commonly mechanical ventilation) are classed as intensive care and not high dependency care patients. Currently, to meet local hospital needs, some high dependency care areas do offer short-term mechanical ventilation. If this does occur, it is vital that suitably trained and skilled staff are available, and that there is an appropriate level of equipment resource.

Patients requiring more detailed observation/monitoring

Category 2 can be an ambiguous category and there are a number of possible scenarios within it:

- High dependency patients do not necessarily require monitoring equipment to be available as part of their care but invariably require close observation. An adequate number of staff with the appropriate skills are necessary and this

■ **BOX 1.2** Categories of organ system monitoring and support (DOH 1996)

I Advanced respiratory support

- Mechanical ventilatory support (excluding CPAP), or non-invasive ventilation.
- The possibility of a sudden, precipitous deterioration in respiratory function requiring immediate endotracheal intubation and mechanical ventilation.

2 Basic respiratory monitoring and support

- The need for more than 40% oxygen via a fixed performance mask.
- The possibility of progressive deterioration to the point of needing advanced respiratory support.
- The need for physiotherapy to clear secretions at least 2-hourly, whether via a tracheostomy, minitracheostomy, or in the absence of an artificial airway.
- Patients recently extubated after a prolonged period of intubation and mechanical ventilation.
- The need for mask-CPAP or non-invasive ventilation.
- Patients who are intubated to protect the airway, but needing no ventilatory support and who are otherwise stable.

3 Circulatory support

- The need for vasoactive drugs to support arterial pressure or cardiac output.
- Support for circulatory instability due to hypovolaemia from any cause and which is unresponsive to modest volume replacement. This will include, but not be limited to, post-surgical or gastrointestinal haemorrhage or haemorrhage related to a coagulopathy.
- Patients resuscitated following cardiac arrest where intensive or high dependency care is considered appropriate.

4 Neurological monitoring and support

- Central nervous system depression, from whatever cause, sufficient to prejudice the airway and protective reflexes.
- Invasive neurological monitoring.

5 Renal support

- The need for acute renal replacement therapy (haemodialysis, haemofiltration or haemodiafiltration.

may not be possible within the constraints of a busy general ward, particularly at night.

- If, as part of their care, the high dependency patients do need to be monitored with specific equipment:

    (i) the ward may not have that equipment; or
    (ii) the ward may have the equipment but there is an insufficient number of nurses to observe the 'results' yielded by that equipment; or
    (iii) the ward may have the equipment, but the nurses may be inexperienced in its use or in the analysis of the 'results' yielded, e.g. ECG monitors and arrhythmia recognition, or arterial blood gas machines and arterial blood gas analysis.

Patients who no longer need intensive care but are not well enough for the general ward

Patients who have been in intensive care move as part of their recovery process through a phase of being highly dependent, physiologically, physically and often emotionally as well. As with the first category, it should be fairly easy to identify these patients.

Post-operative patients who need close monitoring for more than a few hours

These are patients who expectedly or otherwise require an extended recovery period post-operatively. Although all patients in the immediate post-operative period are highly dependent and should be cared for in a designated recovery area, a patient would not be identified as being in this category until that period had extended beyond what is considered 'normal' or 'usual' for the particular surgery or anaesthetic.

In 1995, the results of a study which prospectively assessed high dependency needs was published (Leeson-Payne & Aitkenhead 1995). Over a 2-week period, the acute medical and surgical wards of a major teaching hospital were visited to identify any patients who might be considered for admission to an HDU. Prior to the commencement of the study, a list of admission criteria was designed and this provides an excellent and comprehensive guide to the identification of a high dependency patient.

High dependency care

There are a number of requirements which need to be in place in order to provide a high dependency service. The following four elements are key, and in some ways provide a foundation for the service, for without them, no amount of equipment or purpose-built surroundings will provide effective high dependency care.

The key elements of high dependency care are:

- A nurse-to-patient ratio which allows the close observation of patients 24 hours a day
- A nurse-to-patient ratio which allows observation of specific monitoring tools and the information provided by those tools 24 hours a day
- A skillmix and competency base within that nursing ratio which enables those observations to be understood, analysed and acted upon 24 hours a day
- Ready access to suitably experienced and qualified medical staff 24 hours a day.

> No amount of care or equipment is sufficient – if it is not there 24 hours a day.

There should be evidence of these key elements, or a plan to enable their future provision, in clinical areas which routinely undertake high dependency care.

It is clear from understanding the physiological, physical and emotional needs of the high dependency patient that nursing is key to effective high dependency care. In order to provide the level of observation and care, there has to be a corresponding ratio of nurses. It is a logical progression that for any given number of patients, as the nurse : patient ratio falls, the capacity to observe/input care for each individual patient also falls. Throughout the literature, there are many references to nurse : patient ratios and it is generally agreed that a ratio of one nurse to two patients, i.e. each patient requiring 0.5 of a nurse's time, should be the minimum. That is not to say that all high dependency patients will require 0.5 of a nurse's time, some will require more and some less. The patient who is confused and hypoxic may well require more than 0.5 of a nurse's time. A key characteristic of high dependency patients is the need for close observation. Many of these patients are physiologically 'vulnerable' and potential problems should be anticipated, prevented or detected early to allow timely intervention. Commonly this may be facilitated by the use of monitoring equipment, such as continuous ECG monitoring, pulse oximetry or non-invasive blood pressure recording (NIBP). But this type of equipment is only of benefit if the information it provides is also closely observed and acted upon. It is implicit then that nurses in high dependency care must understand how the equipment works and what its limitations are. Equally, a level of underpinning knowledge and skills is required for the nurse to deliver informed and effective care.

The importance of direct and indirect patient observation must never be under-estimated and the presence of monitoring equipment should not detract from this important nursing activity. It is highly dangerous to assume a sense of security because a patient is connected to numerous pieces of equipment and to rely on that equipment to 'sound the alarm' if and when the patient's condition deteriorates. It is the accumulation of nursing observations and the information gained from monitoring equipment which provide the mainstay of high dependency care.

Regardless of the presence of monitoring equipment, an extremely important part of nursing practice is the visual (and auditory) observation of the patient. It may often be discreet and gradual changes in the behaviour or appearance of a patient which signal the advent of more ominous physiological changes. For example, the patient who is gradually becoming more restless and agitated may be uncomfortable in bed, or be in pain or perhaps have a blocked urinary catheter. Of graver concern would be the possibility that the patient is becoming increasingly hypoxic or is haemorrhaging. The need for close observation dictates that high dependency care should provide a level of nursing resource (the number and the skillmix of nurses) which can provide this central element of the service.

This enhanced provision of nurse-to-patient ratio must be maintained through-out a 24-hour period and this is one of the most commonly stated reasons why high dependency care should not occur on general wards, with their associated level of nursing resource, particularly during the night.

Equally, medical input should always be readily available, again throughout a 24-hour period.

In addition to physiological needs, the high dependency patient will usually, but not always, also be physically dependent to varying degrees. A simple example of how patients become less physically dependent as their physiological condition improves can be seen on the general surgical ward. Take for example a post-operative patient in relation to basic hygiene requirements:

Day 1: Intravenous infusion in progress, intravenous pain management
        Bed bath
Day 2: Intravenous infusion in progress, intravenous pain management
        Assisted wash by the bed
Day 3: Intermittent intramuscular pain management
        Assisted wash in the bathroom
Day 4: Intermittent oral pain management
        Independent wash in the bathroom
Day 5: Discharged from hospital.

It is important to differentiate between the high dependency patient and the patient who is only *physically* dependent. The latter may require a high input of nursing care but may not require *high dependency care* as discussed in this context. It would be an inappropriate use of acute high dependency facilities if patients were admitted as a result of their need for physical nursing care (Vandyk 1997).

Individuals vary in their response to illness. A linear relationship does not exist between levels of anxiety and levels of illness. In addition to the humani-tarian need to alleviate anxiety, there are also sound physiological principles

Be familiar with the formulae, but remember that every patient's needs will be as individual as he is himself.

which underpin this important nursing role. Anxiety and stress can activate the sympathetic nervous system, increasing the levels of circulating catecholamines. These catecholamines exert many effects including an increase in heart rate and peripheral vasoconstriction. These manifestations – which can increase myocardial oxygen demands and jeopardise tissue perfusion – may not be desirable within the physiological environment of the high dependency patient.

Where should high dependency care be undertaken?

High dependency care can occur in many different areas within the acute hospital setting; both informally, and formally, in designated areas.

The unpredictable nature of healthcare means that 'unlikely' venues for high dependency care may suddenly be faced with a highly dependent patient: for example, a patient who collapses while in the outpatient or X-ray department. The environment, together with the sporadic occurrence, dictates that high dependency care should not be undertaken in such areas. There is a requirement however, for *all* patient areas to have staff, equipment and the relevant protocols to deal with such eventualities.

There are clinical areas where the probability of high dependency care is higher: for example, a medical admission or assessment ward. Many acute hospitals have developed such facilities to relieve the accident and emergency services and/or to maintain a more consistent workload pattern in the general ward areas. The clinical condition of a patient may not be fully appreciated until arrival on the ward, and once admitted, that condition may change rapidly. There is a requirement in these areas for staff to be competent in the principles of high dependency care either to stabilise the patient and prevent further deterioration, or to care for the patient until transfer to a more appropriate location. This should be available (along with access to suitably experienced medical staff) throughout a 24-hour period.

Accident and emergency departments and post-operative recovery rooms are well known examples of areas where highly dependent patients are a more common and predictable feature of the workload pattern. This is reflected by the enhanced nurse : patient ratios, the skillmix of the nurses, access to medical staff and the utilisation of monitoring equipment. These areas, while regularly undertaking high dependency care, would normally only do so for short periods of time, after which, if still required, the patient would be transferred to another location.

Formally designated high dependency areas can take many different forms. Broadly, these can be described in three categories:

- Attached to a general or specialised ward; either geographically within the ward, perhaps as a bay of beds, or in close proximity to the ward. This could also include renal units or CCUs.
- Attached to the ICU, either geographically within the ICU or in close proximity to it, or in another part of the hospital but still managed by the ICU.
- Stand-alone, but managed by surgical or medical teams. This could also include specialised high dependency areas such as CCUs or renal units.

There are advantages and disadvantages associated with all of these categories and this will vary in that an arrangement which proves effective in one hospital may not be so in others. Thompson and Singer's survey of HDUs in UK hospitals (1995) revealed the wide range in function, size, structure, venue and services available. Regardless of the geographical venue for high dependency care, however, there are principles which can underpin the effectiveness of a high dependency area.

High dependency care is part of a continuum of care for patients within a hospital; it should not be a completely segregated or isolated facility (Fig. 1.1).

Fig. 1.1 High dependency as part of the continuum of care.

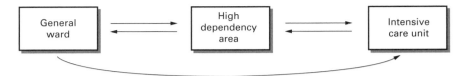

This also serves to illustrate an important function of high dependency care, which is to provide a 'Step-Up' facility (i.e. patients who become too sick for a general ward yet are not sick enough for intensive care) and a 'Step-Down' facility (i.e. patients who progress such that intensive care is no longer required, but they are still too sick for a general ward).

Patients move along the continuum according to the severity of their illness and that movement should be as smooth as possible. Protocols that ensure effective written and verbal communication must be in place between the high dependency facility and the other clinical areas. This applies to all aspects of communication, but of particular importance is the clear handover of information which directly relates to patient care and management. It is extremely unlikely that all of the clinical areas involved in the continuum of care will be managed by the same directorate or department; the need for effective communication is therefore heightened.

Another important factor in the successful movement of patients between levels of care, and to ensure the appropriate use of facilities, is the presence of admission and discharge facilities. The Department of Health report (1996) contains a useful flow diagram for the admission of patients to high dependency care, which could be used as part of a local policy. Of vital importance when developing such policies is the involvement of healthcare professionals who may need to admit patients to and accept patients from the high dependency area.

One of the key elements of high dependency care, as already discussed, is the availability of suitably skilled nursing and medical staff during the day and at night; the venue for high dependency care may have some influence upon this. Many high dependency areas have been developed as part of general or specialised wards. Commonly nurses rotate from the ward area through to the high dependency area, which maintains some continuity for patients and helps to prevent the deskilling of staff. It is essential in these circumstances that staff are provided with the appropriate training and level of supervision which will prevent any feelings of inadequacy or vulnerability when caring for highly dependent patients. Although part of a ward, the levels and skillmix of staff, particularly at night, should be differentiated for the high dependency area.

A potential problem which can result from the development of a number of high dependency areas within one hospital (as opposed to a single, central facility) is that the caseload of highly dependent patients is diluted as the patients are spread throughout a number of areas. For staff to maintain competency the individual high dependency areas must have a sufficient number of patients and activity pattern (Department of Health 1996). Although many acute hospitals utilise the directorate system of organisation, a 'cross-directorate' or 'whole-hospital' approach should be taken during the development stages of high dependency facilities.

Evidence of need will undoubtedly be required initially to set up a high dependency area, and once operational, checks should be in place to ensure the appropriate and effective use of the service. In addition, the future direction and shaping of the service should be informed decisions. For these reasons, data collection and an audit plan should be integral to the management framework of a high dependency area.

CONCLUSION

Many factors have related to the development of high dependency care. The progression of medical technology combined with an ageing population and the ability to control chronic illness have contributed to a greater proportion of high dependency patients in hospital.

The hospital patient population has also been influenced by reduced lengths of stay. Today, the low dependency patient (for example pre-operatively and in the later post-operative stages) is cared for elsewhere, often at home. Previously, those patients (rightly or wrongly) served to 'dilute' the acuity in any given ward, and without them acuity has been concentrated with a resultant increase in the proportion of higher dependency patients.

Nurse recruitment, retention and training, and changes in medical working patterns, have impacted on the suitability of the general ward environment for the high dependency patient. The removal of such patients to designated high dependency areas may well be an appropriate move, but does exacerbate the deskilling of ward staff.

Up to 50% of an ICU budget may be consumed by nursing costs (Kilpatrick et al 1994) because of the high nurse-to-patient ratios (at least 1 : 1). This and the increased demand for intensive care also acted as drivers for the development of high dependency facilities. This may have had an impact on the demand for intensive care but it also revealed a hitherto unquantified patient population in general wards requiring high dependency care. As high dependency services increase, it is a logical progression that a greater proportion of these patients will be treated in such facilities, with the associated higher nurse-to-patient ratios (at least 1 : 2). The overall cost of patient care could therefore increase.

High dependency care has developed significantly, but there are issues which remain unresolved in the wake of that development (such as the deskilling of ward nurses). The future of high dependency will be shaped by the successful resolution of these issues, by the continuing changes in healthcare needs and by changes in the methods of healthcare delivery within acute hospital settings.

REFERENCES

Association of Anaesthetists 1988 Intensive care services – provision for the future. Association of Anaesthetists of Great Britain and Ireland, London

Association of Anaesthetists 1991 The high dependency unit – acute care in the future. Association of Anaesthetists of Great Britain and Ireland, London

Bion J 1994 Cost containment Europe. United Kingdom Critical Care Medicine 2: 341–344

Carnall D 1996 UK reviews intensive care and emergency services. British Medical Journal 312: 655

Department of Health 1996 Guidelines on admission to and discharge from intensive care and high dependency units. NHS Executive, London

Department of Health 1997 Intensive and high dependency care data collection – users manual for the augmented care period (ACP) dataset. NHS Executive, London

Franklin C M, Rackow E C, Mamdani B et al 1988 Decreases in mortality on a large urban service by facilitating access to critical care Archives of Internal Medicine 148: 1403–1405

Hopkinson R 1996 General care units. In: Tinker J, Browne D, Sibbald W (eds) Critical care – standards, audit and ethics. Edward Arnold, London, ch 4

Intensive Care Society 1990 The intensive care service in the UK. Intensive Care Society, London

Jennett B 1990 Is intensive care worthwhile? Care of the Critically Ill. 6(3): 85–88

Kilpatrick A, Ridley S, Plenerleith L 1994 A changing role for intensive therapy: is there a case for high dependency care? Anaesthesia 49: 666–670

King's Fund Panel 1989 Intensive care in the United Kingdom: report from the King's Fund Panel. Anaesthesia 44: 428–31

Leeson-Payne C, Aitkenhead A 1995 A prospective study to assess the demand for a high dependency unit. Anaesthesia 50: 383–387

Metcalfe A, McPherson K 1995 Study of provision of intensive care in England. Revised report for the Department of Health. School of Hygiene and Tropical Medicine, London

Mohan J 1995 A national health service? The restructuring of health care in Britain since 1979. St Martins Press, London

Oh T 1996 The development, utilisation and cost implications of intensive care medicine: strategies for the future. In: Tinker J, Browne D, Sibbald W (eds) Critical care – standards, audit and ethics. Edward Arnold, London, ch 2

Peacock J, Edbrooke D 1995 Rationing intensive care. Data from one high dependency unit supports their effectiveness. British Medical Journal 310: 1413

Rennie M 1995 Strengthening the case for high dependency care. British Journal of Intensive Care, January:p 5

Royal College of Anaesthetists, Royal College of Surgeons of England 1996 Report of the Joint Working Party on Graduated Patient Care. London

Ryan D W 1995 Rationing intensive care. High dependency units may be the answer. British Medical Journal 310: 682–683

Thompson F, Singer M 1995 High dependency units in the UK: variable size, variable character, few in number. Journal of Postgraduate Medicine 71: 217–221

Vandyk R 1997 Cash and carry. Health Service Journal, 1 May: 28–29

The management of high dependency care

Mike Wright

CHAPTER 2

Key learning objectives

- To explore the resource implications (human, financial and other) that are required in order to run a safe, effective and successful high dependency area.
- To consider ways in which nursing staffing requirements can be calculated for high dependency areas.
- To consider the nursing and medical management requirements of high dependency areas.
- To gain insight into the part that high dependency areas play in the continuum of care provision and the need for effective interdepartmental and interdisciplinary communication.
- To discuss the importance of admission, transfer, discharge and bed management policies.
- To develop an understanding regarding the data collection and information requirements of high dependency areas.

INTRODUCTION

Whether designing and developing a brand new high dependency unit or establishing a high dependency service within an existing hospital department or ward, the principles of development and management remain the same. In order to provide appropriate, cost effective and quality patient care, it is essential that the high dependency area is appropriately designed, adequately resourced and efficiently managed. The purpose of this chapter is to identify the major principles for consideration by nurses, doctors and managers, when developing, delivering and managing a high dependency service. It will provide insight into these considerations and the preparatory work that needs to take place before embarking upon delivering such a service, and offer suggestions with regard to the systems that need to be in place for the service to be a success, once it has been established.

Prerequisite knowledge

There are no specific prerequisite knowledge requirements before reading this chapter and useful references are provided throughout it. However – and specifically if you yourself are embarking upon the development of a new high dependency service – it may be useful to try and visit other high dependency units, as this is one of the best ways of gaining insight into what your specific requirements are going to be. Most hospitals will be more than happy to share their experiences with you, pointing out the problems and pitfalls to avoid. This is also one way of developing a network of contacts that may be useful to you later on.

SETTING UP A HIGH DEPENDENCY FACILITY

Perhaps the best position to be in is with a *'carte blanche'* to design and develop a unit or area to your specific requirements. This can be an extremely daunting and difficult thing to do, especially if you have no previous experience of such an undertaking. You only need to speak to people who have been through the process and it is likely that they will probably be only too pleased to share with you what they would do differently if they had their time again! New projects invariably take a great deal of time, often years, to get from the ideas stage to the operational stage. As a result, it would seem to be a common opinion that many hospital buildings are considered to be out of date before they have even been completed! Nevertheless, the opportunity to design and develop a new high dependency facility does not arise very often and it should be relished as an opportunity to commission dedicated and high quality patient care services.

It is more likely that, where the introduction of a new high dependency facility or service is concerned, there will be a need or desire to progress quickly with its development, often resulting in limited time and resources for completing the task. This will most likely be in response to factors such as bed crises, lack of intensive care facilities and an increasingly complex casemix of hospital inpatients (Metcalf & McPherson 1995, Wells 1995, Department of Health 1996a, b, Leifer 1996).

As has already been mentioned, the term 'high dependency' is a nebulous one, meaning different things to different people and has a variety of applications and connotations. Some examples of high dependency areas are:

- Stand-alone high dependency units (e.g. medical, surgical, oncology, obstetric, coronary care, intensive recovery, cardiac surgical, liver, neurosurgical, burns)
- High dependency facilities within/adjacent to intensive care units;
- High dependency facilities within/adjacent to general ward settings.

Irrespective of the driving forces behind the development of a high dependency facility, the involvement of nurses in its design, development and commissioning is essential (Lee 1996). It is after all the nurses who will spend the greater proportion of time working in and utilising the area.

There are many fundamental considerations with regard to the design, layout, aesthetics and development of such a facility, and these should represent the cumulative expectations and needs of patients, relatives and healthcare staff (Dyson 1996). The design of a new unit could be the subject of a book in its own right and, clearly, needs will differ according to the specific type of unit or facility that is being developed. However, Box 2.1 details some of the more common 'environmental' factors that may need to be considered when designing and developing a new high dependency facility.

It is important to give careful consideration to the numbers of patients who are likely to require access to such a facility, the potential for expansion and the future needs of the organisation. A useful analogy to consider is the current proposal to expand the width of the M25 motorway in London from three to six lanes. The proposal is aimed at reducing traffic congestion; however, many consider it likely that increased numbers of people will use the new, wider motorway, and that it will attract those who would have liked to have used it in the past, but could not get access, or chose not to because of the competition for space. It is a common concern that this principle will also be the case where new high dependency facilities are developed within hospitals (Leifer 1996).

Pressure to establish a high dependency unit quickly may impinge on development of an 'ideal' unit. Which do you consider the more important – being safe or being perfect?

The need for cost effectiveness

The National Health Service has come under increasing scrutiny over the years with regard to the way in which it is managed, not least as a result of the increasing

---

■ **BOX 2.1** Environmental factors to consider when a designing and developing a new high dependency facility (Dyson 1996, Lee 1996)

- National Health Services Building notes minimum requirements (details available from local engineering/works departments). These include:
    - bed space/area requirements (with enough room to manoeuvre equipment, beds, trolleys, etc)
    - number and location of electrical sockets, piped gases and suction:
    - location of washbasins, fire exit routes
    - air conditioning
    - lighting (daylight/artificial)
    - acoustics.
- Site, size (see below), location and shape
- Proximity to other areas and essential support services (e.g. operating theatres, main wards, intensive care unit, X-ray, laboratories, A&E, etc)
- Storage requirements (never underestimate)
- Proximity of support services, telephones, sluice, emergency resuscitation equipment, staff rest rooms, linen stores, drug cupboards
- Health and safety and ergonomic requirements:
    — space to utilise, manoeuvre and store manual handling devices, e.g. lifting hoists
    — the position of monitors and shelving to avoid stretching and hyperextension
    — colours of walls, ceilings, etc
- Infection control issues
- Visitor accommodation/waiting area
- Accommodation for resident/on-call medical/nursing staff

---

cost of the service. By virtue of the fact that it is funded out of public resources (general taxation) and the government's need to control public spending, efficiencies are constantly being sought. This problem is further compounded by the fact that demand for NHS care only ever increases at a time when medical intervention and hospital care become more expensive. Butler (1992) summarises this nicely by describing the scale of the problem as being attributable to three factors:

- Demographic changes, including an increasingly ageing population
- Advances in medical science giving rise to new demands
- Rising public expectations resulting in those who use services demanding higher standards of care.

Harrison and Pollitt (1994) take the issue further by mentioning that the NHS is in competition for expenditure with other public sector areas. In addition, they describe the political ideology of Aneurin Bevan and the philosophy of 'National Health Service free at the point of delivery' as being politically untouchable. Nonetheless, as a result of its high profile, the NHS and its spending will come under close scrutiny for many years to come. In view of this, the application of sound business management principles to the NHS has never been more prevalent than it is now. There is now a greater awareness within the NHS of the importance of managing this complex service organisation more efficiently and effectively.

In today's increasingly expensive health service, the costs of patient care are never far away from any healthcare agenda or debate (Department of Health 1996a, Cullen et al 1974a, Keene & Cullen 1983, Cullen et al 1974b, Endacott 1996). The reasons for this are many, not least of which is the justification of how public money is being spent. It follows then that the cost of developing high dependency facilities will come under close scrutiny.

Cost implications of running an HD area will never go away. On a daily basis, HD areas will be asked to justify why they exist, what they do and how much it costs to provide that level of patient care.

When considering the development of such facilities, it is important to be constantly thinking about cost effectiveness and how the budget is to be allocated and managed. It is useful to make regular 'spot checks' throughout the development of any new project in order to ensure that the funding is adequate and that the money is going where it should. Once the high dependency area has been designed, the next consideration is with regard to the equipment that may be needed.

Equipment

Equipment needs will vary according to the type and speciality of patients to be catered for. Some examples of the sorts and types of equipment that may be needed are summarised in Box 2.2. This list is not meant to be exhaustive; it is provided merely to stimulate thinking about some of the possible requirements.

It is important to record all capital purchases within the local departmental or organisational Asset Register. This should include details of original capital cost, date of purchase, serial number, safety and commissioning tests, depreciation

---

■ **BOX 2.2** Potential resource requirements considerations (subject to level of care to be provided within the unit)

- Specialist high dependency/intensive care beds (e.g. electric, adjustable height, split segment, knee bend, traction, X-ray screening)
- Specialist mattresses and pressure-relieving devices
- Manual handling devices (hoists, sliding sheets)
- Piped gases and suction (low [thoracic/wound] and high regulators)
- Monitoring system (preferably modular/expandable) to include:
  — invasive monitoring (BP, CVP, RA, LA, PA, ICP)
  — pulse oximetry and plethsymography
  — ECG analysis (+/– respiratory waveform) and (+/– dysrhythmia analysis)
  — non-invasive blood pressure (NIBP)
  — temperature (invasive and non-invasive) and (single/dual)
  — information download/data transfer/trend analysis
  — compatibility across critical care areas (where possible)
- Portable monitoring for patient transfer/transport
- Emergency resuscitation facilities: defibrillator (internal/external) and portable resuscitation equipment for transportation purposes
- Cardiac pacing boxes
- Artificial ventilation facilities (if indicated):
  – ventilators
  – nasal Intermittent positive pressure ventilation systems (NIPPV)
  – continuous positive airway pressure systems (CPAP)
  – humidifiers (Heat–moisture exchange/H_2O)
- Syringe drivers: to include PCA devices, anaesthesia pumps and enteral feeding pumps
- Access to:
  – rewarming devices
  – theatres/emergency surgery and/or chest opening facilities (cardiac surgery units)
  – blood gas analysis machine/laboratory/facility
  – 12-lead ECG machine
  – portable X-ray facilities
  – pathology laboratories
- Chart trolleys and writing areas
- Data sockets for clinical information systems (to include the practicalities of access to terminals, wire/cable location versus bed movements, etc.)

period (and method), revenue implications and maintenance costs (and record). This information will help with future planning for equipment replacement (including a record of the depreciation of capital resources) and may also be necessary as a medico-legal record of equipment maintenance and servicing, particularly in the event of equipment failure. Advice regarding the compilation of such records should be obtainable from a hospital's capital accountants and/or medical physics departments.

Maintenance costs and revenue consequences

No debate about the procurement of new or additional capital equipment requirements should take place without giving due consideration to the revenue implications of running such equipment. As most new equipment is only usually covered by a manufacturer's guarantee for a maximum period of a year, maintenance costs soon become a reality. It is easy to forget to factor in an allowance for these costs into the overall budget projection, especially beyond the first year. However, maintenance costs, replacement parts, 'call-out' fees and extended warranties should all form part of any discussions and negotiations that take place with equipment suppliers and distributors.

> Buying a piece of HD equipment is the tip of the iceberg. Day-to-day running costs, unless knowledgeably budgeted for, can make equipment unusable as a result of high running costs.

The same applies to the day-to-day revenue implications associated with using the capital equipment. For example: in order to be able to measure invasive blood pressure, the unit will require a pressure transducer (usually disposable), a pressure infuser bag, a drip stand, transducer mount and transducer leads to connect to the monitoring system. All disposable and single-use items have a 'per unit' cost associated with them and the cumulative costs of these will clearly mount over time. Some other examples of potential revenue considerations are described in Box 2.3 although, again, needs will vary according to the type and location of the high dependency area.

It may seem pedantic to mention some of the items in Box 2.3; however, unless an allocation or allowance has been made for them, they can become significant and unfunded cost pressures later on. It is also worthwhile to retain records pertaining to how original costs were calculated and what they comprised. This will provide useful data against which to compare changes in clinical practice and cost pressures in the future, as well as assist with the often difficult task of calculating

> Costs which aren't budgeted for can accumulate over years – and make a unit unviable.

■ BOX 2.3 Potential revenue considerations associated with high dependency care

- Pressure transducers (disposable or reusable)
- Temperature probes (disposable or reusable)
- ECG dots/stickers, 12-lead ECG and monitor paper
- External pacemaker electrodes
- Continuous positive airway pressure (CPAP)/nasal intermittent positive pressure ventilation (NIPPV) circuits
- Incentive spirometers
- Ventilator and humidifier circuits
- Resuscitation circuits
- Heat and moisture exchange filters
- Pharmacy costs, e.g., cost of anaesthetic agents, sedatives, antibiotics, antifibrinloytic and haemostatic agents
- Blood gas analyser agents
- Rewarming blankets/blood and solution warming sets
- Specialist beds (where this has not been previously considered)
- CSSD and general medical and surgical supplies

the overall costs of clinical care. Some clinical information and management information systems now include resource utilisation and materials management functions. While these systems are only currently in their infancy within NHS hospital settings, they are becoming increasingly popular and it is likely that we will see a significant rise in their usage in the future.

The cost pressures associated with both maintenance and revenue requirements will also need to be included as part of the strategic and business planning process for directorate managers, nurse managers and business managers.

HUMAN RESOURCE IMPLICATIONS

A continuous source of debate and discussion is the level and skillmix of nursing and non-nursing personnel required to staff hospital wards and departments. High dependency units are no exception to this debate. There are many factors to consider when looking at the number of nurses required to provide a safe, high quality and risk-averse service. This is particularly pertinent in view of the example of intensive care units, where nursing staffing costs can represent up to 75% of the total operating budget of the unit (Metcalf & McPherson 1995).

The calculation of nurse staffing establishments is a complex undertaking, particularly in areas or units where activity either fluctuates or is unpredictable, and demand is uncertain. One of the difficulties associated with nurse staffing establishments – particularly in critical care areas – is that if there are too many nurses, this is considered as wastage. If there are too few, conversely, it is considered that there is a crisis. This makes it extremely difficult to get the balance right.

Many attempts have been made to try and establish indicators and mechanisms whereby nurse : patient ratios can be accurately calculated. These have included attempts to use patient dependency scores and illness severity scores as predictors of the level of nursing care required. However, while the report of the working group on guidelines on admission to and discharge from intensive care and high dependency units (Department of Health 1996a), acknowledges the usefulness of severity scoring systems because of their importance in intensive care medicine, it does not support the use of severity scores to determine nursing establishments or for other uses for which they were clearly not designed.

The guidelines that arose from the findings of the working group (Department of Health 1996b) mention:

A key distinguishing feature between intensive care, high dependency care and ward care is the nursing activity required. Nursing activity will vary with patient dependency and there is usually an association between patient dependency and nursing activity. As a result, in general, intensive care patients require the highest nursing activity. There are times, however, when a patient who has a lower dependency requires greater nursing activity, such as the spontaneously breathing, hypoxic patient who is admitted to high dependency care for close observation and may require more nursing activity than the fully ventilated and sedated patient in intensive care.

These Guidelines suggest the *minimum* recommended nurse : patient ratios in intensive care and high dependency units as shown in Table 2.1.

Table 2.1 Recommended nurse : patient rations			
Area	Number of nurses	Number of patients	Ratio
Intensive care units	1	1	1:1
High dependency areas	1	2	1:2

While the Department of Health recommendations provide useful guidance, nurse managers should review their nursing establishments on a regular basis, for the following reasons:

- To continue to ensure the delivery of safe and high quality patient care (including flexibility for contingency/emergency arrangements)
- To provide the necessary level of support, training and development required by all grades of clinical staff
- To accommodate changes in clinical practice and the role that nurses play in this
- The need to balance costs with efficiency by reducing wastage and unnecessary expenditure
- In order to justify staffing expenditure
- To ensure an appropriate balance between nursing and non-nursing personnel, including skillmix reviews
- The need to change establishments according to shifts in activity and patient dependency (e.g. changes in contract volumes, seasonal adjustments)
- In accordance with sound managerial practice.

Endacott suggests that the 1:1 nurse-to-patient ratio required for intensive care, as stipulated by the Department of Health, is not research based and that 'nurses need to be ready to answer the critics who suggest that such levels of staffing are not necessary' (Endacott 1996). Consider the following working example, however. There are four patients in a post-surgical high dependency unit: two after cardiac surgery, the other two as a result of other surgery that day. Two of the patients require continuous positive airway pressure (CPAP) support, the other two have only recently been extubated following long surgical procedures. There are four nurses working in this unit: one sister and three staff nurses. The sister has worked in the unit for 5 years, one of the staff nurses for 2 years, one for 6 months and the third for 6 weeks (newly qualified).

If we are to class this area as a high dependency area, then the nurse-to-patient ratios could be considered excessive if the recommended ratios are accepted as reasonable and taken at face value. There is, however, more to this scenario that requires consideration, for example:

- The current clinical condition of each patient.
- The level of drug and therapeutic support required for each patient, the proposed plan of care for each and the complexity of that care.
- The level of passive, as well as active, care and observation that each patient needs.
- The fact that two patients have had cardiac surgery and are at increased risk of cardiac dysrhythmias and cardiac tamponade. Such complications can present spontaneously and, when they do, require more comprehensive and resource-intensive care (if that expertise is not immediately available, then consideration needs to be given as to where it would be obtained from, should the need arise).
- The patients receiving CPAP therapy may be hypoxic and could therefore be confused and/or disorientated.
- Two patients have only recently been extubated (with a whole range of associated potential problems).
- The current level of expertise and knowledge of the nurses (and previous experience in this area or with these sorts of patients). This includes allowing each nurse time to gain the necessary background and current knowledge about his/her patient.

- The level of clinical supervision required and training needs of each nurse.
- The support systems that may or may not be in place to aid the delivery of care and decision making, e.g. medical support, healthcare assistant support, technician support.
- The situation with patients' relatives and friends and the level of support and care that they may need.
- The likely administrative and managerial responsibilities of the sister and nurses, not least of which includes the provision of meal and rest breaks for the staff.

> Statistics about ratios need to be remembered as facts about people – ill people and their families—who have needs, expectations and the right to high-quality care.

There are many other factors to consider with such an example. Nonetheless, it is used to highlight that just 'playing a numbers game' is highly subjective without giving due consideration to the needs of the patients, their relatives and friends, as well as to the nurses responsible for their care and management.

It is clear that further and more comprehensive research is required into this area in order to establish whether models can be developed that consider all the comprehensive variables of nursing care. It is arguable as to whether such models could ever be developed because of the intensely variable and intangible nature of many aspects of nursing care (Needham 1997).

Consider attempting, for example, to measure the nursing workload requirement when emptying a patient's urinary catheter drainage bag. In one situation, this may take the nurse only a minute to perform. On another occasion, however, this could take 20 minutes if, for example, the patient enquires as to what the nurse is doing. Furthermore, such discussions often expand into other aspects of care and can occupy a significant amount of a nurse's time, all of which could be entirely relevant to that patient's care. How do you apply an equivalent 'measure' to each of these examples?

Arguably, it should be up to the multidisciplinary healthcare team responsible for the delivery of care to decide upon the level and comprehensiveness of that care, and nurses have a key part to play in this decision-making process. After all, it is they who will be held professionally accountable for the level of care that they give (UKCC 1992) – although the Department of Health guidelines form a useful basis upon which to start. An additional consideration, particularly in view of the current national nursing recruitment crisis, is the concern among many nurses about deteriorating levels of permanent nursing staff within some wards and departments (Nursing Times Editorial 1997, 1998a,b Thomas 1998).

Once the healthcare team has decided upon the level and comprehensiveness of care that is likely to be required in the high dependency area, the calculation of the overall numbers of staff is fairly straightforward. One of the best ways to look at the implications of various care options is to design a simple template via the use of a spreadsheet. Tables 2.2 and 2.3 show examples of how this might be achieved and how the same model can be reworked according to various care and patient dependency options.

The example in Table 2.2 assumes the following:

- There are four beds in the high dependency area.
- There are two shifts per day (day and night) [this can be easily modified to include the number of shifts relevant to the local area].
- The unit is operational 7 days per week.
- All patients require 1:1 care.
- A supervisor is required for each shift.
- Shifts are 12.5 hours long (nurses' working hours are 10.75 per shift after deducting non-statutory break allowances).

Table 2.2 Template for calculating nursing staffing establishment requirements

A	B	C	D	E	F	G	H	I	J	K	L	M	N	O	P
	Monday		Tuesday		Wednesday		Thursday		Friday		Saturday		Sunday		Total
Beds/patients	Day	Night	Day	Night	Day	Night	Day	Night	Day	Night	Day	Night	Day	Night	Total
1	1	1	1	1	1	1	1	1	1	1	1	1	1	1	14
2	1	1	1	1	1	1	1	1	1	1	1	1	1	1	14
3	1	1	1	1	1	1	1	1	1	1	1	1	1	1	14
4	1	1	1	1	1	1	1	1	1	1	1	1	1	1	14
Supervisor/float	1	1	1	1	1	1	1	1	1	1	1	1	1	1	14
Total nurse shifts (sum rows 3 to 7)	5	5	5	5	5	5	5	5	5	5	5	5	5	5	70
Hours equivalent (multiply row 8 figure by shift working hours, in this case 10.75)	53.75	53.75	53.75	53.75	53.75	53.75	53.75	53.75	53.75	53.75	53.75	53.75	53.75	53.75	752.50
Whole time equivalent (WTE) (row 9 figure divided by 37.5)	1.43	1.43	1.43	1.43	1.43	1.43	1.43	1.43	1.43	1.43	1.43	1.43	1.43	1.43	20.07
											22% mark up for sickness. a/l, days off, etc. (22% of cell P10)				4.41
											Total no of nurses (WTE) (Sum of cells P10 and P11)				24.48

The template works as follows:

- The number of nurses per patient, per bed, per shift are entered (the total area of cells B3 to O6 inclusive).
- The number of supervisors required per shift are entered (cells B7 to O7 inclusive)
- The totals of the various rows (3 to 7) and columns (B to O) should be calculated. The results are then placed in row 8 and column P.
- Row 9 represents the number of nurses in row 8 multiplied by the number of hours worked by each nurse (in this case 10.75 hours per nurse).
- Row 10 represents the figure in row 9 divided down by the number of full-time hours worked by a nurse (in this case 37.5 hours) to give the 'whole-time equivalent (WTE) rating' for each shift.
- Column P represents the sum total of each row.
- Cells P9 (752.50 hours) and P10 (20.07 WTE) represent the total nursing hours and whole-time equivalents per week required to deliver a 1:1 service, 7 days per week, with one supervisor on duty for each shift.
- These figures take no account of days off, annual leave, study leave requirements, staff sickness, maternity leave, etc. An allowance for these has to be 'factored in' before the final establishment is calculated. This is achieved in cells P11 and P12.
- Cell P11 represents 22% of the number in cell P10. (This percentage will vary according to the way in which leave, etc., is accounted for. Figures between 19% and 22% are, however, common for this calculation.)
- Cell P12 represents the sum total of cells P10 and P11. This is the final indicator of overall staffing requirements, allowing for staff leave and days off, etc.

To summarise this example, in order to provide a four-bedded unit that is open 7 days a week, with 1:1 care for each patient, an additional supervisor for each day and night shift, and provide for annual leave, days off, etc., requires 24.48 WTE staff. Once this figure is known, the nursing team will then need to decide upon the skillmix requirements within the calculated requirement. This will vary according to the type and level of care to be given.

The cells within rows 8, 9, 10, 11 and 12 and column P are all what is known as 'formula' cells. These cells have been programmed within the spreadsheet to automatically calculate the numbers entered for each patient/bed and day of the week (across each row and column). Once these cells have been programmed, the model may then be used repeatedly to calculate staffing requirements based upon various different scenarios (any accountant/business manager will assist you in the development of formula cells, if you are unfamiliar with spreadsheets). Table 2.3 has been modified to accommodate another scenario.

As can be seen from this example:

- Only two of the patients require 1:1 care, with patients three and four only requiring one nurse to two patients (1:2 care).
- While a supervisor is indicated for each day shift, there is no additional requirement for the night shift, nor at the weekends.
- All shift times remain the same as in Table 2.2.

The results of this example indicate a requirement of 16.44 WTE nurses, a difference of 8.04 WTEs. This is an important difference, because the costs of the 8.04 extra nurses to accommodate the first option will be significant and anything in the region of £120 000 to £180 000, depending upon the skillmix and grades of staff used. The issue of skillmix is, again, a matter for the local healthcare team to decide. This is likely to vary according to the type of high dependency area, the available support mechanisms (nursing, medical and other), the level of clinical

Table 2.3 Template for calculating nursing staffing establishment requirements

	A	B	C	D	E	F	G	H	I	J	K	L	M	N	O	P
1		Monday		Tuesday		Wednesday		Thursday		Friday		Saturday		Sunday		Total
2	Beds/patients	Day	Night	Day	Night	Day	Night	Day	Night	Day	Night	Day	Night	Day	Night	Total
3	1	1	1	1	1	1	1	1	1	1	1	1	1	1	1	14
4	2	1	1	1	1	1	1	1	1	1	1	1	1	1	1	14
5	3	1	1	1	1	1	1	1	1	1	1	1	1	1	1	14
6	4	0	0	0	0	0	0	0	0	0	0	0	0	0	0	0
7	Supervisor/float	1	0	1	0	1	0	1	0	1	0	0	0	0	0	5
8	Total nurse shifts (sum rows 3 to 7)	4	3	4	3	4	3	4	3	4	3	3	3	3	3	47
9	Hours equivalent (multiply row 8 figure by shift working hours, in this case 10.75)	43.00	32.25	43.00	32.25	43.00	32.25	43.00	32.25	43.00	32.25	32.25	32.25	32.25	32.25	505.25
10	Whole time equivalent (WTE) (row 9 figure divided by 37.5)	1.15	0.86	1.15	0.86	1.15	0.86	1.15	0.86	1.15	0.86	0.86	0.86	0.86	0.86	13.47
11	22% Mark up for sickness, a/l, days off etc (22% of cell P10)															2.96
12	Total no. nurses (WTE) (Sum of cells P10 & P11)															16.44

supervision and clinical teaching required, etc. This helps to understand how important it is to try and get the calculation right from the start. Another factor that needs to be taken into account when calculating nurse staffing establishments is the likely availability of and access to bank, agency and 'pool' nurses. Access to such facilities can be useful during busy and peak periods and provides additional extra flexibility when needed. However, it is also important not to become over-dependent upon agency or bank staff sources, as this could affect standards and continuity of care.

The development of nursing staff

As has been previously mentioned, it is imperative that nurse training, development and clinical supervision requirements are given due consideration, in order that high quality patient care services can be delivered in the high dependency area. The amount of time and resources required to train and develop advanced clinical and assessment skills in nurses should not be underestimated. For example, it is wholly unacceptable for nurses to be expected to care for patients requiring artificial ventilation if they have not had the necessary training, development and assessment to carry out this care safely and effectively. Acquiring such skills takes time, commitment from all members of the multidisciplinary team and investment, both in financial terms and with regard to access to study resources, research, etc.

The growth of high dependency areas has brought with it the requirement to consider the specialist educational needs of the nurses working in them. Until recently, nurses working (or wishing to work) in high dependency areas have had to access general intensive care courses, as these have represented the nearest thing to the training and development they need. This has led to two problems:

1. The skills learned and developed on such courses are not fully tailored to the requirements of high dependency areas, nor the needs of high dependency nurses – although clearly there is overlap and commonality in certain areas; and
2. Increasing competition for a scare resource with the unfair potential to displace other candidates who, otherwise, ultimately wish to specialise in general intensive care work.

> It is indefensible for hospitals to expect nurses to provide high-quality care if the hospital cannot provide access to high-quality training.

This has led to the development of specific graduate/diploma nurse training programmes such as the English National Board course number A75 – Care and Management of Patients requiring High Dependency Nursing – particularly for high dependency areas that fall outside the management of intensive care directorates. In view of the wide variety and diversity of high dependency units, there is however a need for local areas to develop their own educational curricula in partnership with local schools of nursing and universities, in order to meet their own specific needs. In addition, it is important that such courses are given appropriate academic accreditation and recognition (Chaboyer et al 1997). This is in order to be both useful to the nurse as part of his or her personal and professional development and career progression and also a recognition of the actual level of complexity of the skills and knowledge that have been obtained and developed.

Academic courses form only part of the process of developing nurses in high dependency areas. Box 2.4 highlights some of the additional factors that need to be considered when compiling professional development programmes for nurses.

It is only reasonable that nurses who are expected to take responsibility for the care of patients in high dependency areas are given the appropriate support and

■ **BOX** 2.4 Additional factors to consider when compiling professional development courses

- The level and complexity of care to be provided which should, in turn, inform any indicative course content.
- The level of pre-existing knowledge, qualifications and skillmix within the nursing and multidisciplinary teams in order to support staff development.
- Access to learning and teaching resources (library, lecture/seminar rooms, word processing, Internet, etc).
- Due consideration of the level of study leave and study support required (particularly where nurses are working full-time in busy clinical areas). This requirement should not be underestimated.
- The level and type of clinical teaching that is to be given in the clinical area
- Access to and structure for clinical supervision (Kohner 1995. McCallion & Baxter 1995, Fish & Twinn 1997).
- The importance of the following developmental tools:
  — performance management process (or individual performance review)
  — the use and importance of reflective practice
  — the compilation of a personal and professional portfolio.
- Assessment strategies and standards to be used
- The training and development of supervisory and assessment skills in others
- The level of ownership, commitment and involvement of the multidisciplinary team members, particularly at managerial level.

training to do so effectively and efficiently. Conversely, it is indefensible for hospitals to expect nurses to provide such high level care for patients, if they have not had access to the necessary training, development and other non-paying resources in order to be able to deliver that care safely and effectively.

Further to the development of nursing skills and education, there is an additional need for research into what nursing is and what nurses do in high dependency areas. This concept of research by nurses, midwives and health visitors has been given further encouragement by the production of a set of guidelines by the Department of Health (1997a) entitled 'Achieving effective practice: a clinical effectiveness and research information pack for nurses, midwives and health visitors'.

MEDICAL MANAGEMENT

Access to regular medical care, advice and assessment is an essential requirement of any high dependency area. The Department of Health guidelines (1996b) suggest the following:

- Wherever possible, the referral of patients for high dependency care should be by a consultant.
- Decisions on admissions and discharges should rest with consultants, or their designates.
- Where care decisions are delegated, this should only be to appropriately qualified and trained personnel.
- Adequate consultant sessions are a prerequisite for the provision of effective intensive care and high dependency care. The guidelines cite similar recommendations by the Intensive Care Society (1990) and the Association of Anaesthetists (1988);

- High dependency care should provide a designated consultant as director with continuous consultant cover from either the admitting speciality or intensive care.

(Department of Health 1996b)

The allocation of consultant and junior medical cover is likely to vary according to the size, location and level of care being offered or provided. The precise level of cover is, ultimately, a matter for the local multidisciplinary healthcare team to decide. This is particularly important, bearing in mind that it is they who will be held to account for the level and quality of that care and also justify the decisions that they have taken. Nonetheless, if the principle of high dependency care is to optimise the treatment of patients so as to prevent further deterioration, where possible, the medical care of these patients should not be left to junior doctors alone. Access to regular consultant sessions and continuous consultant cover or advice outside of the regular session times are likely to be critical success factors. This is with particular regard to both the delivery of high quality patient care and the effective management of any high dependency area.

Admission, discharge and bed management policies

The topics of admission, discharge and bed management policies for high dependency areas can be highly subjective and often provoke emotive and conflicting responses from different stakeholders. This is particularly likely to be the case where there is competition for a limited resource, for example, in a post-surgical high dependency area that serves many different surgical specialties. The best way to try and resolve this problem is by involving representatives from as many of the various stakeholder groups as is reasonably practicable in the development of operational guidelines for the management of the facility. Box 2.5 lists some of those who may form part of the decision-making team.

Box 2.6 details some of the factors to consider when developing an operational policy and/or operational guidelines. These are not meant to be prescriptive, but are provided to stimulate thought as to who and what may be useful and/or important to consider.

■ BOX 2.5 Some potential decision-making team members

- Nurses responsible for the day-to-day operational management of the area (to include):
  — nurse manager(s)
  — nurse educators
- Medical staff (to include):
  — those responsible for consultant cover for the area
  — representation from 'user directorates' (e.g. surgeon, cardiologist, physician)
- Directorate/business/operations manager
- Physiotherapists
- Radiographers
- Laboratory staff
- Healthcare purchaser/local health authority representation
- Accident and emergency representative
- Intensive care representative (if separate team)
- User ward/department representation
- Clinical audit
- Patient/relative groups

■ **BOX 2.6** Some factors to consider when compiling operational guidelines/operational policy for a high dependency area

- The type of facility that is to be provided, e.g.:
  - Standard and minimally invasive monitoring facilities (e.g. maximum two invasive pressures – normally BP and CVP/RA)
  - Non-invasive artificial ventilation, e.g. CPAP/NIPPV (+ intensive, physiotherapy)
  - Low-dose drug support, e.g. low dose inotropes, antiarrhythmics
  - Sophisticated analgesia management (epidural/patient-controlled analgesia)
  - A ratio of one nurse to two patients maximum (and any contingency arrangements in the event of an unforeseen situation or emergency arising).
- The type of facility that is **not** to be provided, e.g.:
  - Invasive artificial ventilation
  - Haemodialysis/haemofiltration (unless this is a renal high dependency area)
  - High-dose drug therapies, e.g. cardiac inotropes
- A statement regarding the expected usage of the area/facility, to include, for example:
  - Where patients will be accepted from (to include restrictions on admission, e.g. a surgical high dependency area may not accept medical admissions).
  - Those patients who are likely to benefit from high dependency care (+/–local restrictions, e.g. terminally ill patients who, it is considered, are unlikely to gain any benefit from admission to the area. However, these should clearly represent the collaborative opinions of the multidisciplinary health care team +/– patients and relatives, where appropriate).
  - Any limitations with regard to the expected time periods (e.g. maximum 48-hour stay) and the procedure to follow should patients require further high dependency care and/or transfer to other areas/hospitals.
- Details of the overall purpose of the high dependency area, to include:
  - Procedures for referral to the high dependency area, including who can make referrals (to include the grade/level of experience of the personnel), who can accept referrals, contact personnel, bleep numbers, who the lead clinician is).
  - Where medical responsibility for the care of the patient lies, e.g., with referring consultant or intensive care consultant.
  - The local procedures for documenting care requirements/parameters of care and subsequent changes to that care.
  - The times and procedures by which patients should have their care reviewed each day. This is particularly important when considering the time of morning admission and discharge rounds as this can affect the operational efficiency of the high dependency area. This particular aspect needs to be managed firmly.
- When the facility will be available, e.g., 7 days per week, 5 days per week, etc.
- The nursing and medical management arrangements for the area.
- Where responsibility for clinical/activity audit lies.
- The procedure to follow when demand supersedes supply.
- The procedure in the event of disputes over bed allocation and who should arbitrate when these undesirable, yet possible, situations arise.
- The costs of the service and any internal financial re-charges, between departments or directorates, that may be incurred as a result of using the high dependency service.

It is important and prudent to review any such guidelines regularly. This is particularly important where guidelines are being developed for a new facility where utilisation might not have gone according to the original plan. It is also important as new developments in clinical care become apparent over time.

PATIENT DEPENDENCY AND NURSE WORKLOAD SCORING

The use of patient dependency and nurse workload scoring systems in high dependency areas would appear to be significantly less well developed than in intensive care units. Acute physiology and intervention scoring systems include:

- Acute Physiology and Chronic Health Evaluation (APACHE III)
- Simplified Acute Physiology Score (SAPS II)
- Mortality Prediction Model (MPM II)
- Therapeutic Intervention Scoring System (TISS).

While these are useful research and audit tools for critical care environments with regard to the prediction of care and treatment outcomes (Ridley 1994, Collins 1995), they are not designed to predict nurse-to-patient ratios, nursing workload or for determining admission to, or discharge from, an intensive care or high dependency area (Chellel et al 1995, Department of Health 1996a,b, Endacott & Chellel 1996, Viney et al 1997).

It would seem that there is no patient dependency or nurse workload scoring system currently in existence that encompasses all aspects of nursing care and work in both high dependency and intensive care areas. With reference to Needham's work (1997), it is questionable as to whether a model will ever be developed that will become a single predictor of nursing care and work. However, it is important, in the absence of anything else, that physiological scoring systems and intervention scoring systems are not used as predictors of nurse workload and patient dependency.

DATA COLLECTION, INFORMATION TECHNOLOGY AND AUDIT

As has been previously mentioned (see Ch. 1) there are undoubtedly large populations of patients who could be classed as requiring high dependency care or as high dependency patients but who, due to lack of access to formal high dependency facilities, have not been cared for in such a setting. In the past this has led to these patients never being 'captured' in data management terms as ever having needed or required access to specially trained staff or other high dependency resources. This resulted in the development of the augmented care period (ACP) dataset (Department of Health 1997b). The ACP dataset has been developed in an attempt to capture standardised data pertaining to both intensive care and high dependency patients on a national basis. This has important implications, for the following reasons:

- It informs the strategic and business planning processes for each local hospital.
- The dataset assists with calculating and measuring resource utilisation, particularly useful for the healthcare contracting process.
- It provides useful management and service utilisation information.
- The dataset helps to monitor trends in utilisation (type of patients, seasonal adjustments, changes in clinical practice/clinical emphasis).
- It develops a national and comparative database for the first time. This will help to identify the scale of delivery of this type of care.

The ACP comprises the measurement of 13 items including such information as the length of stay in high dependency areas, type of high dependency or intensive care area and the number of organs supported. This data collection has become mandatory for all high dependency and intensive care areas (and other areas where such specialist care is being delivered) from 1st October 1997.

Depending upon the type of high dependency area, it may be useful to expand upon the range of audit data that is recorded and collected for each patient. The type and range of data that will need to be collected are a matter for the local multidisciplinary healthcare team to decide. However, there are two types of audit that should be given consideration. The first type is the demographic-style audit, for example:

- Age and sex of patients
- Length of stay
- Source of admission (e.g., ward, A&E, GP).

The second type is concerned with the frequency of certain events and occurrences, for example:

- Numbers of patients requiring continuous positive airway pressure (CPAP) support, inotropes
- Returns to theatre for bleeding
- Cardiac arrests (plus outcomes)
- Critical incident analysis (problems, faults, accidents, incidents, etc.).

Whatever the type of high dependency area, it is important that a comprehensive system for data collection exists.

In some ways, audit data is more likely to be useful retrospectively. This is because things cannot always be changed immediately or at the time at which problems or issues arise. Audit data is often more useful, or more relevant, as a source of reflection. Furthermore, each high dependency area should have a quality monitoring strategy. This is important for the development and furtherance of clinical standards, policies and procedures and can be implemented in many ways. 'Quality circle' groups for example, could be developed to critically examine methods of working, procedures, incidents, etc. This is becoming increasingly important, particularly in relation to the concept of 'Clinical Governance', as described in the Government White Paper, The New NHS – Modern, Dependable (1997). Clinical Governance requires NHS Trusts to:

> Audit data is useful as a source of reflection: what can be done better, or differently.

ensure that clinical standards are met and there are processes to ensure continuous improvement, backed by a new statutory duty for quality in NHS Trusts.

(Department of Health 1997c)

THE NEED FOR EFFECTIVE COMMUNICATION

The development of high dependency units or areas is likely to introduce yet another tier or department to the hospital setting. It is therefore vital that effective communication systems are established from the outset, particularly as it is likely that a patient may move between many different departments or wards during his hospital stay. In the majority of cases, the high dependency portion of that care represents only a part of the whole and is likely to be transient in nature. The aims and objectives of all of those involved with that care should be with regard to delivering a seamless service. This is not just with regard to the delivery and continuance of clinical care but also the ways in which that care is communicated and documented. It is not just in the patients' best interests that effective communication takes place (history, progress, etc.), it is also important for those who are accountable for care delivery that full and complete details are communicated. This has particular implications where care is being transferred from one department to another – for example, from the high dependency area to the ward. With this in mind, it is important and helpful for wards and departments to work together in establishing standardised ways of communicating. In order to save time and energy and to prevent wastage, it is helpful if documentation can be standardised wherever possible.

CONCLUSION

The development and management of any high dependency area represents a significant challenge to all involved and should not be entered into lightly nor half-heartedly. It is something that requires planning, consultation and consideration if it is to meet its full potential as a safe and high quality patient care area. In addition, it will only be successful and able to provide the necessary level of comprehensive medical and nursing care if it is appropriately resourced, staffed and financed.

High dependency care is often, however, practised outside formal high dependency areas or units. At a time when hospital inpatients are becoming more highly dependent and medical and nursing care is becoming more dependent upon technology, the development of appropriate high dependency facilities has never been more crucial than it is now.

Such care is expensive and it is important to monitor costs and utilisation, in both human and material resource terms. However, if established and managed appropriately, with supportive nurse and medical staff development programmes, the high dependency area can be an extremely rewarding and motivating environment in which to work. In addition, such an environment can offer invaluable professional development opportunities to nurses at all levels, while providing the opportunity to deliver a high quality and appropriate patient-care service.

REFERENCES

Association of Anaesthetists of Great Britain and Ireland 1988 Intensive care services provision for the future. AAGBI, London

Butler J 1992 Patients, policies and politics. Open University Press, Miton Keynes

Chaboyer W, Theobold K, Pocock J, Friel D 1997 Critical care nurses' perceptions of their educational needs. Australian Journal of Advanced Nursing 14:3

Chellel A, Dawson D, Endacott R, Andrews I 1995 Patient scoring systems in critical care – can they be used as measurements of nursing workload? British Journal of Intensive Care 5: 250–254

Collins A 1995 MPM II and SAPS II: a review of easy to use severity systems. Care of the Critically Ill. 11(2): 73–76

Cullen D, Civetta J M, Briggs B A 1974a Therapeutic intervention scoring system: a method for quantitative comparison of patient care. Critical Care Medicine 2: 57–60

Cullen D J, Nemeskal A R, Zaslavsky A M 1974b Intermediate TISS: a new therapeutic intervention scoring system for non-ICU patients. Critical Care Medicine 2: 57–60

Department of Health 1996a Report of the working group on guidelines on admission to and discharge from intensive care and high dependency units. NHS Executive, London

Department of Health 1996b Guidelines on admission to and discharge from intensive care and high dependency Units. NHS Executive, London.

Department of Health 1997a Achieving effective practice – a clinical effectiveness and research information pack for nurses, midwives and health visitors. NHS Executive, London

Department of Health 1997b Intensive and high dependency care data collection – users manual for the augmented care period (ACP) dataset. NHS Executive, London

Department of Health 1997c The new NHS – modern dependable. Executive summary. HMSO, London

Dyson M 1996 Modern critical care unit design. Nursing in Critical Care 1(4): 194–197

Endacott R 1996 Staffing intensive care units: a consideration of contemporary issues. Intensive and Critical Care Nursing 12: 193–199

Endacott R, Chellel A 1996 Nursing dependency scoring: measuring total care workload. Nursing Standard 10(37): 39–42

Fish D, Twinn S 1997 Quality clinical supervision in the health care professions. Butterworth Heinemann, London

Harrison, S, Pollitt, C 1994 Controlling health professionals. Open University Press, Milton Keynes

Intensive Care Society 1990 The intensive care service in the UK. ICS, London

Keene A R, Cullen D J 1983 Therapeutic intervention scoring system: a method for quantitative comparison of patient care. Critical Care Medicine 11: 1–3

Kohner N 1995 Clinical supervision in practice. King's Fund Centre: Nursing Development Units, London

Lee S 1996 Designing and developing a new high dependency unit – here's one I prepared earlier. Nursing in Critical Care 1(4): 198–201.

Leifer D 1996 Creating demand – new guidelines on intensive care and high dependency units may lead to problems. Nursing Standard, 10(26): 13.

McCallion H, Baxter T 1995 Clinical supervision – take it from the top. Nursing Management 1:10

Metcalfe A, McPherson K 1995 Study of intensive care in England 1993. Department of Health, London

Needham J 1997 Accuracy in workload measurement: a fact or fallacy? Journal of Nursing Management 5: 83–87

Nursing Times Editorial 1997 The recruitment crisis. 93(26): 3.

Nursing Times Editorial 1998a Supernurses will not solve the recruitment problem. 94(37): 3

Nursing Times Editorial 1998b Solve the recruitment problem. 94(50): 3

Ridley S 1994 Scoring systems and prognosis for critical illness. Care of the Critically Ill. 10 (2)

Thomas L 1998 Pay, recruitment and conditions of service for nurses continue to hit the headlines. Nursing Standard 13(1): 1

United Kingdom Central Council for Nursing, Midwifery and Health Visiting 1992 Code of Professional Conduct, 3rd edn

Viney C, Poxon I, Jordan C, Winter B 1997 Does the APACHE II scoring system equate with the Nottingham Patient Dependency System? – can these systems be used to determine nursing workload and skill mix? Nursing in Critical Care 2(2).

Wells W 1995 Investigation into neurosurgery patient transfers. South Thames Regional Health Authority, 1995

FURTHER READING

Best D, Rose M 1996 Quality supervision – theory and practice for clinical supervisors. W B Saunders, London

Franklin K, McClune B 1987 The Mead ward care plan, based upon the Mead model – part 2. Intensive Care Nursing 3(4): 141–156

Hayes E 1991 Matching demand and resources in an intensive care environment: Intensive Care Nursing 7: 206–213

Rundell S 1991 A study of nurse-patient interaction in a high dependency unit. Intensive Care Nursing 7: 171–178

Wardle B 1997 Dependency scoring in a critical care area: a direct nursing assessment method. Intensive and Critical Care Nursing 5: 282–288

CHAPTER 3

Interpersonal issues in high dependency care

John Allen Wilkinson

Key learning objectives

- To understand that good communication practice is essential to good clinical practice.
- To consider factors which influence the quality of communication which occurs within a healthcare setting.
- To recognise that communication in critical care situations has the potential to be particularly effective when it is integrated into a therapeutic partnership.
- To analyse the quality of communication in practice to ascertain the extent to which it is accessible, understandable, attended to and perceived appropriately, remembered and motivating to be acted upon.
- To explore the potential of different concepts of stress to guide the assessment and management of anxiety provoking situations.

INTRODUCTION

Almost 150 years ago the most authoritative voice of professional nursing included the following advice:

> *I have often been surprised at the thoughtlessness (resulting in cruelty, quite unintentionally) of friends or of doctors who will hold a long conversation just in the room or the passage adjoining to the room of the patient, who ... knows they are talking about him ... [I]f friends and doctors did but watch, as nurses can and should watch, the features sharpening, and eyes glowing almost wild, of fever patients ... these would never run the risk again of creating such expectation, or irritation of mind. Always sit within the patient's view ... never speak to an invalid from behind, nor from the door, nor from any distance from him, nor when he is doing anything* (Nightingale 1859: pp 34, 35, & 37).

This chapter will address a number of topics which are relevant to interpersonal aspects of high dependency nursing. In doing so, there are recommendations of ways in which professionals, patients and their visitors may more effectively communicate.

COMMUNICATION AND HEALTHCARE

In her *Notes on Nursing*, Florence Nightingale seems to have captured the essence of good patient communication, as relevant now as when it was first published in 1859. Nightingale's observations of interpersonal relationships with patients led her to a number of conclusions which are summarised in Box 3.1.

It could be claimed that the principles of good communication are one of the few aspects of healthcare to remain unchanged in a context of rapidly changing technology, such as is found in a high dependency setting. Given the establishment

> Whatever their level of consciousness, people have a degree of awareness of their environment. Never assume a patient cannot hear what is said about him.

■ **BOX** 3.1 Communication advice offered by Florence Nightingale (summarised from Nightingale 1859)

• You should avoid talking about a patient, without including them, within their sight or hearing.
• Nurses have skills in non-verbal communication to enable them to assess patient distress in response to poor communication.
• Ensuring eye contact is an important aspect of good communication.
• Physical proximity enhances human interaction.
• Communication demands attention and should be practised in the absence of other activities to be most effective.

■ **BOX** 3.2 Summary of communication deficits between hospitals and their patients (summarised from the Audit Commission 1993)

• Patients tend to be poorly prepared on how to cope with the specific effects of illness or treatments.
• Information when offered or requested is frequently unclear and jargon-laden.
• In the case of sensory, physical or cognitive difficulty there is poor indication of special provision to address specific needs.
• Inconsistencies in information provided suggest that there is inadequate communication both within and between the various professional groups involved in a particular patient's care.

---

of the importance of effective communication to patient care and the identification of strategies to achieve this since the inception of professional nursing, it would perhaps be reasonable to expect that this is an aspect of care which requires little further attention. A review of the evidence suggests that this is not the case.

The topic of communication is well documented – see for example Hargie et al (1994), who focus upon the skills required to enhance communication in a diverse range of settings, while Pearce (1994) applies the principles of communication to critical care nursing. The Patient's Charter (Department of Health 1995) expresses the UK government's expectations of the National Health Service in the light of its healthcare policies. Within the Patient's Charter are rights and standards in relation to communication and the provision of information which patients can expect from healthcare professionals.

Despite health policy, however, and the value placed upon communication by most healthcare professionals, there is evidence that communication between hospital staff and patients is poor. The Audit Commission (1993) investigated communication from the patient's perspective. Their findings revealed communication deficits in a number of areas which are summarised in Box 3.2.

This is a somewhat bleak picture and clearly merits consideration by all hospital staff. It is, however, necessary to view these factors in context. MacAlister (1994) summarises and supports the recommendations suggested by the Audit Commission (see Box 3.3) but additionally comments that workload pressure might well be the key factor in preventing the implementation of good communication practices. She suggests that part of the solution may lie in adequate funding to enable the problems to be tackled. Clearly, clinicians have a role to play in ensuring that their practice facilitates good communication. However, the context in which an individual practises must also be conducive to the implementation of appropriate strategies. Although the recommendations offered in this chapter focus upon nursing practice, it is essential that local and national policies are supportive of the implementation of such practice.

More recently Martin (1997), the nursing adviser to the Health Service Commissioner, has highlighted that poor communication has led to an increase in complaints to the NHS Ombudsman. All healthcare professionals need to explore possible reasons behind any increase in complaints. If the service has deteriorated, then steps need to be taken to address this. If consumer expectations have risen, then the reasonableness of this needs to be ascertained. Martin suggests a number of factors which would improve patient communication and lead to a reduction in complaints which are included in Box 3.4.

■ **BOX 3.3** The Audit Commission (1993) recommendations (adapted from MacAlister 1994 p 5)

- Hospital staff should view communication from the patient's point of view in order to gain an understanding of their priorities.
- Managers and clinical staff should work together to resolve communication problems.
- Audits and complaints procedures should enable patients to focus on the issues that concern them. They should not be constrained by the design of forms used.
- Senior medical staff should receive training in communication skills.
- Professionally produced written information should be available to ensure that all patients receive good quality information concerning their admission, treatment and discharge from hospital.
- Interpreters should be available to ensure that non-English-speaking patients are kept informed of all issues concerning their treatment and care.

■ **BOX 3.4** Recommendations to reduce communication-related complaints to the NHS Ombudsman (adapted from Martin 1997)

- Co-ordinate multidisciplinary care and involve patients and their families.
- Avoid the use of jargon when communicating with lay people.
- Be aware that even good communication strategies can be blocked by the effects of stress and anxiety.
- Written information which is patient-friendly is a good supplement, but not an alternative to oral communication which should also occur.
- More training is required to assist nurses to communicate simply and directly.
- Ambiguous phrases such as 'comfortable' are vague and do not indicate improvement or deterioration, and hence should be avoided or explained further.
- Good record-keeping is essential to communication between healthcare professionals and to satisfy the requirement of professional accountability (this is of particular importance when patients are transferred, e.g. from a high dependency unit to a ward).
- Patient assessment, progress and evaluation of care must be recorded and communicated within the multidisciplinary team.

COMMUNICATION IN HIGH DEPENDENCY SETTINGS

It might be imagined that in a high dependency care setting there would be a sufficient mix of staff who are skilled in communication to avoid some of the problems encountered by patients in clinical specialties where the staffing levels and expertise are less favourable. An anecdotal account of a personal experience of high dependency care, which makes shocking reading, is offered by Barber (1997) who is a nurse himself. Some of Barber's claims are controversial, but the conclusions he draws from his own perceptions of the care he received should provide food for thought for all high dependency care nurses. Barber found that:

- Many nurses gave the impression of being focused upon technology rather than people.
- Nursing notes reported a pain-free status although the patient was never directly asked about this.
- Decisions about his own care were not encouraged, and when attempts were made to take control of some of his care this was not welcomed.
- The patient – Barber – felt that he should not complain through fear of being labelled as uncooperative.
- His own anxiety and that of his family about his transfer to a lower dependency area were poorly recognised and not addressed.

Since the seminal work of Ashworth (1980), communication in intensive care settings has been the subject of much attention and ongoing research (e.g. Pearce 1994). Rundell (1991) comments upon the wealth of literature that refers to both hospital wards and intensive care units, but draws attention to how little research has been conducted to investigate communication specifically within high dependency areas. Rundell makes the point that while there are similarities between the needs of intensive care and high dependency unit patients in terms of critical illness, there is however a key difference in that patients in the former are generally unconscious while in the latter they are more likely to be aware of their circumstances. It must be remembered that irrespective of their state of consciousness many people have a degree of awareness of their surroundings. A person with restricted mobility and unable to communicate may yet be able to hear perfectly and, in the absence of other stimuli, is likely to attend closely to what is said about them by others in close proximity.

What kind of nurse does the high dependency patient want?

Calnan (1987) comments that patients will make demands of those that provide care which reflect their personal agenda, and that they will evaluate care according to the extent to which their demands are met. This calls into question the kind of nurses that patients want. It can be argued that when a person is critically ill, both they themselves and their significant others need to rely heavily upon healthcare professionals because of their expertise in dealing with critical illness. While it is often difficult for lay people to ascertain what is desirable physical care, it is usually easier for them to evaluate interpersonal care, given that interaction is a familiar aspect of human experience. Hence a key area in which high dependency nurses can address the expressed needs of their patients and their visitors is through the provision of client-centred communication which has an underpinning relationship as its basis.

A research study which set out to investigate the relationship between nurses and patients is reported by Webb and Hope (1995) who sought to evaluate an aspect of 'new nursing' which Salvage (1990) considers to have an ideology of partnership between nurse and patient at its heart. New nursing, through its focus upon communication, perhaps has the potential to counter the problems highlighted by the Audit Commission (1993). Specifically, Webb and Hope were interested in Salvage's assertion that information provision is a key aspect of the nursing role, and as they anticipated, they found that acute care patients' considerations of the most important nursing activities are focused around technical competence, communication and education about specific worries. Porter (1994) conducted a study of nurses' understanding of their relationships with patients which was also informed by the notion of new nursing. He found that nursing practice which has shifted from a stance of authority to one of empowerment and partnership in the context of clear lines of communication is perceived as beneficial by both nurses and their patients.

It seems, therefore, that there is research evidence to suggest that the physical aspects of high dependency care can be complemented with attention to the development of a sense of partnership in practice related to skilled communication. To be able to communicate effectively it is essential to be accessible to the other parties involved. In a setting which is likely to be dominated by extremely important attention to physical care needs, it is perhaps necessary to raise the profile of interpersonal care. Conducting her research in an intensive care setting, Leathart (1994a) found that although many nurses were aware of the important contribution that good communication can make to patient recovery, it was often the case that this understanding was not acted upon in practice. An important way of implementing practice is through making interpersonal aspects of care a key component of a patient's care plan and including the needs of visitors as part of this area of care, the importance of which is stressed by Scullion (1994). Not only will this stress the importance of communication, but it will also demonstrate the value given to such care.

Fundamental processes in good communication are:

- being sensitive to the messages being conveyed by others (verbally and non-verbally); and
- responding in a way that is clear and understandable.

This is particularly relevant in high dependency settings where professionals, patients and their significant others are having to exchange information in a context which is potentially stressful for all parties.

> Information empowers. Nursing practice which has shifted from authority and silence to partnership and communication benefits everyone.

GETTING THE MESSAGE ACROSS

The importance of utilising communication skills has been emphasised, and the challenges facing the use of these in a high dependency setting has been explored. The processes involved in information exchange are analysed below in order to illustrate the application of skills as part of a process (see Fig. 3.1).

It must be appreciated that the relationships between the components highlighted is complex, being idiosyncratic to each interaction, and not in the linear and sequential format presented. Consideration of each element in turn will indicate the contribution of each component to the whole process.

Ensuring that information is accessible

Nurses need to ensure that they are accessible to the patient and his or her visitors by overtly demonstrating their willingness to communicate. Detailed accounts of how to demonstrate an open posture and how to listen actively are well documented elsewhere (e.g. Argyle 1994).

> Nurses cannot communicate if they are not physically present. Open body posture, accessibility and eye contact are vital in conveying that you are free to talk – and there to listen.

Fig. 3.1 The process of interpersonal communication.

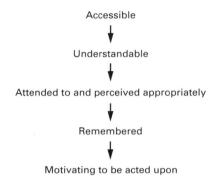

Using communication skills to ensure that the message is:

Accessible

↓

Understandable

↓

Attended to and perceived appropriately

↓

Remembered

↓

Motivating to be acted upon

As important as what is said is the accompanying behaviour of the skilled communicator (Egan 1994). High dependency nursing demands time-consuming practical nursing skills such as observation, assessment, physical care and the operation of complex equipment. Patient safety is clearly of utmost importance and of course should not be unnecessarily compromised. It has, however, been well documented by Menzies (1970) and more recently by Barber (1993) that many nurses perceive the practical aspects of care to be less emotionally demanding upon themselves than interpersonal care. An implication of this is that attention can sometimes be directed away from the communication aspects of practice by overly rigorous attention to practical care.

Consider a situation where a nurse is paying great attention to technology, charts or notes. How accessible is this nurse being to patients and their visitors? The more insecure a nurse is with a piece of equipment, the more it is likely to dominate her attention. Equally, the less comfortable a particular nurse is with working in a high dependency setting, the less comfortable she may be working under the scrutiny of any visitors who are present. A nurse who appears underconfident will communicate this to patients and their visitors. In such circumstances, a coping mechanism may well be to 'cut off' from the patient and his visitors and to overly concern oneself with the technology. Junior staff have a responsibility to be sufficiently self-aware of any such tendency within themselves, and more senior staff need to take steps to provide education and support so that confidence through better understanding is facilitated.

In effective communication, the process is necessarily valued as much as the information being exchanged. It is therefore essential to make the time required to enable skills to be used effectively. It is accepted that practice which focuses upon unthinking adherence to routine often occurs without the conscious awareness of the individual (Stevens 1983). It is recommended by Barber (1993) that enhanced self-awareness is required in order to challenge such habitual practice. In professional nursing, this sort of critical enquiry into practice has achieved prominence in the context of reflective practice (Atkins & Murphy 1993) often in combination with clinical supervision (Johns 1993).

In addition to being accessible to their patients and significant others, it is important that nurses ensure that the nursing agenda is accessible to other healthcare professionals. It is recognised that nursing in high dependency, as in other settings, is practised in the context of a multidisciplinary team approach. Niven and Robinson (1994) suggest that a group perceived as powerful or high status may be intimidating unless an individual has the necessary assertion skills to present

Are you confident enough with the technology you use to look at the patient and not the machine? If not, what strategies or training would help you achieve this?

■ **BOX 3.5** Model of assertion (summarised from Egan 1994)

People tend to take action if two conditions are satisfied:
- They see that certain behaviours will most likely lead to certain desirable conse-quences (outcome expectations).
- They are reasonably sure that they can successfully engage in such behaviour (self-efficacy expectations).

		Outcome expectations	
		yes	no
	yes	assertive	non-assertive
Self-efficacy expectations	no	non-assertive	non-assertive

their arguments. A model to represent assertion is offered by Egan (1994) which is summarised in Box 3.5.

According to this representation, it is only possible to ensure the dissemination and hence accessibility of a nursing voice if nurses are confident of the positive outcomes of their practice, and of their ability to implement their recommendations. Confidence stems from training and experience, and Leathart (1994b), writing about intensive care nursing, argues that there is a need for improved training in the use of communication skills for critical care practitioners which she recommends occurs in both classroom and work settings.

Ensuring that information is understandable

Evidence of the existence of professional and lay theories in a range of domains including healthcare is presented by Furnham (1994) whose research demonstrates that there are differences in the way that health is interpreted between professionals and the laity. He comments that it is important to appreciate that whatever view of health is held, it must be recognised that the view is valid for the holder. Support for this claim is the work of Davidson, Smith and Frankel (1991) who draw attention to a process termed 'lay epidemiology' which refers to an activity whereby individuals make use of their routine observations, discussion of illness and death in personal networks and information from the media in order to interpret health risks. It is claimed that lay epidemiology has the potential to moderate and block official health beliefs conveyed in the form of health promotion. In high dependency care, nurses should be aware that their own values and understanding of a given issue or situation are likely to be different to those of a patient under their care. To enhance this nurses should have the resources and skills to assess their patients, and to get their message across in a way which is sensitive to the values held by the patient and their significant others.

The Audit Commission (1993) and Martin (1997) both drew specific attention to the inappropriate use of jargon and deficits in patient information literature. Arthur (1995) comments upon the generally poor quality of such materials with respect to both content and presentation. This she attributes to a dissonance in the perspectives of the authors of such materials and the intended recipients. Although printed materials have the potential to disseminate sound information in a time and cost effective fashion, it seems that their design needs careful consideration in order to match the perceived needs of the readers to the values of the authors.

> Focus on the language you use every day — words like tumour, heart failure, high dependency, pain management. Imagine these words used in connection with someone close to you. Be aware of the distressing and alienating effect of jargon.

Attending to information and perceiving its meaning

Attention is a skill which can be learned and developed. It is an active process, and you can choose how to allocate it.

Attention is the ability to focus on different aspects of the flood of incoming information from the senses (Slack 1990). Attention is an active process which can be flexibly allocated, sometimes being divided between several tasks and sometimes focused on a single activity. The selectivity of human attention is sometimes illustrated in a high dependency unit when a nurse may not be distracted by general background noise, but will be alert to the specific sounds of patient distress or monitoring alarms. The flexible nature of attention suggests that it is a skill which can be learned and developed. Crow, Chase and Lamond (1995) review research which demonstrates that experts and novices in a range of specialties attend to problems in their field differently. Expertise usually arises through knowledge, practice and experience. Hence a nurse who is experienced in a different specialty and moves into high dependency nursing will need time to regain the level of expertise enjoyed in a different field of practice.

Knowledge of attention is of relevance to nurses for two reasons. Firstly, the nurse needs to be aware of any personal sensory difficulties as well as those of the patient and the patient's visitors. A number of authors have shown that sensory impairment or distortion can affect critically ill people (e.g. Kloosterman 1991). Secondly, it is important to remember that the mere provision of information by a nurse or a patient does not necessarily mean that it will be attended to by the intended recipient of that information. These issues are of extreme importance considering the significance of good communication skills to all fields of nursing. However, they are particularly relevant in high dependency care because of the attentional demands made upon nurses, patients and visitors due to the presence of monitoring equipment and the diversity of symptoms often accompanying critical illness.

Clarity of information substantially enhances human attention. Child (1996) categorises factors which influence attention as external or internal. External factors include strategies such as the use of vibrant colours, novelty and humour which have been used to good effect in health education literature, or in the design of complex comprehensive observation charts. Internal factors are associated with the disposition of the person attending to the stimuli and this is linked to their level of understanding, fatigue and motivation to attend.

'Perception is the process by which we organise and give meaning to sensory information by forming some mental representation of it' (Clark & Keeble 1990: p 59). Perception is a complex information processing activity which is described by Gross (1996) as having two elements: the physiological functioning of the sensory organs (sight, smell, taste, hearing and touch), and a predisposition to conceptualise sensory stimuli in a particular way which is likely to be influenced by personality, culture and experiences. These elements of perception combine to facilitate interactive processing. How a person perceives the world is reflected in attitudes and behaviour, and this in turn shapes perceptions of the world. Hence perception is a dynamic and evaluative process, in which the individual is considered to make judgements based upon their sensory information and their way of making sense of the world (Gregory 1990).

Expectations are the product of life experiences such as education, life events, gender and socialisation. Many interpretations overlap with those of others, while some are highly individual. The influence of expectations helps to explain those situations when perception is distorted. From a nursing perspective, consider the administration of medicines and the similarity of the drug names *prednisolone* and *prednisone* or *dipyridamole* and *disopyramide*. Consider also the abbreviation PID which can represent both 'prolapsed intervertebral disc' and 'pelvic inflammatory disease'. It would be potentially disastrous if nurses relied on an automatic and passive mode of attention. In high dependency nursing the unexpected can, and often does, occur and it is necessary to actively pay attention to this. From a patient or client perspective we may speculate what the use of technical jargon such as 'heart failure' or 'tumour' may mean. It is essential to anticipate that patients will not necessarily view healthcare, nor interpret its terminologies, in the same way as healthcare professionals.

The 'halo and horns' effects refer to a self-fulfilling prophecy characteristic of person perception. In the halo effect, a positive impression of a person leads to that person being consistently perceived in a favourable way. This in turn acts in a cyclical fashion, providing positive feedback that further promotes the original notion. The horns effect is the same process occurring with unfavourable impressions. In a classic study, Stockwell (1972) has drawn attention to the hazards of being labelled as an 'unpopular patient' which suggests that nurses have considerable influence upon the treatment and self-concept of those for whom they care. Despite communication being a feature of nursing curricula during the intervening years, Walsh (1995) has shown that some patients are still perceived by nurses to be less popular than others. In a high dependency setting a patient may be perceived as unpopular because of poor response to treatment, which may provoke a sense of failure. The code of professional conduct for nurses, midwives and health visitors (UKCC 1992) is very clear regarding the importance of nursing people without favour or prejudice and it would be unprofessional to do otherwise knowingly. However, Mackellaig (1990) cautions that in a critical care setting, unpopular long-term patients may be overly allocated to temporary agency nursing staff, and this may convey an underlying message to patients or their visitors.

> Reflect on patients who have been given 'labels' such as 'unco-operative'. Is it possible to trace back to the lack of communication which may have led to this?

Attribution theory is considered by Davies (1996). There is experimental evidence that we tend to attribute our own actions to situational determinants and the actions of others to dispositional determinants. This has plausible application in nursing practice. For example, it may be perceived that a patient is angry because that is a feature of his personality (dispositional determinant) when in fact he is angry because a member of the nursing team has failed to keep a promise about something important to him (situational determinant). There are two important points to note from this. Firstly, it is important not to overlook situational determinants of behaviour as they are frequently more addressable than dispositional elements. Secondly, it is often a mistake to draw conclusions about personality and its determinants from behaviour. Nursing observations inform assessment more accurately if a stream of behaviour is reported as it occurs, rather than the conclusions drawn. 'Reluctant to follow advice, poor attention span, expresses a pessimistic outlook and lack of interest in recovery' is likely to be more helpful than 'poorly motivated'.

Remembering information

Many nurses have experienced situations where a patient or visitor asks the same questions on several different occasions. A significant part of communication in nursing practice is that the information presented is remembered. In high dependency nursing this is of particular importance for two reasons. First, when a patient is critically ill, there is frequently a great deal of information which the patient and his significant others will request. Second, when a patient is highly dependent upon healthcare professionals a key aspect of care is to give the information necessary to restore independence as quickly as is practicable to empower patient participation in recovery (Cahill 1996). These issues pose challenges upon memory, and nurses need to understand this in order to assist the enhancement of the process. Memory is frequently conceptualised as a dynamic

> Even clear information lucidly conveyed is inevitably reflected through the patient's own anxiety and distress, and that of his family. Don't assume you only need give information once if you give it clearly. You may need to repeat and repeat again, in a variety of ways.

process which involves encoding, storage and retrieval components (Eysenck & Keane 1996).

Encoding is the process by which memories are accessed from our experience and organised. Information which needs to be remembered must be attended to and perceived accurately. Remembering is easier if the new information can be related to existing memories and understanding, and therefore it is helpful if nurses can make use of their knowledge of this in communicating with others. A common way of doing this is by the use of analogies, for example in likening the heart to a pump or the kidneys to filters, if it can be established that the recipient of the information can relate to these parallels. Cognitive learning theory suggests that encoding in memory will be enhanced if information is processed actively and deeply (McKenna 1995). This can be promoted if patients and their visitors are encouraged to link what is known with that which is new and complex material is associated with that which is perceived to be simpler and already understood. Giving information in stages allows time for assimilation and hence this is a recommended approach.

Storage occurs when encoded memories are maintained as long-term files of information, often referred to as schemas. The storage of memories is not usually considered to be problematic in the absence of neurological damage. What is often blamed as being a failure of memory storage is frequently a problem associated with either ineffective encoding or retrieval.

The process by which information is accessed from memory is termed retrieval. When attempting to retrieve memories, it is important to make use of the same filing (that is, schema) system as was used for encoding. It is important for nurses to appreciate that the schema used for encoding is likely to be idiosyncratic to the patient and hence may differ from that of the professional schema which they themselves have developed as a consequence of their expertise in high dependency care. To avoid interference between these two potentially different modes of memory storage, it is recommended that questions are posed which enable the patient to contextualise the required information. For instance, it is often better to ask patients to use examples of a good diet than to outline the underpinning principles. If it is difficult for a patient or their visitors to remember important information, this can be a source of anxiety for them. In such circumstances it is useful to consider that recognition is considerably easier than unprompted recall, and that the use of cues retains a degree of independence and achievement which may be important to self-confidence.

Being motivated to act upon information

Motivation is concerned with the relationship between beliefs, values, attitudes and behaviour (Kent 1996). A belief is a representation of knowledge which is rightly or wrongly held by an individual, a value being a related judgement. It is the inter-linkage of beliefs and values which combine to form attitudes, which consequently may be positive or negative predisposition towards an issue. This in turn contributes to choices about behaviour. For example, a patient may decide that he requires total rest to recover (a belief) and hence evaluate nursing insistence upon participation in a degree of contribution to his care as inappropriate (a value). In this instance the patient's attitude towards contribution to his own care would be one of resistance to behaving co-operatively. The relationship between attitudes and behaviour is not one of simple causation, as it is a complex function of many variables. An understanding of this complexity is key to the motivation of self and others.

Motivational theories can be divided into two types, push theories and pull theories. Under push theories we find such terms as drive, motive or even stimulus. Pull theories use such constructs as purpose, value or need. In terms of a well-known metaphor these are the pitchfork theories on one hand, and the carrot theories on the other. But our theory is neither of these. Since we prefer to look at the nature of the animal himself, ours is best described as a jackass theory

(Kelly 1958: p 58).

Using Kelly's eloquent analogy a number of strategies which nurses may utilise to motivate high dependency patients will be explored.

Push theories are associated with responding to some form of external drive to perform a given set of behaviours. Nurses or a patient's visitors may supply such stimuli in the form of verbal encouragement which is often repeated regularly. Two issues arise from the use of this approach to motivation. Firstly, the importance of consistency in information provision. Asch (1952) has demonstrated the effect of the consistent opinions of others upon the promotion of compliance in individuals. Secondly, the message should be acceptable to the recipient. Lewin (1947) demonstrated experimentally that if a message is perceived to be unacceptable it will simply be ignored, even if the source of the message is accepted as being credible and trustworthy. However, if the same message is presented to a group in the form of a discussion topic it was shown that the acceptability of the message increased and that this was accompanied by a tenfold increase in behaviour change. This research suggests that nurses should work closely with visitors to present a co-ordinated strategy of information provision so that the message is consistently reinforced. Asking visitors to nominate a link person through whom all information can be related is often a useful way of ensuring consistency of message between named nurse, patient and visitors.

Pull theories of motivation are centred on the notion of goal acquisition. Myles (1993) has used the hierarchy of needs model presented by Maslow (1970) to demonstrate how nursing care can be structured around this classic representation of human needs. It is important to acknowledge that the ascending sequential and linear presentation of Maslow's model is not an accurate reflection of the reality of human motivation, but is more a useful checklist of factors which may be motivational at a given time. It is therefore recommended that the taxonomy of needs, (physiological needs, the need for safety, for love, esteem and a sense of belonging, cognitive needs and the goal of self-actualisation) is used as a basis for assessment rather than a prescription for care. In doing so, the model yields the potential to highlight factors which are important goals for an individual patient. If goals for nursing practice can be matched to patient-generated goals there is an enhanced basis for the uptake of health promotion (Dines 1994).

'Jackass' or person-centred theories of motivation combine elements of push and pull theories in the context of the person's understanding of their experiences. This notion of the interaction between internal and external factors in influencing attitudes to health issues and their relationship to behaviour is exemplified by research into how individuals process information in the contexts of their social circumstances and emotions (Ogden 1996). The term social cognition model of health behaviour is used by Connor and Norman (1996) to identify a group of theories which seek to explain and predict health-related behaviour in order to indicate how a person might be motivated to select healthier options. The main recommendations to emerge from research into social cognition are summarised in Box 3.6.

In a high dependency setting the potentially unstable nature of the patient's condition could result in changed attitudes as circumstances alter. This is therefore a challenge to nurses who need to frequently reassess a patient's level of motivation in order to respond with a range of motivating strategies.

■ **BOX 3.6** Summary of concepts considered to determine health behaviour (summarised from Connor & Norman 1996)

- Demographic variables, e.g. young males tend to be higher risk-takers and hence should be particularly targeted.
- Health promotion cues which are understandable and deemed relevant tend to alter behaviour, so every opportunity should be taken to offer advice about a healthier lifestyle.
- External locus of control in terms of powerful others is influential and healthcare professionals should take advantage of the fact that many patients and their significant others will perceive them in this way.
- External locus of control in terms of luck, fate or religion may be influential to some patients, and so must be acknowledged or challenged as appropriate.
- Internal locus of control in terms of self-efficacy is influential through fostering a personal sense of self-efficacy.
- Intentions in terms of attitudes are likely to be shaped by significant others as well as rational argument and hence it is important to muster the support of those whom the patient values to reinforce health advice.
- In motivation, consider employing push, pull and person focused factors.
- The perceived benefit of adopting a behaviour pattern should be stressed.
- The perceived cost of adopting a behaviour pattern should be stressed.
- Severity of threat evaluation related to continuing present behaviour should be stressed.
- Social support is important – get the relatives and all other significant others involved.

STRESS AND HIGH DEPENDENCY SETTINGS

Foxall et al (1990) compared the frequency and sources of stress in a range of clinical settings and came to the conclusion that nursing the critically ill is stressful. Specifically, Tyler and Ellison (1994) have reported the stressful nature of high dependency nursing. From a patient perspective, Soehren (1995) has reviewed literature which suggests that critical illness is a stressful experience. A study by O'Malley et al (1991) identifies the significance of stress upon the relatives of the critically ill. It is clear from the literature that, for many of those involved, high dependency care settings are associated with stress.

The concept of stress is classically delineated and represented by three models, i.e. stimulus, response and cognitive–phenomenological–transactional (Baily and Clarke 1989). Each explanation will be considered in turn as issues relevant to high dependency nursing arise out of each approach.

The stimulus model of stress

In the stimulus model, stress is defined as something external to the individual in the environment, which impinges upon the person. Examples are factors that can be perceived by the senses, such as unpleasant sights, sounds, smells, temperatures and tastes. The dominance of environmental stressors such as nursing acutely ill patients, nursing 'heavy' long-term patients, prolongation of life in the critically ill, lack of time and inadequate patient : staff ratios were identified by White and Tonkin (1991) in their investigation of stressors in Australian intensive care units.

A number of high dependency units are being set up on general wards that may not be of an ideal design to facilitate both the technical and interpersonal aspects of care. In addition, a high dependency unit which is attached to a less acute practice setting may not have the appropriate nurse staffing establishment, in terms of

numbers or levels of expertise, to satisfy the patient care demands of either specialty. Stressors imposed by such an environment have the potential to compromise communication because of inadequate time, unreasonable workloads and
staff with an inadequate knowledge of the specialty in which they are working.

A strength of the stimulus explanation of stress is that it can direct attention to
such stress-provoking factors. Nurses clearly have a responsibility to monitor the
environment in which care is delivered to ensure that it is safe and conducive to
recovery. The advice of Nightingale (1859) that hospitals should do patients no
harm is as relevant in modern healthcare settings as it was when it was first suggested. Stressful environmental stimuli which are generally accepted as undesirable, such as excessive noise, bright lights, heavy workloads and inadequate
knowledge base are measurable and steps should be taken to address potential
causes of patient, visitor or staff stress.

Some environmental factors, however, are less clearly identifiable as stressful.
Ashbury (1984) argues that there is an increase in public awareness of the use of
technological equipment in healthcare settings such as a high dependency unit,
although the consequences of this are unclear. Familiarisation with technology
may help to mentally prepare patients and their visitors who witness its use,
although Clifford (1986) comments that exposure to 'life support' machinery on
television may be entirely different to experiencing its use on oneself or a relative.
Hence for some individuals the presence of equipment may be reassuring, while
for others it may act as a source of stress. Clearly, the best way of ascertaining this
is to assess people as individuals. The importance of this is exemplified by
Bergbom-Engberg and Haljamäe (1993) who found that the same stressors are perceived differently by different nurses. From this research it seems that the way that
potentially stressful stimuli are interpreted is more important that the nature of the
stimuli themselves.

Thus an interpretation of stress as being attributable to stimuli alone is reduc-
tionist and static. This is a limitation as it fails to acknowledge individual differences in the perception of what might be stressful. The assumption of linear and
progressive causality of stress is additionally flawed because there is poor
acknowledgement of human capacity to adapt and cope.

The response model of stress

The response model defines stress as the individual's physiological responses to
perceived threat in an effort to maintain homeostasis. This is mediated princi-
pally through the release of catecholamines which have been considered in other
chapters and is clearly highly relevant to the management of critical illness. The
strength of this understanding of stress is that there is the establishment of a relationship between stress and disease, although the nature of this is unclear (Ogden
1996). Like the stimulus model, the response model can be criticised for being an
overly deterministic explanation of stress which fails to fully allow for individual
interpretation and response to circumstances which might yield stress.

The cognitive–phenomenological–transactional model of stress

The cognitive–phenomenological–transactional model of stress is a consequence of
the work of Lazarus and colleagues between the 1960s and the 1980s (Sarafino
1994). According to this approach, stress is defined as the result of an interaction
between the individual and his understanding of his own situation. The key to the
model is the idiosyncratic interpretation of threat and the perception of what can
be done in response in the form of coping strategies. The model has three phases.
Primary appraisal involves the initial assessment of challenge or demand. In this

phase the person may ask themselves questions such as 'what's happening?' or 'how will this affect me?' In other words it is suggested that each individual makes an assessment, and evaluates whether he feel threatened or not. Secondary appraisal is an estimation of personal resources to counter, or coping resources to deal with, any perceived threat. In this phase the person may ask questions such as 'what can I do?' or 'what help do I need?' Coping in response to appraisal may be to address a problem directly, or to seek emotional release of tension (Clarke 1984). Finally, the reappraisal phase is an evaluation of the subsequent outcome in the light of the primary and secondary phases. Here the questions asked may be 'how am I coping?' or is the situation better or worse now?'

The strengths of this model lie in its highly individualistic and dynamic representation which allows for differences and change both within and between people. It offers an explanation for stress in the absence of an apparent stressor, such as in the case of covert phobias or anxiety states. The model serves well to remind nurses that the way they interpret a given situation may differ from that of those they care for, or their colleagues. Practice can be guided by the model if the questions associated with each phase are used as a basis for assessment. A limitation in the application of the cognitive–phenomenological–transactional model of stress is that it requires a degree of articulacy to be able to voice the thought processes linked to each phase, and not all individuals will be able to express this.

> What can be stressful to one patient may not be stressful to another. Assumptions about a patient's state of stress are as invalid as any other assumptions a nurse can make without checking with reality.

A composite explanation of stress

In summary, all representations of stress are relevant to high dependency nursing. Assessment of the environment will indicate avoidable stress-inducing factors. Assessment of the patient will indicate physiological responses which will potentially confound other physical pathology. It has been suggested that at the heart of stress, however, are the interpretations and responses made by each individual linked to their perception of their situation. In this context communication skills are as important as an environmental audit or physical examination. It is important to remember this in a care setting which, for very good reasons, is likely to be dominated by environmental and physical demands upon human attention.

CONCLUSION

> Good communication is part of therapy – just as much as drugs or interventions.

An important aspect of high dependency care which should be borne in mind is its transient nature. This has substantial implications for communication, as patients rarely undergo all of their illness management exclusively within a high dependency setting. It is more usually the case that the rapid movement in and out of a high dependency unit leads to different teams of staff becoming involved in care and this is a potential source of deficits in the continuity of information. The management of severe illness often requires the contributions of a diverse range of healthcare professionals, both within and outside the high dependency care multidisciplinary team. The experience of being critically ill, and being at the centre of activity is likely to be extremely frightening for the patient and his relatives. Good communication is the key to making sense of the complex activity which defines high dependency practice. A number of recommendations to this end emerge from the chapter and are summarised in Box 3.7.

A central theme to arise from this chapter is the importance of practising skilled communication which is sensitive to the particular needs of the patient, his significant others and the context in which care is practised. It is hence timely that the UK Council for Nursing, Midwifery and Health Visiting recently disseminated new guidelines for professional practice which include the following:

■ **BOX 3.7** Summary of key interpersonal issues related to high dependency nursing

- Consider the context in which high dependency nursing is practised in relation to communication.
- Develop expertise in the use of a range of communication skills.
- Practise in a way which is conducive to partnership with each patient and his visitors.
- Understand that people are individuals with specific and idiosyncratic needs and be rigorous in assessment to identify these.
- Plan care in the light of your assessment.
- Be aware that needs will be dynamic and will require frequent reassessment.
- Work collaboratively with other care workers and develop a consistent approach to care for each individual.
- Strive to make your message one which is accessible, understandable, attended to and perceived appropriately, memorable and motivating to be acted upon.
- Assess and manage stressful situations proactively using an eclectic interpretation of the concept.

Communication is an essential part of good practice. The patient or client can only make an informed choice if he or she is given clear information at every stage of care. You need to listen to the patient or client ... use language that is familiar to them and make sure that they understand the information you are giving

(UKCC 1996 : p15)

REFERENCES

Argyle M 1994 Psychology of interpersonal behaviour, 5th edn. Penguin, London
Arthur V 1995 Written patient information: a review of the literature. Journal of Advanced Nursing 21: 1081–1086
Asch S 1952 Effects of group pressure upon modification and distortion of judgements. In: Swanson G, Newcombe T, Hartley E (eds) Readings in social psychology. Holt, Rinehart & Winston, New York
Ashbury A 1984 Patients' memories and reactions to intensive care. Care of the Critically Ill 1(2): 12–13
Ashworth P 1980 Care to communicate. Royal College of Nursing, London
Atkins S, Murphy K 1993 Reflection: a review of the literature. Journal of Advanced Nursing 18: 1188–1192
Audit Commission 1993 What seems to be the matter? Communication between hospitals and their patients. HMSO, London
Baily R, Clarke M 1989 Stress and coping in nursing. Chapman & Hall, London
Barber P 1993 Who cares for the carers? Distance Learning Centre, South Bank University, London
Barber P 1997 Caring: the nature of the therapeutic relationship. In: Perry A, Jolly M (eds) Nursing: a knowledge base for practice, 2nd edn. Edward Arnold, London
Bergbom-Engberg I, Haljamäe H 1993 The communication process with ventilator patients in the ICU as perceived by the nursing staff. Intensive and Critical Care Nursing. 9: 40–47
Cahill J 1996 Patient participation: a concept analysis. Journal of Advanced Nursing 24: 561–571
Calnan M 1987 Health and illness: the lay perspective. Tavistock, London
Child D 1996 Psychology and the teacher, 5th edn. Cassell, London
Clark E, Keeble S 1990 Introduction to psychological knowledge. Distance Learning Centre, South Bank University, London
Clarke M 1984 Stress and coping: constructs for nursing. Journal of Advanced Nursing 9: 3–13
Clifford C 1986 Patients, relatives and nurses in a technological environment. Intensive Care Nursing 2: 67–72
Connor M, Norman P (eds) 1996 Predicting health behaviour. Open University Press, Milton Keynes

Crow R, Chase J, Lamond D 1995 The cognitive component of nursing assessment: an analysis. Journal of Advanced Nursing. 22: 206–212

Davidson C, Smith, G, Frankel S 1991 Lay epidemiology and the prevention paradox: the implications of coronary candidacy for health education. Sociology of Health and Illness. 13: 1–19

Davies M 1996 Explaining people and events. In: Aitken V, Jellicoe H (eds) Behavioural sciences for health professionals. W B Saunders, London

Department of Health 1995 The patient's charter and you, 2nd edn. HMSO, London

Department of Health 1996 The National Health Service: a service with ambitions. HMSO, London

Dines A 1994 A review of lay health beliefs research: insights for nursing practice in health promotion. Journal of Clinical Nursing. 3: 329–338

Egan G 1994 The skilled helper: problem management approach to helping, 5th edn. Brooks/Cole, Pacific Grove

Eysenck M, Keane M 1996 Cognitive psychology: a students handbook, 2nd edn. Lawrence Erlbaum Associates, Hove

Foxall M, Zimmerman L, Standley R, Bene B 1990 A comparison of frequency and sources of nursing job stress perceived by intensive care, hospice and medical–surgical nurses. Journal of Advanced Nursing 15: 577–584

Furnham A 1994 Explaining health and illness: lay perceptions on current and future health, the causes of illness and the future of recovery. Social Science and Medicine 39: 715–725

Gregory R 1990 Eye and brain, 4th edn. Weidenfield & Nicholson, London

Gross R 1996 Psychology: the science of mind and behaviour, 3rd edn. Hodder & Stoughton, London

Hargie O, Saunders C, Dickson D 1994 Social skills in interpersonal communication, 3rd edn. Routledge, London

Johns C 1993 Professional supervision. Journal of Nursing Management. 1: 9–18

Kelly G 1958 Man's construction of his alternatives. In: Lindzey G (ed) Assessment of human motives. Holt Rinehart & Winston, New York

Kent V 1996 Attitudes. In: Aitken V, Jellicoe H (eds) Behavioural sciences for health professionals. W B Saunders, London

Kloosterman N 1991 Cultural care: the missing link in severe sensory alteration. Nursing Science Quarterly. 4(3): 119–122

Leathart A 1994a Communication and socialisation (1): an exploratory study and explanation for nurse–patient communication in an ITU. Intensive and Critical Care Nursing 10: 93–104

Leathart A 1994b Communication and socialisation (2): perceptions of neophyte ITU nurses. Intensive and Critical Care Nursing 10: 142–154

Lewin K 1947 Group decision and social change. In: Newcombe T, Hartley E (eds) Readings in social psychology. Holt, Rinehart & Winston, New York

MacAlister L 1994 Stuck in a time warp: communication between hospitals and patients (editorial). British Journal of Nursing 3(1): 4–5

Mackellaig J 1990 A review of the psychological effects of intensive care on the isolated patient and his family. Care of the Critically Ill 6(3): 100–102

McKenna G 1995 Learning theories made easy: cognitivism. Nursing Standard 9: 29–31

Martin L 1997 Talking point. Nursing Standard 11: 19

Maslow A 1970 Motivation and personality. Harper & Row, New York

Menzies I 1970 The functioning of social systems as a defence mechanism against anxiety. Tavistock, London

Myles A 1993 Psychology and health care. In: Hinchliff S, Norman S, Schober J (eds) Nursing practice and health care 2nd edn. Edward Arnold, London

Nightingale F 1859 Notes on Nursing. Harrison and Sons, London (Republished 1980 by Churchill Livingstone, Edinburgh)

Niven N, Robinson J 1994 The psychology of nursing care. British Psychological Society/Macmillan, Leicester

Ogden J 1996 Health psychology: a textbook. Open University Press, Milton Keynes

O'Malley P, Favaloro R, Anderson B 1991 Critical nurse perception of family needs. Heart and Lung 20: 189–201

Pearce J 1994 Communication in critical care nursing. In: Miller B, Bernard P (eds) Critical care nursing. Baillière Tindall, London, p 313–330

Porter S 1994 New nursing: the road to freedom. Journal of Advanced Nursing 20: 269–274

Rundell S 1991 A study of nurse–patient interaction in a high dependency unit. Intensive Care Nursing 7: 171–178

Salvage J 1990 The theory and practice of 'new nursing'. Nursing Times 86: 42–45

Sarafino E 1994 Health psychology: biopsychosocial interactions, 2nd edn. Wiley, New York

Scullion P 1994 Personal cost, caring and communication: an analysis of communication between relatives and intensive care nurses. Intensive and Critical Care Nursing 10: 64–70

Slack J 1990 Attention. In: Roth I (ed.) Introduction to Psychology, vol 2. Lawrence Erlbaum Associates, Hove

Soehren P 1995 Stressors perceived by cardiac surgical patients in the intensive care unit. American Journal of Critical Care 4(1): 71–76

Stevens R 1983 Freud and psychoanalysis. Open University Press, Milton Keynes

Stockwell F 1972 The unpopular patient. Royal College of Nursing, London

Tyler P, Ellison R 1994 Sources of stress and psychological well-being in high dependency nursing. Journal of Advanced Nursing 19: 469–476

United Kingdom Council for Nursing, Midwifery and Health Visiting 1992 The code of professional conduct. UKCC, London

United Kingdom Council for Nursing, Midwifery and Health Visiting 1996 Guidelines for professional practice. UKCC, London

Walsh M 1995 Why patients get the blame for being ill. Nursing Standard 9: 38–40

Webb C, Hope K 1995 What kind of nurses do patients want? Journal of Clinical Nursing 4: 101–108

White D, Tonkin J 1991 Registered nurse stress in intensive care units – an Australian perspective. Intensive Care Nursing 7: 45–52

Social issues in high dependency care

Paul Mulligan

> ### Key learning objectives
>
> - To be aware of the many social factors that influence the patient in high dependency care.
> - To explore through case example and reflection how an understanding of these factors may improve the quality of care.

Prerequisite knowledge

- Understanding of basic sociological terminology
- Understanding of the concepts of interpersonal skills

INTRODUCTION

We all have a medical history, but outside of a GP's surgery or hospital ward it is not something we dwell on too much. Our personal histories are more important in our daily lives. It is only when we are admitted to something like a high dependency unit that our medical histories come into play. But for the nurse working in a hospital environment, dealing with patients every day, it is easy to lose sight of the fact that each patient is a person with his own unique story.

The fact that the patient might have been admitted urgently, with a severe, life-threatening condition means that the nurse tends to concentrate on dealing with medical priorities rather than anything else. She has to get the treatment, the technology and the drugs right, and, of course, there are other patients to care for. So the patient may become a chart, a set of responses to monitors and machines. Personality can get submerged in the paraphernalia of treatment.

So it is not surprising that it can be hard to deal with the patient as a person, with a social background, a family, an ethnic heritage and personal needs. The length of time they will be within our care is often short. Our aim on a busy unit is to reduce the patient's need for high dependency services and so 'step down' as quickly as is practical.

Yet our professional duty is much broader than that. The UKCC code of professional conduct is clear about what a nurse's duty is: '…to recognise and respect the uniqueness and dignity of each patient and client and respond to their need for care irrespective of their ethnic origin, religious beliefs, personal attributes, nature of their health problem or any other factor' (UKCC 1992: Clause 7).

The nurse is there to respond to the patient's need for care. In the high dependency setting that care is complex and concentrated in terms of the medical condition of the patient, but a professional nurse needs to be able to balance those aspects with insight, understanding and empathy for all the 'human' needs of the patient. In other words we have to take a 'holistic' approach to the patient. Understanding the patient's ethnicity or religion, for example, may have an effect on their family's response to their illness, their need to interact with their family while in hospital, and their attitude to life and death issues. Brykczynka (1992) put it thus: 'The most important and significant aspect of caring however is that delicate reintegration and synthesis of knowledge, skills, commitment, professional integrity and love, manifested each time a professional nurse consciously undertakes to nurse a patient or client. This is done because the nurse cares.'

The aim of this chapter is to give the reader information and generate questions about some of the social factors that influence a patient's stay during their experience of high dependency care. Secondly the aim is to help the reader integrate that knowledge by short case studies in order to bring theory to practice and challenge the way that care is delivered.

THE FAMILY

The patient in your care will be part of a social grouping: the most common of these is the family.

The family is a concept most people will be instantly familiar with. We are nearly all born into one and will probably die a member of one. Its influence is very powerful and yet it is vulnerable to the effects *of* social change as much as it is an agent *for* social change. It has been called variously an agent of social control and an agent of the state and yet at no other time has the family undergone such radical and fundamental change as in the latter part of the 20th century. Understanding these changes will help to understand more about the patient.

The family has been described as being 'nuclear' or 'extended'. The classic distinction is that the nuclear family is of our current experience: it is small in number, self-reliant, economically self-fulfilling, geographically mobile, often with only one parent, possibly with both parents working. It is the creation of the industrial/technological age.

The extended family used to be the norm. It consists of wider kin relationships living in close proximity, giving financial and social support. It undertook many of the caring, nurturing and healing roles that have been taken over by health professionals.

To some, the extended family may be an idealised construction. Nurses may judge the value of the patient's family by the degree of their involvement in caring for the patient. The important point is to try and understand the patients' own experience of family and how they live within their social grouping, what that means for them, and who is important to them.

> - Reflect on a family disaster – how has that changed the dynamics in your family?
> - What sort of social roles do you perform and how do they affect your relationship with other members of your family?
> - What personal experience have you had of hospitals – either when you were a patient, or a member of your family?

> ### CASE EXAMPLE 4.1
>
> *Danny at 16 was the eldest son of a travelling family. He suffered a subarachnoid haemorrhage. His mother and twin elder sisters accompany him on admission. He came to HDU for stabilisation prior to transfer to a neurosurgical unit. His condition deteriorates. He is ventilated and is making no respiratory effort. It seems that he is probably brain dead and the first set of brainstem tests confirm this. The father is unable to visit Danny but stays outside the unit. However, the 'family' have been informed. Over the next 2 days nearly 100 'uncles', 'aunts' and 'cousins' visit Danny. The nurses are upset as this appears to be a show of curiosity. The family are spoken to and his mother says that when someone is near to death the whole family must visit.*

What is your idea of the ideal family? How do you project that idea onto the families of patients? What happens when your idealised view doesn't match the reality of the experience?

CASE EXAMPLE 4.1 – RESOLUTION

Relations between the nurses and the family come to a head and the ward manager allows only the immediate family to visit. There is a great deal of shouting and arguing for a few hours. The visiting ceases except for close relatives, who are much happier with this arrangement but felt powerless to stop the traditional response of the extended family. The father asks for a priest and Danny is baptised. Removed from the scrutiny of the 'wider family' Danny's father is able to sit with his son and say his goodbye.

It can be stressful for the nurse dealing with the patient's family and relatives. This may be due to the fact that so much nursing energy is taken up looking after the patient. Our expectation is that the family should be coping and that they should be able to care for themselves, or that we don't understand the effects on the family that hospitalisation causes.

Millar (1989) talks about the physical and biological crises that patients experience when admitted to intensive care – for intensive care read also high dependency care. The consequence is that their families are thrown into emotional turmoil due to the real and perceived threat to the wellbeing of the patient and of themselves. This may put overwhelming pressure on their abilities to cope.

CASE EXAMPLE 4.2

Gordon aged 28 is a self-employed motorcycle courier. He is married to Sally and they have a 2-year-old daughter. Gordon is admitted following an RTA in which his left leg is badly crushed. He is admitted to the HDU as surgical amputation is a high priority. He is denying the seriousness of his condition and says he has been in dozens of accidents before. Sally is very upset and keeps saying she knew something like this was going to happen. She talks about the financial consequences of his impending unemployability as a motorcycle courier and anticipates that she will have to give up her part-time work to care for him as both their families live far away.

Who is providing social support? What can be done to alleviate fears anxieties and worries? How can nursing care help all parties cope?

CASE EXAMPLE 4.2 – RESOLUTION

Gordon undergoes a below-knee amputation and is transferred to the surgical ward 24 hours post-op. The nurses encourage the wider family to visit and suggest ways in which they can help. Both Gordon and Sally's parents visit and offer help and support. This enables Sally to work full-time initially so that outstanding bills can be paid. The nurses contact the social service department and a social worker is sought and takes up their case.

SOCIAL CLASS AND SOCIAL STRATIFICATION

An analysis of social grouping is provided by descriptions of social class and social stratification.

■ **BOX 4.1** Categories of social stratification (Social Trends 1996)

I	**Professional**	Higher managerial, administrative or professional
II	**Intermediate**	Intermediate management, administrative or professional
IIIn	**Skilled non-manual**	Supervisory or clerical and junior managerial administrative or professional
IIIm	**Skilled manual**	Skilled manual workers
IV	**Partly skilled manual**	Semi-skilled and unskilled manual workers
V	**Unskilled manual**	State pensioners or widows (no other earners) or Lowest grade workers or long-term unemployed.

• What social class do you think you belong to?
• Why do we generally feel uncomfortable talking about class?

The patient requiring high dependency care will be categorised statistically within a social class. Understanding its broad outlines will help understand specific individuals. When admitting a patient we take note of their occupation. This is represented by the categories of social stratification (Box 4.1).

These are the categories used by *Social Trends* when analysing social data. Social class is a term that often creates strong feelings. It is sometimes used to categorise people in prejudicial stereotypes, and high dependency care is not immune from this.

Each unit will receive patients from across the social spectrum. The nursing and medical team will also reflect a wide variety of social backgrounds. Both patients and staff will have their own prejudices. For example, the patient who considers himself traditionally working class may feel socially isolated in a unit where the staff are overtly 'middle class', since he may feel the staff are judgemental about his lifestyle, manner, pattern of speech and mode of understanding the world.

CASE EXAMPLE 4.3

Colonel Grouse, 82, is admitted from the medical ward with bilateral pneumonia. He is to have continuous positive airway pressure (CPAP) for his respiratory failure. He is hypoxic, hypercarbic and pyrexial. He has moments of confusion. He is orientated to time and person but insists he is in a different place. The patient in the bed opposite, Joe O'Reilly, is on TPN following major abdominal surgery. Colonel Grouse becomes convinced Joe is in the IRA. He believes the TPN bag is Semtex explosive and that Joe's family is plotting a bombing or terrorist campaign. The Colonel talks to all nurses as if they are private soldiers and the doctors as junior officers. Despite explanation his anxiety is not dissipated.

How does an understanding of class explain the Colonel's behaviour? What can be done to remove his misapprehensions? Is there anything in nursing behaviour which may exacerbate the scenario?

CASE EXAMPLE 4.3 – RESOLUTION

On such a small unit it was not possible to separate the patients. The nurses tried to calm the Colonel down and tried to get Joe O'Reilly's family to pop over and talk to him. Nothing seemed to work. One nurse 'played the game' and acted like a deferential soldier. The Colonel responded and felt that at last someone was listening to him. The nurse defused the situation by distracting the Colonel during visiting time and by ignoring his most bizarre misapprehensions. A combination of antibiotics, good oxygenation and ventilation and adapting responses to the situation helped return the patient to normal.

A particularly significant report in 1982 (The Black Report) considered health inequalities across the UK. It came to the conclusion that social class determines disease and ill health, and that the risk of death for those in groups IV and V was much greater than those in groups I and II at every stage of life. Poverty was a major determinant of ill health. There is evidence that those in poor health move down the social scale, since unemployment often follows, creating economic instability and loss of status. The idea of access to healthcare as determined by class suggests that some groups are disadvantaged by illiteracy, ignorance or lack of power to achieve the same health outcomes as those in higher socioeconomic groups. The authors of the report acknowledge there is no simple explanation but that: 'much of the evidence on social inequalities in health can be adequately understood in terms of specific features of the socioeconomic environment ... work accidents, overcrowding, cigarette smoking, which are strongly class related in Britain and also have clear causal significance (Townsend & Davidson (1982)).

In terms of ill health encountered in high dependency care it would be very difficult to pinpoint specific factors of social inequality in many patients. The vaguer the explanation the more difficult it is to relate to practice. But it appears that poverty, deprivation and ignorance are the most significant factors – these may be inferred from the patient's socioeconomic group and they may be a result of ill health.

RACE

Another aspect of inequality is race. British society is multicultural, composed of many ethnic groups of people of both pure and mixed race.

Race is a biological concept whereby people may be categorised by physical criteria. Skin colour, for example, is the most obvious and widely used, but so are nasal shape, lip form, eye colour and hair type. Of course this categorisation does not explain any of the real differences between people. The idea that inequality could be removed if the immigrant population was integrated into the host population is described as assimilation: the onus being on the immigrant to assimilate the host culture, to 'join the club' and succeed. This however ignores class divisions and prejudices within the host and immigrant populations. A criticism of this approach, which could be termed Marxist, suggests that there is a vested interest for the host culture not to achieve integration, as the immigrants provide the workforce for the national economies of Western society as cheap labour. This creates a climate of revolt where the host population believes '*they* are taking over': this in turn may create an underclass where the indigenous (host) working class splits from the immigrant working class. This may create racism, which is discrimination solely on the grounds of race. Where discrimination enters the social structure of an organisation, for example, then this is termed institutional racism. The health service, as part of society's social structure, is not immune from the effects of this and has been criticised as a mediator of racism through its employment practices. Most organisations, including the NHS, have antiracism policies such as equal opportunity practices. As a workable concept we talk about ethnicity, a description of people's experience and expression of common culture, language, diet, history, art, music. These groupings may contain cultural groups and subgroups.

Understanding cultural and ethnic variations will improve the care of patients and their families receiving high dependency care. However it is dangerous to make assumptions about people based on knowledge received from books, previous experience, or personal prejudices. The patient who calls himself a Muslim, Jew, or Hindu may not behave in the way that textbooks suggest. The starting point must be the person's own experience.

- Reflect upon any personal experience of prejudice that you have had.
- What do you honestly feel about the religious beliefs of others?

CASE EXAMPLE 4.4

Mr Aziz has been keeping a lonely vigil at his wife's bedside from early morning to late at night. By the second day, having refused food and drink, he begins to behave oddly. He appears to drop off to sleep over his wife's bed, but when roused he gets agitated after a nurse insists he leaves the unit for a break or a drink and something to eat. On questioning it becomes clear it is Ramadan and he is fasting and he is going to do what he has to do, not what someone who is not a Muslim is telling him to do. Relations with the nursing staff are in a standoff position.

How could an assessment have prevented this? How can Mr Aziz be helped while still retaining his cultural and religious expression?

CASE EXAMPLE 4.4 – RESOLUTION

The nurses consider it very odd that the children don't visit their mother. There are two adult daughters and a son who are seen in the hospital but not in the high dependency unit. One nurse talks to them and discovers that Mr Aziz is feeling very guilty about his wife, is ignoring everything at home and is not looking after the youngest child, who is 10 years old. At the nurses' suggestion, the family decide to bring Mr Aziz's brother in to talk to him and he realises that he is ignoring the rest of the family and stopping them from caring. This seems to work during the patient's stay in the unit.

HEALTH BELIEFS

It may be easy to identify early on that some people will have a different way of looking at and experiencing the world. This will have a bearing on how the nurse cares for them in terms of dietary requirements, gender issues when giving intimate nursing care, and the variations on religious requirement when caring for a deceased patient. However, there are whole areas of belief that are not bound by cultural or racial expression but all the same will influence the way that a patient and his family makes sense of his illness and their experience of high dependency care. These are the patient's own health beliefs.

These beliefs relate to how the patient describes the illness in his own words, including the 'special' words that people use to describe medical conditions and secondly, the cultural, social and emotional labels that they may attach to it. For example, when we consider the variety of words we use to describe pain – crushing, niggling, stabbing, aching, burning, searing and so on – we are making a judgement on the patient's pain by the words he uses to describe it. If the words the patient uses and the words the nurse uses have different meanings then effective communication has not taken place. Whenever we as nurses explain anything to patients or their families, we have to ensure that they understand what we are talking about. The discussion about social class and ethnicity has introduced some subtle concepts that may hinder understanding. The issue of lay health beliefs is, perhaps, even more subtle. People do not generally think about their health in universally similar ways. They may not have had a medical education but they will have received ideas passed down through the generations and have particular experiences of health and ill health which will affect the way they think. Sayings – such as 'feed a cold and starve a fever' – are an example of a lay health belief. In

- What remedies do you or your family rely upon in ill health?
- Are they 'scientific' remedies?
- Have you ever been dissatisfied with an explanation regarding an illness or treatment from any health professional, and, if so, why?

some cultures this is more formalised – for example, the Hindu culture believes that some illnesses are hot and some are cold and that they have to be treated in this 'hot' and 'cold' manner. The way that illness is explained is often mechanistic and this is a common belief within Western society. If the machine is broken then there has to be a way of fixing it. It has a blockage, so it needs flushing out. If there is a leak it needs plugging. The mechanistic model has its limitations, however.

CASE EXAMPLE 4.5

Sara is 7 years old and is admitted following emergency bowel surgery and the creation of a temporary colostomy. Her parents are very protective, both spending as long as possible with Sara apparently to the exclusion of the other children in the family. The parents are very quiet and do not relate to the nurses very well except to criticise the lateness of the doctor's round, the level of noise or the lack of clean sheets. The nurse caring for Sara discovers that she had diarrhoea for 2 weeks before admission and had been given large amounts of kaolin mixture to stop it. The side effect was to cause a blockage of nearly 'pure clay' as the surgeon wrote, which caused the bowel to become inflamed and rupture. As the relationship develops between the parents and the nurse, they say that they feel so guilty but they thought they were doing the right thing.

How can an understanding of lay health beliefs help in understanding this situation? How can Sara's parents begin to overcome their guilt?

CASE EXAMPLE 4.5 – RESOLUTION

Sara's parents remained very distant throughout her stay and although the nurses had identified their feelings of guilt and shame they were not able to address them in the HDU. However communication between them and the paediatric surgical ward, and the use of family-centred care, meant that the problem was documented and a plan of care created to address the problem.

When something is explained to a patient it is important that their understanding is checked. It is also very important to listen to the words that patients use, because words are often the key to the beliefs that patients express either consciously or unconsciously. The words that health professionals use are often taken for granted. Take the term 'high dependency care'. Patients may understand the term intensive care but may not have heard of high dependency care. Dependency may mean something to do with alcohol or drug addiction and the patient may think they are going to a 'drying out' clinic. If it is explained that high dependency is a little like intensive care then it is important to find out what patients understand by intensive care. Many people experience hospital as a place of pain and suffering and particularly believe that ITUs are places where people die. This belief has to be dealt with carefully and honestly. The challenge is to identify whether or not health beliefs are a significant factor in misunderstanding between patient and health professional.

IATROGENESIS

Patients' past experience of hospital may have been threatening, frightening, painful and distressing. Occasionally the experience of hospital may have caused further pain on top of the admitting illness. The patient may have contracted an infection in hospital. He may have undergone unnecessary treatments, and may have become more unwell as a direct result of treatment. The term used for this is iatrogenesis: it comes from the Greek words *iatros* meaning doctor and *genesis* meaning origin, and is used to describe the harmful effects of medical and surgical treatments. Most treatments will have some degree of risk. This may be due to the side effects of the drugs used, the inexperience of the practitioner delivering the treatment, or as a consequence of the treatment being more painful and disfiguring than the disease itself. All these factors could apply to the patient requiring high dependency care.

The term iatrogenesis was coined by Ivan Illich (1977a) in his work *Medical Nemesis*. He criticised medicine and the healthcare system for creating three types of iatrogenesis:

- Medical: where treatments cause actual harm to patients
- Social: where the power of medicine has so increased that it has 'medicalised' natural events such as birth and death
- Cultural: which is a consequence of the above, as complex urban industrialised communities give up caring for themselves and each other and relinquish that care to the 'professional' carers.

It has long been recognised that hospitals are dangerous places: Florence Nightingale (1859) said that 'hospitals should do the patient no harm'. However some of the sickest patients require high dependency care, and they often require some of the riskiest, most highly invasive interventions such as chest drains, arterial lines, urinary catheters, intravenous catheters, central venous lines, biopsy and mechanical ventilation. Iatrogenic risks may be due to:

- The nature of the procedure
- The inexperience of the operator
- The appropriateness of the treatment.

CASE EXAMPLE 4.6

Gwen Teal, aged 83, is 24 hours post-op following total right hip replacement after a fall at home. She is underweight and appears a little malnourished. She lives alone and has some help from social services but has not been coping well. This is compounded by recently diagnosed mild dementia. She has developed a productive cough with green sputum. Her chest X-ray shows a consolidation in the right lung. She is admitted for high dependency care for chest physiotherapy, pulse oximetry and observation. The locum doctor says that the ward cannot cope with her. On admission, her condition is very poor. The locum doctor insists on siting a central line. The first attempt is unsuccessful. On the second attempt Gwen becomes very breathless, and cyanosed. The doctor is again unsuccessful, and he leaves the unit saying he has to see another patient and will return later to put the line in again. The registrar is called, and a tension pneumothorax is diagnosed. A chest drain is inserted. The registrar reassesses Gwen's resuscitation status and decides she can return to the ward for palliative care. There are now no beds on the ward so she has to stay in the unit.

Which categories of iatrogenesis can be identified? How could the events have been predicted and prevented?

CASE EXAMPLE 4.6 – RESOLUTION

Gwen remained very confused and repeatedly pulled out her i.v. cannula. Fortunately she could not pull out the chest drain despite repeated attempts. The feeling in the unit was that she was 'blocking a bed' and that she was just a nuisance making so much noise.

It is not just doctors who are responsible for iatrogenic incidents. Giraud et al (1993), in a study on incidents in French intensive care units, found that nurses committed twice as many errors as physicians. The main reasons cited were a heavy workload, and a nurse : patient ratio of 1 : 4. This may also be true for high dependency units.

The power and influence of medicine in the Western world is widespread. Illich's (1977a) idea of social iatrogenesis is that birth and death have been medicalised. More births occur in hospital than elsewhere and a higher percentage of these births are by caesarean section. The reasons for this are complex, but there is compelling evidence that the reduction in infant and maternal mortality and morbidity is a direct result of greater medical intervention. As regards death and dying, it is now the 'norm' for people to die in hospital, compared with 50 years ago. People who require high dependency care may be at greater risk of death from the effects of their disease process. How the process of death and dying is handled has immense significance for the patient and his family. The hospital environment is a very alien place. High dependency care relies upon technology, but technology can be very alienating.

> - Think about the ways that caring for one of your patients has led to them getting worse, not better.
> - Who and what were the factors involved?
> - How is society becoming more medicalised?

CASE EXAMPLE 4.7

Mrs Black is dying. Her husband has been told her diagnosis and her prognosis and appeared to take it in. She has a morphine intravenous infusion and seems pain free but is only semi-conscious. She has a cardiac monitor, CVP monitor, temperature, blood pressure and oxygen saturation monitor recording her vital signs. Her husband is with her, but he seems to have lost sight of his wife as his eyes are inexorably drawn to the machines. One alarms, the other bleeps. He reacts. He calls the nurse. The nurse resets the monitor. They alarm again. The nurse resets it again. There is an unusual trace, and Mr Black is becoming expert in observing the machines. He calls another nurse over.

How can we 'demystify' the technology in high dependency care?

CASE EXAMPLE 4.7 RESOLUTION

The nurse sits down alongside Mr Black and asks him how he is feeling. He talks about his anxiety over all the monitoring. She again tells him the truth about his wife and says that his wife doesn't need the monitoring any more. When the monitoring is taken away, Mr Black is able to hold his wife's hand. This gives them the opportunity to talk and the possibility of eventually saying goodbye.

The hospice movement has responded to the needs of dying people. It attempts to demedicalise death, by giving greater choice and control back to the patient and their family and allowing patients to die at home. What can we learn from the values of the hospice movement in high dependency care?

Cultural iatrogenesis is perhaps more difficult to pin down. It has to do with the power and influence that the profession of medicine and to some extent that of nursing have within society. The professions seem to have cornered a niche market in terms of their knowledge and skills. This is reflected in the length and breadth of training and the status that the individual members accrue within society (social groups I and II). The argument runs that the family may have abrogated its responsibility for looking after their sick relative, and may have lost the caring, nurturing and healing skills. The power of the professions grows stronger.

Illich (1977b) says that the only way forward is to: demystify medical matters. The laity, he argues, must be consulted on all decisions, and the individual must be assisted in developing autonomy, and be responsible for their coping ability.

How far has the development within nursing moved towards meeting the above aims?

ADVOCACY

- Think of an occasion when you have disagreed with a patient's medical or nursing treatment.
- What did you do about it?
- If you were not happy with what you did, why do you think that was and what would you do differently next time?

One of the approaches that assists the individual is the concept of advocacy. The UKCC Code of Professional Conduct (1992), the Patients' Charter (1990) and the 'named nurse' initiative, all reflect the use of the concept of advocacy. The advocate is a 'voice for' – someone to take the place of, someone who will speak for you whether you are present or not. This could present a picture of the nurse benignly standing alongside the patient during their illness and hospitalisation. The idea is very appealing. Within the UK legal system, however, we have an understanding of advocacy based upon adversarial conflict. This image presupposes the nurse standing between the patient and whoever he is in conflict with – the physician, the family, other nurses, hospital management, society at large. This presents a more complex picture of the role of the nurse. It can be argued that there are many things preventing nurses from executing their role such as their own professionalism, their duty to the organisation and their obligations to the other patients in their care.

One approach to care that has explored these avenues is primary nursing. Meutzel (1988) sees the relationship between the nurse and patient as a therapeutic relationship. It has three main elements:

- *Reciprocity*, where the nurse may receive support and care
- *Intimacy*, a closeness which has meaning and value
- *Partnership*, which suggests a balance of power and an equality in the nurse/patient relationship.

The expression of the partnership of the nurse/patient relationship is, however, complex. Salvage (1991) says that it is not straightforward as there is insufficient evidence that the patient explicitly wants this type of relationship. The situation where it appears to be most fruitful – but also most complex – is where patients are unable to speak for themselves. The patient who is unconscious is without a voice. How is his autonomy and freedom to make choices respected? The nurse, with her skills, can anticipate, plan and deliver care to meet his needs, but what happens when there is disagreement between the patient's family and the medical team?

CASE EXAMPLE 4.8

Brian Fuller is 72 years old. He has always spoken about 'living wills' and 'advanced directives', saying he 'didn't want to be a vegetable' and that he didn't want any Tom, Dick or Harry having any of his organs. His relatives have been persistent in trying to get him transferred to the local private hospital. Brian is none too fussed. He keeps asking about the patient in the next bed who is awaiting transfer to a specialist centre for transplantation. He is very moved by the plight of this patient and tells the nurse that he would give his organs if he died, saying that this has gone against everything that he has said before but that seeing the pain of a real situation has changed his mind. Later that day Brian suffers a cardiac arrest in the high dependency unit and resuscitation is unsuccessful. His family are distraught. The doctors decide that it is not worth asking the family for organ donation because of the brittle relationship between them. The nurse knows, however, that Brian has changed his mind and broaches the subject. The family initially react badly, and one of the doctors is angry that the nurse has gone against their wishes.

How can you continue to be an advocate for the patient after their death? Where is your responsibility to maintain the partnership: with the patient, the family or the doctors?

CASE EXAMPLE 4.8 – RESOLUTION

The family can't believe that Brian has changed his mind so radically, but left with some literature and the opportunity to come back and ask questions they give it some thought. The nurse stands by her principles and the doctor becomes more isolated in his opinions. The family agree to heart valves and corneal retrieval.

SICK ROLE

Advocacy draws to our attention an approach about how the nurse should act. But how do we expect patients to behave, especially during their experience of high dependency care? The Sick Role (Parsons 1951) is a theory of 'ideal behaviour' that people who become patients exhibit when they are ill. It defines the behaviour as rights and duties (Box 4.2).

This may be or simplified as:

- Excused
- Blameless
- Autonomous
- Compliant.

■ **BOX 4.2** Rights and duties of the sick role (Parsons 1951)

Rights
1. The sick person is exempt from normal work and family duties.
2. The person is not held responsible for their illness, and has a right to sympathy and support.

Duties
3. There is an obligation to get well as quickly as possible.
4. There is a duty to co-operate with competent medical help in order to achieve wellness.

There is a reciprocal relationship with doctors:

- They must act in the interests of the patient and not in self-interest.
- They must apply a high degree of skill and knowledge.
- They must be objective, emotionally detached and professional in attitudes and behaviour.

- Who do you know who is chronically sick and unable to work? What is your attitude to him, and what is his attitude to those who are in work?
- Think of the last time you were off sick from work.
- How did you feel about this and did your behaviour change in any way?
- What process did you have to go through to return from sick leave?

The rights and obligations of both sides maintain the social relationship in the healthcare setting and in society at large. This theory has been criticised because it is paternalistic, as the patient is seen as a passive recipient of care. People do not always behave in this way. The theory is by no means universal, and there are many exceptions: for example, the patient who has a chronic illness, or the patient with depression who has lost the motivation to get better, or the patient who is considered to have a self-induced illness through smoking or alcohol abuse. They will not be considered 'blameless', and it follows that they may not comply with their treatment. When a patient is admitted needing high dependency care it is often unplanned, and this makes the experience a more anxious one. Parsons (1951) suggests that the patient role is a universal one and people understand how to behave even in this emergency situation. Rotter (1966) saw personality traits to be a significant factor in how people perceive a situation. This can be translated to the high dependency setting. Sudden illness, severe illness and emergency care create great stresses both biological and emotional within the individual. These can be both real and imagined. It also depends on how the person 'perceives' the threat or experience and, in terms of high dependency, the seriousness of admission. Rotter grouped people into whether they had an *internal* locus of control or an *external* one. Internals have a high perception of individual control over a given situation. In terms of illness, they feel that they can have some power or control over their illness, and their compliance with treatment and care would best be achieved through a partnership between them and the health professionals. Those with an external locus of control believe they have little influence upon the situation: they may experience events as being beyond their control and influence. Externals are likely to be compliant and more open to persuasion. These patients may, on the surface, be easier to care for because they appear to go along with what medical or nursing action is prescribed. However, they may also appear as passive recipients. Take, for example, the patient who has been diagnosed as an insulin-dependent diabetic. In the high dependency setting, where there is greater nursing and medical contact, he may appear to comply with his dietary restrictions and insulin treatment. But the time spent there may be very short. When the patient returns to the ward with a reduced dependency, and reduced nurse and medical contact, he may have problems complying with ongoing treatment, since the external 'force' will be diminished. This is one theory of how personality traits may influence health behaviour. It is unlikely that patients will define themselves in this way but it is a useful tool in attempting to understand behaviour that is either too compliant or not compliant.

The issue of compliance is one that is central to all healthcare relationships. As Parsons suggested, in order to fulfil the responsibilities of the sick role, the patient would have to comply with his treatment. This is dependent upon the relationship with the doctor (and the nursing staff), the wish to get well (and the ability to do so) and the ability to co-operate.

Central to the issue of compliance is the issue of consent. The patient must be free and able to give consent to treatment. This consent must be informed and the patient must have understanding for the consent to be valid. The difficulties arise with those patients who do not comply.

At one end of the spectrum is the unconscious patient who cannot make a decision. Such patients are of course explicitly unable to give consent, so the decision is made for them until such time as they are able to make it for themselves. At the other end are those patients who are fully informed but refuse to give their consent: for example, the Jehovah's Witness who refuses a blood transfusion, the patient with operable cancer who refuses surgery, or the patient with arterial disease who refuses to stop smoking. Unless there are factors to the contrary, these patients are free to choose not to comply with treatment. There is always a grey area in between. The patient who has deliberately harmed himself or who is suicidal is a danger to himself; there a is duty to care for him – if necessary with coercion – until he is free of any impediment to making a clear, fully informed decision. Here the issue of compliance can be the most difficult for health carers to deal with. A great deal of sensitivity and understanding is required in caring for such patients. The amount of time nurses can spend with each patient is at a premium in high dependency care, and great tensions can arise when trying to balance the needs of the individual with the needs of the whole unit.

CONCLUSION

Nurses in the high dependency unit will often find themselves undertaking a number of activities using many aspects of their role. There is the patient's condition to treat, their own personal needs to address, and the needs of the family to meet. This may require that the nurse responds with technical skills at one moment and listening skills the next. While taking the patient's personal history, the nurse may require the insights of sociological theory and an understanding of how different cultural groups express themselves, in order to understand the patient in their care.

A broad understanding of the issues that determine the medical imperatives of the situation, as well as its human aspects, will enable the nurse to reflect in the situation and on the situation. This may help in decision making, by bringing to the fore the expertise needed to help, and the ability to perform quality nursing care.

It is important to know what to do at a time of medical emergency, but it is also vital not to lose sight of the fact that nursing skills are being used in the care of a human being: a person with a unique history, a place in society, a family and a set of needs which transcend the purely medical. The demands of the UKCC (1992: Clause 7) to provide holistic care may at times be daunting. Each patient is unique; no amount of tubes, wires, drugs, and flashing screens should obscure that truth. The worried family, eager for news, will be a reminder that the person being cared for is not simply a patient.

The case examples in this chapter have highlighted some of the many factors which affect the patient who requires high dependency care. They have only scratched the surface of some of the main issues which come into play with every hospitalisation. The patient, ill or injured, has a personality that was formed, in most cases, long before the illness or injury. Sometimes the condition affects the personality of the patient, and it also sometimes affects the reactions and opinions of the family. The nurse may have to deal with the consequences of the interaction of such events.

Taking the time to weigh up the patient's needs, based on his social position, familial circumstances, ethnic background and traditions, his beliefs and personal opinions, will make the responsibility of caring for the patient much easier, and more satisfying, within the context of high dependency care.

REFERENCES

Brykczykna G 1992 Caring: a dying art? In: Nursing care – the challenge to change. Edward Arnold, London, ch 1

Giraud T, Dhainaut J F, Vaxelaire J F et al 1993 Iatrogenic complications in adult intensive care units: a prospective two centre study. Critical Care Medicine 21(1): 40–51

Illich I 1977a Disabling professions. Marion Boyars, New York

Illich I 1977b Limits to medicine. Medical nemesis: the expropriation of health. Pelican Books, London

Meutzel P 1988 Therapeutic nursing. In: Pearson A (ed.) Primary nursing: nursing in the Burford and Oxford nursing development units. Croom Helm, London

Millar B 1989 Critical support in critical care. Nursing Times 85 (16): 31–32

Nightingale F 1859 Notes on nursing. Churchill Livingstone, Edinburgh

Parsons T 1951 The social system. Routledge & Kegan Paul, London

Rotter J 1966 General expectancies for internal versus external control of reinforcement. Psychological Monographs 80(1): 1–28

Salvage J 1991 The new nursing: empowering patients or empowering nurses. In: Robinson J, Gray A, Elkin R (eds) Policy issues in nursing. Oxford University Press, Oxford

Social Trends 1996 HMSO, London

Townsend P, Davidson N (eds) 1982 The Black Report. Pelican Books, London

UKCC 1992 Code of professional conduct. UKCC, London.

FURTHER READING

Bond J, Bond S 1995 Sociology and health care. Churchill Livingstone, London

Kikuchi J F, Simmons H (eds) 1992 Philosophic inquiry in nursing. Sage, London

Porter R 1997 The greatest benefit to mankind. HarperCollins, London

Robinson K, Vaughan B 1992 Knowledge for nursing practice. Butterworth-Heinemann, London

Clinical issues in high dependency care

Respiratory care

CHAPTER 5

Debbie Field

Key learning objectives

With prerequisite knowledge of respiratory physiology, the reader of this chapter will be able to:

- Identify the causes, signs and symptoms of respiratory failure, recognising those patients who are at greater risk of developing respiratory distress and who may require high dependency care.
- Describe and give a rationale for patient assessment in relation to optimising and maintaining effective breathing in these patients.
- Identify and give a rationale for the main principles of respiratory care, nursing interventions and prevention of complications for these patients.
- Demonstrate greater awareness of the drugs most commonly used in respiratory care and their effects on the patient.
- Identify and be aware of the usefulness and limitations of those technological interventions used in respiratory care and observation on these patients.

INTRODUCTION

The purpose of this chapter is to demonstrate the importance of the nurse's role in relation to the delivery and effectiveness of respiratory care for those patients who are at risk of developing respiratory failure and require high dependency care, whether within the ward environment or in a designated high dependency unit (HDU). In both areas nurses need to be able to apply their knowledge and skills in order to extrapolate, analyse and critically evaluate the data observed, the interventions and treatment being initiated and the nursing care implemented. This chapter is, therefore, designed to give nurses a greater understanding of the concepts of patient assessment, nursing care, therapeutic and technological intervention, treatment options and pharmacological agents in order to prevent complications and to optimise and maintain effective respiration for those patients who require high dependency care in any setting. With greater understanding of respiratory care, nurses will ultimately effect a quality patient outcome by reducing morbidity and mortality in those patients who require high dependency care.

Prerequisite knowledge

It is essential that the reader has an understanding of normal respiratory anatomy and physiology before studying this chapter. This knowledge is summarised in Box 5.1. However, a brief overview of the main concepts of respiratory physiology will be presented in order to enhance the reader's application of these to patient assessment, intervention, treatment and care.

■ **BOX 5.1** Prerequisite knowledge

Anatomy
- Major structures: mouth/nose, trachea, bronchi, lungs, diaphragm, pleura
- Blood supply
- Micro structures: alveoli, goblet cells
- Anatomical deadspace

Physiology
- Lung volumes
- Carriage of gases
- Aerobic and anaerobic cellular respiration
- Oxyhaemoglobin dissociation curve
- Physiological deadspace
- Ventilation/perfusion match (V/Q)
- Control of breathing
- Boyle's law, Dalton's law

Acid–base balance
Determinants of work of breathing

■ **BOX 5.2** Respiratory components

1. Mechanical movement of gases into and out of the lungs. This includes atmospheric air/lung pressure gradient, airway resistance, muscular function, lung compliance, intrapleural pressures, neural control.
2. Exchange of these gases across a membrane by diffusion.
3. Carriage of gases to and from the tissues.
4. Metabolic process of the cell to produce energy.

CONCEPTS OF RESPIRATORY PHYSIOLOGY

The primary function of the respiratory system is to supply adequate oxygen (O_2) to the tissues for the oxidation of respiratory substrates (carbohydrates, fats and proteins) in order to yield energy (cellular respiration) and to remove the waste product, carbon dioxide (CO_2). This is represented in Fig. 5.1 below. This function is interdependent with the circulatory system's prime role of blood transport.

Fig. 5.1 Representation of respiratory function

$$O_2 + fuel = energy + CO_2 + H_2O$$

Normal respiratory physiology and function can be divided into four components (see Box 5.2).

Movement of gases

In order to move air or O_2 from the atmosphere to the lungs, a pressure gradient is created between the mouth and the alveoli (trans-airway pressure) through the movement of the chest wall and diaphragm during inspiration. During spontaneous breathing (that is, unassisted) this pressure gradient is negative and initiates the flow of air from the atmosphere to the alveoli.

Movement of gases is therefore dependent upon the factors listed in Box 5.3.

Surfactant decreases the surface tension of the alveoli in order to aid the diffusion of gases. A reduction in the production of surfactant will directly affect alveolar gas exchange (see Box 5.4).

This negative pressure also enhances venous return which contributes to an adequate cardiac output.

■ **BOX 5.3** Spontaneous inspiration and expiration: dependent factors

- Atmospheric pressure
- Chest wall compliance
- Respiratory muscle function
- Neural control
- Negative pressure gradient between mouth and alveoli
- Resistance of the airway to flow of air
- Elasticity of the lung tissue
- Surfactant production

■ **BOX 5.4** General causes of reduced surfactant production

- Acidosis
- Hypoxia
- Hyperoxygenation
- Atelectasis
- Pulmonary vascular congestion
- Starvation

Gas exchange

Gas exchange only takes place within the functioning units of the alveoli and where there is adequate alveolar capillary blood flow in order to allow movement of gases across the pulmonary capillary membrane by diffusion (see Fig. 5.2). Once there has been an exchange of gases at alveoli level O_2 is transported to the tissues (see Fig. 5.3 on p. 72) and CO_2 is excreted via the lungs during expiration.

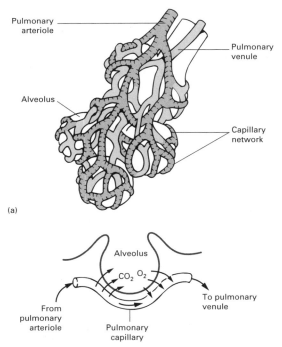

Pulmonary arteriole

Pulmonary venule

Alveolus

Capillary network

(a)

Alveolus

CO_2 O_2

From pulmonary arteriole

Pulmonary capillary

To pulmonary venule

(b)

Fig. 5.2 Gas exchange in the lungs. (From Hinchliff & Montagu 1988)

Fig. 5.3 Gas exchange in the tissues. (From Hinchliff & Montagu 1988)

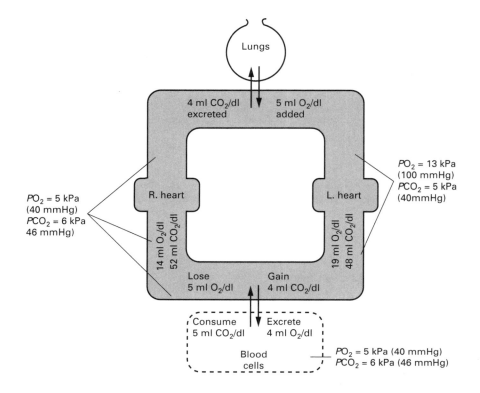

Ventilation/perfusion match

Another important determinant of gas exchange is the relationship between pulmonary perfusion (Q) and alveolar ventilation (V). There is normally a small degree of mismatch between ventilation and perfusion in different areas of the lungs. This is due to the effect of gravity which increases the amount of work required to force blood through the vessels further above the heart.

Hypoxaemia causes a pathological V/Q mismatch and is seen as a right to left shunt (venous admixture). This is where poorly ventilated areas of lung continue to be perfused (see Fig. 5.4). Causes of right to left shunts can be seen in Box 5.5.

Carriage of gases

This process is also dependent on an adequate cardiac output (see Ch. 6). The majority of O_2 is carried in combination with haemoglobin and only 0.3 ml O_2 is carried dissolved in plasma. At a normal level of haemoglobin (15 g/dl), 20 ml O_2 is carried per 100 ml of blood.

One important aspect in relation to the carriage of O_2 is the oxyhaemoglobin dissociation curve (see Fig. 5.5 on p. 74), that is, the detachment of O_2 from haemoglobin. The actual chemical structure of haemoglobin allows for varying affinity to O_2 molecules which is dependent upon the partial pressure of O_2 (PO_2) within the capillary. A fit individual with normal lung function, therefore, who has a PO_2 of 13.3 kPa will have used almost all of the O_2 binding capacity of haemoglobin and the haemoglobin is said to be approximately 98% saturated.

Where O_2 is extracted at tissue level haemoglobin saturation is reduced to about 75% and O_2 is released to the tissues. This leaves about three-quarters of the

A patient with a low haemoglobin will therefore carry less O_2 per 100 ml blood. This means that there is less available O_2 at tissue level for adequate cellular metabolism.

■ **BOX 5.5** Causes of right to left shunts (V/Q mismatch)

- Hypoventilation for any reason (e.g. excess sedation, pain, respiratory muscle weakness, abnormal thoracic anatomy)
- Atelectasis (e.g. following general anaesthesia)
- Alveoli consolidation
- Pulmonary oedema
- Obstructive lung disease (emphysema, bronchitis, asthma)
- Restrictive lung disease (pneumonia, fibrosing lung disease, adult respiratory distress syndrome)

> When demand exceeds supply – for example when a patient has an acute asthmatic attack – cellular metabolism changes from aerobic metabolism to anaerobic metabolism which results in lactate production and metabolic acidosis thus reducing the patient's O_2 reserve further.

haemoglobin oxygenated which provides a reservoir for conditions when there is an increased demand for O_2 (e.g. during excerise or illness), in order to maintain aerobic metabolism.

Several important factors affect the oxyhaemoglobin curve (see Box 5.6 on p 75) which can 'shift' the curve to the right (i.e. for the same level of arterial PO_2 the haemoglobin saturation is lower therefore more O_2 is available to the tissues); or to the left (that is, for the same amount of arterial PO_2 the haemoglobin saturation is higher and there is therefore less O_2 available to the tissues). These shifts in the curve will have minimal effects on O_2 availability and physiological homeostasis if the PO_2 remains within normal range.

> Shifts in the oxyhaemoglobin curve become highly significant for those patients who present with a low PO_2 as their O_2 reserve is already compromised.

Physiological deadspace

Ventilation but no perfusion
$\dot{V}_A/\dot{Q}>1$

Causes

Pulmonary embolism
Pulmonary arteritis
Necrosis of fibrosis
(TB, Fibrosing
alveolitis
– loss of capillary
bed)

Physiological shunt

No ventilation but perfusion
$\dot{V}_A/\dot{Q}<1$

Causes

Airway limitation (asthma and chronic bronchitis)
Lung collapse or consolidation

Loss of elastic tissue (emphysema)

Diseases of the chest wall

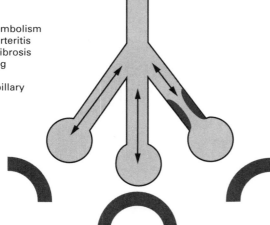

Normal

Ventilation and perfusion
$\dot{V}_A/\dot{Q}=1$

Fig. 5.4 Ventilation and perfusion. (From Kumar & Clark 1990 with kind permission.)

Fig. 5.5 (a) The oxygen–haemoglobin dissociation curve. This curve applies when the pH is 7.4, blood temperature is 37°C and the PCO_2 is 5.3 kPa. It should also be assumed that haemoglobin concentration is 15 g/dl blood.

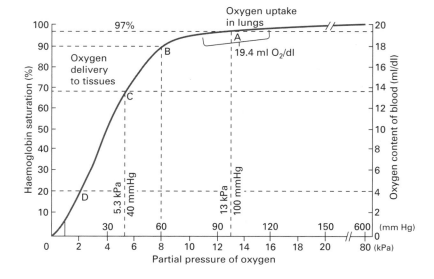

(b) Factors influencing the position of the oxygendissociation curve. L From Hinchcliff & Montague 1988 with kind permission.)

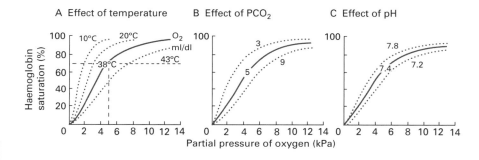

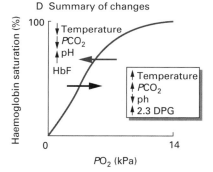

i) Once haemoglobin is fully saturated no further increase in PO_2 will increase the amount of O_2 carried by haemoglobin. Increasing the patient's inspired O_2 will not increase his PO_2 if his haemoglobin is fully saturated.

(ii) A patient's PO_2 can decrease quite considerably before there is any significant fall in haemoglobin saturation. Looking at Fig. 5.5 we can see that a haemoglobin saturation of 90% has a PO_2 of around 8.0 KPA. This is an important point to understand especially in relation to the monitoring of patients using pulse oximetry (this will be discussed later in the chapter).

Carbon dioxide

There are six different mechanisms involved in the carriage of CO_2 (see below).

Plasma

1. As dissolved CO_2 (10%)
2. Protein bound
3. As bicarbonate (HCO_3)

Red blood cells

4. As dissolved CO_2 (10%)
5. Combined with haemoglobin
6. As bicarbonate (70%)

■ **BOX 5.6** Factors causing shifts in the oxyhaemoglobin curve

Factors causing a shift to the right:
- Decreased blood pH (i.e. pH below 7.35)
  – acidosis
- Increase in body temperature
- Increase in $P\,CO_2$
- Increase in 2,3-diphoglycerate (2,3-DPG). 2,3-DPG is a substance contained within the red blood cell formed during anaerobic glycolysis. Levels are increased in response to hypoxia and/or anaemia.

Factors causing a shift to the left:
- Decreased blood pH (i.e. pH greater than 7.45) – alkalosis
- Decreased body temperature
- Decreased $P\,CO_2$
- Decreased 2,3-DPG
- Carbon monoxide poisoning

DEFINITIONS OF RESPIRATORY FAILURE

Respiratory failure may be characterised as:

- Type I hypoxaemia without hypercapnia, in which the PaO_2 is low and the $PaCO_2$ is normal or low. It is usually acute and occurs with diseases that damage lung tissue, with hypoxaemia due to right to left shunts or V/Q mismatch. Common causes include pulmonary oedema, pneumonia and chronic conditions such as pulmonary fibrosing alveolitis.
- Type II hypoxaemia with hypercapnia, in which the PaO_2 is low and the $PaCO_2$ is high. This occurs when alveolar ventilation is insufficient to excrete the volume of carbon dioxide being produced by tissue metabolism.

Inadequate alveolar ventilation is due to reduced ventilatory effort, inability to overcome an increased resistance to ventilation, failure to compensate for an increased deadspace and/or CO_2 production, or a combination of these factors. The most common causes are chronic bronchitis and emphysema.

Risk factors

It is important to identify those patients who are commonly admitted to general clinical areas and who are most at risk of developing respiratory distress or failure (see Box 5.7).

It is beyond the scope of this chapter to address all of the causes listed (see Further Reading) and many are self-explanatory in their effect on respiratory function. It is important, however, for the nurse to identify those patients who are at greater risk of developing respiratory distress and/or failure and who may therefore require a higher dependency of care.

Age and site of operation

Patient age and the site of operation have been well documented as factors which influence the risk of post-operative chest complications, (Giroux et al 1987, Chuter et al 1990). These writers demonstrated that the higher the incision in abdominal surgery the greater the risk of decreased diaphragmatic movement leading to atelectasis. Patients over the age of 60 also have decreased physiological reserve for coping with stress (Foyt 1992).

■ **BOX 5.7** Conditions that increase the risk of respiratory distress/failure

- Chronic lung disease – asthma, chronic airway limitation, emphysema, pulmonary fibrosing alveolitis
- General anaesthetic causing atelectasis and possible pneumonia
- Upper abdominal surgery
- Chest surgery/trauma
- Chest wall deformities
- Nasogastric tube in situ for more than 24 hours (without enteral feeding)
- Depression of respiratory centre including drug-induced depression and neurological injury
- Respiratory muscle weakness including myasthenia gravis, Guillain–Barré syndrome, poor nutritional status
- V/Q mismatch such as atelectasis, pneumonia, pulmonary oedema, hypoperfusion
- Immobilisation

General anaesthetic

General anaesthesia causes a decease in functional residual capacity (FRC) as a result of a change in the shape and position of the diaphragm and chest wall. This alters the distribution of inspired gas without adjustment in pulmonary blood flow. Consequently, this leads to the development of low ventilation–perfusion lung units which cause atelectasis to develop (Matthay & Wiener-Kronish 1989). General anaesthesia may predispose to mild oxygenation defects causing atelectasis and decreased FRC. However, in the absence of chronic lung disease or other pre-existing pulmonary disease, these effects are mild and usually transient if good respiratory management is employed.

Nasogastric tubes and nutrition

Do the patients that you nurse receive adequate daily nutrition? Are meal times given priority in the care and management of patients?

Pulmonary complications may arise if a nasogastric tube (NGT) remains in situ for more than 24 hours and the patient is not being enterally fed. This is possibly due to an increase in reflux and aspiration, or decreased coughing efficacy (McConnell 1991). This may cause translocation of bacteria into the pulmonary system.

Poor nutritional status, in particular low serum phosphate, will directly affect respiratory muscle strength. Phosphate is the major energy source for effective muscle function. The nurse must therefore ensure that the patient who is at risk receives adequate nutrition. As mentioned earlier, starvation decreases surfactant production.

Mobility

When patients increase their mobility after being on bed rest they will increase their energy requirements. This will also increase their oxygen demand. It is important, therefore, to ensure that the patient is receiving the appropriate amount of calories to meet his new energy demands.

Immobilisation may appear to be self-explanatory in relation to reduced respiratory function. It is, however, important to identify the psychological impact that being immobile has in influencing respiratory function. This relates to feelings of depression and lack of control on the part of the patient, resulting in a lack of compliance to nursing interventions and physiotherapy regimes.

PRINCIPLES OF RESPIRATORY CARE

Nursing assessment, intervention and care must be based upon an individual and holistic approach to each patient for whom the nurse cares. It requires continuity of care if the nurse is to optimise and maintain effective respiration with the ultimate aim of making the patient feel comfortable and cared for and to prevent complications. Continuity of care is achieved through:

- Effective communication throughout the team
- Proactive and creative nursing strategies and interventions
- An appropriate and effective framework of care (e.g. team nursing)
- Nursing audit
- Care reviews.

The patient at risk of developing respiratory failure needs continuous physiological and psychological observation and assessment, and well-planned nursing strategies must be implemented. There is therefore an increased patient dependency on nursing care, nursing time and technology such as non-invasive respiratory support, cardiac monitoring and oximetry.

The principle of respiratory care is to optimise and maintain ventilation and perfusion. This is achieved by:

- Continuous observation and assessment of the patient
- Proactive patient-centred comfort care
- Positioning
- Assistance with physiotherapy techniques
- Oxygen therapy and non-invasive respiratory support
- Accurate fluid balance
- Adequate pain-relief
- Temperature control
- Chest drain management
- Appropriate administration and evaluation of drug therapies in relation to respiratory function
- Continuity of care from the whole multidisciplinary team.

NURSING OBSERVATION AND ASSESSMENT

The assessment of patients requires nurses to use their skills of observation, communication, monitoring, analysing and interpreting both objective and subjective data in order to deliver effective care. Observation skills, which include sight, hearing, touch and smell, should not be underestimated. They are important factors in assessing and collecting information about the patient's respiratory function. From such observations the nurse will often gain intuitive perceptions of how the patient is reacting to hospital admission, the hospital environment, the course of treatment and care and his whole sense of being. This intuitive knowledge is just as important as the meticulous collection of empirical data in relation to the patient's physiological status and it should never be trivialised.

Respiratory assessment is an important part of holistic patient assessment and nurses should not regard it as a separate entity.

It has been demonstrated that expert nurses (Benner 1984, Roach 1985) improve patient outcomes when delivering direct care or acting as role models. With this in mind it is important to ensure that those patients who are at risk or have respiratory failure are cared for by an appropriately experienced nurse or that the nurse caring for the patient is facilitated by someone experienced in this area.

Normal respiratory work at rest consumes 2–3% of the total O_2 intake but this increases to 40–50% in respiratory distress leading to cardiovascular and neurological deterioration.

Respiratory work may be increased and ventilation and perfusion may be decreased well before the signs of hypercapnia and hypoxia are present.

Assessment for the signs and symptoms of potential respiratory failure demands that the nurse look for subtle changes in the patient's condition and vital signs. This requires continuity of nursing care.

■ **BOX 5.8** Respiratory assessment

- Respiratory history (see below)
- Respiratory rate, rhythm, depth and facial signs
- Breath sounds
- Sputum and secretions
- Cardiovascular signs
- Neurological status
- Psychological status
- Pulse oximetry
- Blood profiles: Hb, phosphate, urea and creatinine, WBC
- Chest X-ray (CXR)
- Pain assessment
- Pulmonary lung function tests
- Imaging: CT scan, magnetic resonance imaging (MRI)
- Bronchoscopy
- Arterial blood gases

Respiratory history will include the following details:
- Relevant past medical history
- History of dyspnoea – at rest or on exertion. Has the patient's exercise tolerance decreased recently and why?
- History of coughing – productive or dry?
- History of haemoptysis
- History of asthma or other chronic lung disease
- Smoking – has the patient ever smoked and does he smoke now?
- Recent or chronic respiratory infections
- Relevant drug history
- How does the patient cope with stress? (Stress will increase the patient's sympathetic response and therefore increase O_2 demand)
- What is the patient's normal sleeping pattern? In what position does he sleep?
- Nutritional history: has there been any recent weight loss or weight gain?
- Pain strategies: how does the patient cope with acute or chronic pain?
- Base line observations (TPR & BP)

Respiratory assessment should include the information contained in Box 5.8.

Clinical signs

The clinical signs of respiratory distress signify an increase in *respiratory work* which can eventually lead to respiratory failure. The most important and significant signs of respiratory distress are manifested by the respiratory, cardiovascular and central nervous systems.

The normal rate of breathing at rest is about 14–16 breaths per minute. An increase in the patient's respiratory rate of even three to five breaths per minute form the patient's normal respiratory rate at rest is significant. This is an important and *early* danger sign of respiratory distress and consequent hypoxaemia. A rise in respiratory rate initially minimises the increase in respiratory work required as the patient's lung compliance falls. It may initially affect the patient so little that he deries he is breathless. This is a result of the effect of compensatory factors such as mouth opening and increased heart rate. However, together with the small increase in respiratory rate, the nurse's observation of the patient will demonstrate that speech is appreciably impaired at this stage.

A patient whose respiratory rate has increased at rest will begin to talk in short sentences, pausing to take a breath during the sentence spoken.

■ **BOX 5.9** Signs of respiratory distress (respiratory system)

- Mouth opening
- Pursed/tightened lips
- Nasal flaring
- Sweating forehead
- Prominent sternomastoid
- Use of other accessory muscles
- Depth of breathing
- Regularity of breathing
- Chest wall movements
- Cyanosed lips

Gradually, breathlessness may increase and the patient will begin to show further signs of respiratory distress (see Box 5.9).

Mouth opening Commonly, the mouth opens at an early stage of respiratory distress. Initially this is slight and variable, or occurring only during inspiration. It is often difficult to detect, but it becomes more and more obvious as the distress increases. *Even minor changes are significant.* There are two physiological benefits – a reduction in anatomical deadspace and in respiratory work.

Pursed-lips breathing This sign is often combined with open-mouth breathing, where the mouth opens with inspiration and the lips purse with expiration. Obstruction and prolongation of expiration by pursed lips is a natural positive end-expiratory pressure (PEEP) mechanism. It increases functional residual capacity and lung compliance, and benefits respiratory work and gas exchange.

Cyanosed lips and extremities These are not very accurate signs of central cyanosis and consequently arterial desaturation. These two signs are more indicative of decreased perfusion due to sympathetic response.

Central cyanosis, which indicates arterial desaturation, can be more reliably observed in the discolouring of the patient's mucous membranes and buccal cavity. This is an ominous sign and requires immediate attention.

The forehead The patient may sweat and feel cool and clammy to touch. This reflects increased respiratory effort and increased sympathetic nervous system response rather than carbon dioxide retention. It may also signify a failing circulation, and the need for immediate therapy.

The nose Flaring of the nostrils is a late sign of respiratory distress in adults, but not always reliable. Nostril flaring in children and babies is indicative of acute respiratory distress.

The neck The sternocleidomastoids, important accessory muscles of respiration, are often prominent in acute respiratory distress and failure. Patients often hold their head off the pillow to enhance the action of these muscles, despite their tiredness.

Accessory muscles The use of accessory muscles will be observed in patients who develop moderate to severe respiratory distress. The use of these muscles indicates an increase in the work of breathing, with a consequent increase in oxygen demand. Accessory muscle action includes suprasternal retractions, intercostal retractions and diaphragmatic breathing or abdominal breathing.

During severe exercise in the fit individual, he will use open-mouth panting in order to decrease respiratory work and anatomical deadspace as this is an autonomic response.

This manoeuvre is seen following severe exercise. When athletes finish running a race, for example, you will note that they often bend forward, open their mouths to breathe in, then purse their lips when breathing out.

■ BOX 5.10 Flail chest

- Injury to the chest wall produces instability of the thoracic cage and lung contusion.
- Ribs fractured in several places or combined with dislocations of the costochondral junctions or sternum, the negative intrapleural pressure generated on inspiration causes the isolated segment of the chest wall to collapse inwards (flail chest) compromising ventilation. This will be demonstrated by the patient in terms of *paradoxical breathing* (when the thoracic cage moves inward during inspiration as opposed to normal inspiration when the rib cage expands in a symmetrical fashion).
- Chest wall injuries are *extremely painful* which will further compromise the patient's respiratory function – the patient will hypoventilate.

> Patients who have pre-existing lung disease may have chronic use of accessory muscle breathing but this will be further exaggerated if the patient has an exacerbation of chronic lung disease.

Depth of breathing As respiratory distress increases patients will hypoventilate. Breathing gradually becomes laboured and the use of accessory muscles will become even more prominent.

Regularity of breathing Breathing will change from regular to irregular, as respiratory distress worsens. Eventually the patient's breathing may become periodic and the patient exhibits periods of apnoea.

Chest wall movements Movement of the chest wall will change as the work of breathing increases. The rhythm of breathing will become dysynchronous. Movement of the chest wall also relates to the anatomy of the patient and whether his movements are restricted by chest drains, wound site, dressings or chest wall trauma causing a flail chest (see Box 5.10).

Auscultation of chest

Listening to air entry is a difficult observation, as it requires experience to be able to interpret what is heard. It may take time to master the skill but once mastered it will be an important addition to a thorough respiratory assessment of the patient. It is important that nurses seek help and advice from colleagues within the multidisciplinary team (such as physiotherapists and doctors) in order to learn and master this observation.

Listening to air entry and breath sounds is a basic measure to ensure that there is flow of air to all areas of the lung. Common causes of decreased or non-existent air entry in self-ventilating patients are listed below:

- Hypoventilation
- Atelectasis
- Lobar collapse
- Sputum retention
- Pneumonia
- Pleural effusion
- Pneumothorax.

Breath sounds result from air passing over the larynx and vary in loudness and rhythm depending on where the stethoscope is placed. There are three normal types of breath sound heard over different parts of the chest.

Normal breath sounds

Vesicular A gentle rustling noise which is audible all over the periphery of the lungs. It is loudest on inspiration and fades away rapidly during the early part of expiration.

Bronchial High pitch, loud, with a pause between inspiration and expiration. Expiration equals inspiration and should only be heard over the trachea. If these bronchial sounds are heard over any other areas of the lung it is indicative of lung pathology.

Bronchovesicular A combination of the above sounds, heard over major airways in most other parts of the lung.

Abnormal breath sounds

Crackles These are high-pitched rustles heard mainly during inspiration. They occur in diseases affecting the alveoli or terminal airways and often (but not always) when there is an excessive amount of exudate or transudate in these regions. Crackles will be heard in conditions such as pneumonia, bronchiectasis and pulmonary oedema.

Coarse crackles are loud bubbling sounds and are heard during both inspiration and expiration due to copious secretions in the large airways. This can occur in bronchiectasis, bronchitis and where patients are unable to expectorate secretions effectively – also if the patient has left ventricular failure (LVF).

Wheezes These are musical sounds of low or high pitch that can occur on inspiration or expiration. They are due to the passage of air moving through narrowed airways at high velocity. The pitch of the sound varies directly with the narrowness of the airways and the velocity at which air travels through the airways. Wheezes are commonly heard in patients suffering from chronic airway limitation or bronchial asthma when the obstruction is due to secretions and bronchospasm.

Pleural friction rubs Rough, grating, and crackling sounds heard on inspiration and expiration. These are found in areas of pleural inflammation when the normally smooth surfaces of parietal and visceral pleura are roughened and rub on each other.

Sputum and secretions

If the patient is producing sputum it is important to observe the colour, consistency and amount. This observation will also add to a better understanding of the patient's respiratory function (see Box 5.11).

Measurable respiratory signs

Peak expiratory flow rate (PEFR) There will be a decreased PEFR in patients who develop respiratory failure. Those patients who already have asthma or chronic airway limitation will probably experience 'morning dips' in their PEFR as their respiratory failure worsens. These morning dips in PEFR are highly significant and should not be ignored. This will be discussed further in the section on drug therapies.

Vital capacity Observing a patient's vital capacity will demonstrate the strength of the respiratory muscles (directly proportional to the use of the muscle). This is especially important if patients have a history of neuromuscular disorder such as multiple sclerosis, Guillain–Barré syndrome or myasthenia gravis.

Pulse oximetry has established itself as the most convenient non-invasive method of continuously monitoring arterial saturation. Its use is well established

■ **BOX 5.11** Sputum and secretions

- Copious amounts of white bloodstained frothy sputum are indicative of pulmonary oedema which can be seen in some patients who develop respiratory distress. This is due to increasing oxygen debt, anaerobic respiration and sympathetic response leading to an increase in workload on the heart. If the patient already has pre-existing heart disease, then it is quite possible that pulmonary oedema will develop.
- Yellow/green sputum is evidence of infection.
- Rusty sputum is indicative of pneumonia. Thick and tenacious secretions may indicate that the patient is dehydrated or has an acute or chronic chest infection such as bronchiectasis. The patient may find it extremely difficult to expectorate such secretions – this may lead to sputum retention. This in turn leads to bronchospasm and alveolar hypoventilation, with the consequence that the patient develops acute respiratory failure.

within theatres, recovery and critical care areas. There is increasing use, however, within general wards owing to the higher levels of dependency among patients being admitted. A pulse oximeter monitors the saturation of haemoglobin with oxygen in arterial blood (SpO_2). The normal range of SpO_2 for a patient breathing room air and with no significant lung disease is 95–99%.

Pulse oximetry, however, is not foolproof and has its limitations. It requires those who use it to have an adequate understanding of respiratory physiology and basic principles of the management of acute respiratory dysfunction (Stoneham et al 1994). The pulsatile signal is very susceptible to noise, especially in association with poor peripheral circulation and movement all of which will produce a false reading. Stoneham, Saville and Wilson (1994) demonstrated that knowledge of pulse oximetry was poor. Their study found that medical and nursing staff did not always realise that an SpO_2 value below 90% implied that arterial partial pressure of oxygen (PaO_2) is low and that there may be critical hypoxaemia. Pulse oximetry can give a false reassurance of what is seen as a 'normal' SpO_2 especially when a patient is receiving supplementary oxygen.

When using pulse oximetry, the nurse must consider the points listed in Box 5.12 to ensure the patient's safety.

CASE EXAMPLE 5.1

A patient has returned from theatre following repair of a hiatus hernia with a morphine infusion running and oxygen at 45% via a face mask. He is a smoker. A pulse oximeter shows that his saturation is 91%.

Question: *What are the implications of this oximeter reading?*

Answer: *There is critical hypoxaemia because the patient is already receiving supplementary oxygen at a relatively high dose.*

Question: *What interventions are required?*

Answer:

- *Check the pulse oximeter's pulse wave, as it may not be adequate enough to give a reading*
- *Check the patient's conscious level*
- *Check airway, breathing and circulation*
- *Call for medical assistance.*

■ BOX 5.12 Points to consider when using pulse oximetry

- Pulse oximetry is an adjunct to a thorough respiratory assessment and should never be seen in isolation.
- Is there an adequate pulsatile waveform?
- A displaced or detached transducer will give a poor reading.
- Poor perfusion due to peripheral constriction for whatever reason will give a poor reading. It is sometimes preferable to use a transducer attached to the ear or the bridge of the nose.
- The presence of carbon monoxide in blood (e.g. exposure to smoke/fume inhalation) will give erroneously high but false readings.
- Pulse oximetry gives no indication of carbon dioxide levels.
- A low SpO_2 on supplementary oxygen indicates a serious pulmonary complication (unless the patient has significant chronic lung disease).
- Oxygen saturation trends need to be assessed rather than just a one-off reading.
- The SpO_2 value and the inspired oxygen should always be recorded together.

Cardiovascular signs

Attention should be paid to the rate, rhythm, volume and character of the radial pulse.

A bounding pulse and large volume associated with cyanosis and a history of chronic airway limitation suggest carbon dioxide retention due to respiratory failure. Other signs associated with this should also be looked for such as drowsiness, sweating and flapping hand tremor.

Diminished volume of the radial pulse during inspiration (known as *pulsus paradoxus*) is attributed to limitation of venous return to the right side of the heart. This is caused by constrictive pericarditis or restrictive cardiomyopathy but also occurs in severe chronic obstructive airway limitation.

In response to the oxygen debt there will be an increase in heart rate which in turn increases oxygen demand. This then sets up a cycle of events; the oxygen debt increases further and the heart rate increases as a response but with no subsequent increase in oxygen supply. The increase in heart rate will also have an immediate effect on myocardial perfusion, as well as oxygen demand owing to decreased filling time during diastole.

If the oxygen debt increases to the point that the patient becomes hypoxic and therefore has an acid–base imbalance the patient may experience life-threatening arrhythmias. These may include atrial fibrillation, paroxysmal atrial tachycardia, ventricular fibrillation, ventricular tachycardia or severe bradycardia.

Initially there will be a rise in the patient's blood pressure because of the increase in heart rate and subsequent stroke volume, (sympathetic response). However, as respiratory distress increases and oxygen demand is not met, myocardial contractility will be impaired and lead to decreased tissue and cellular perfusion. The patient will in consequence manifest signs of shock due to the sympathetic response of low perfusion (see Box 5.13).

Neurological signs

Levels of consciousness decrease as respiratory distress increases. The patient often stares vacantly, seems drowsy – and apathy is often noticeable. This cannot solely be attributed to derangement of the blood gases but is more likely attributable to decreased cerebral perfusion.

Agitation must always be attributed to hypoxia unless another cause for the patient's agitation can be directly identified. The patient who is agitated must

> ### ■ BOX 5.13 Signs of shock
>
> - Further increase in heart rate and/or arrhythmias
> - Increase in pre-load therefore rise in central venous pressure. The patient's jugular venous pressure (JVP) may be visible on his neck.
> - Increase in after-load
> - Decrease in cardiac output leading to decrease in blood pressure
> - Cooling of extremities
> - Decreased urine output
> - Feelings of anxiety
> - Pallor
> - Further decrease in respiratory function

always therefore be suspected of being hypoxic in the first instance and treatment must be directed to correcting the hypoxia. This is usually achieved initially with the administration of oxygen. The nurse must always stay with the patient.

Pain assessment

Although there is a chapter in this book dedicated to the concept of pain, its importance cannot be overstressed here. If the patient at risk of developing respiratory failure is experiencing pain, whether physiological or psychological, and there is no nursing intervention to alleviate such discomfort, then that patient is put at further risk.

Significant conditions will enhance pain and directly interfere with the patient's respiratory function:

- Chest trauma (including surgery)
- Abdominal surgery
- Severe chest infections
- Pleural rub
- Pericarditis
- Psychological manifestations: feelings of insecurity, loneliness, isolation and depression
- Sleep deprivation.

If the patient remains distressed and anxious a negative cycle of events will ensue and lead to increased shortness of breath and further discomfort (see Fig. 5.6).

It is important that the nurse uses strategies to interrupt this cycle. These may include:

- Analgesia
- Talking calmly and slowly to the patient
- Using biofeedback techniques
- The use of relaxation tapes, massage, music therapy
- Companionship
- Guided imagery.

Temperature

If the patient's core temperature is raised above normal on or during admission or for 24 hours post-operatively it is indicative of infection. A raised temperature will cause an increase in oxygen demand which may lead to decreased respiratory function.

A decreased central temperature will also affect oxygen demand as oxygen will not be so readily released to the tissues from the haemoglobin molecule.

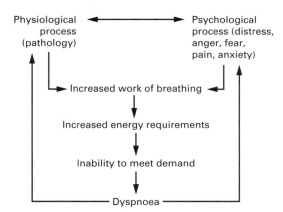

Fig. 5.6 A negative cycle of events.

Therefore, there will be an increase in oxygen debt at tissue level with an increase in anaerobic respiration.

Peripheral temperature is an important but often-overlooked observation, and a very important sign in patients who are at risk of developing respiratory failure. Cooling of the extremities with a gradient between the patient's core temperature and peripheral temperature is indicative of decreased perfusion. There will thus be anaerobic respiration at tissue level.

Blood profiles

Haemoglobin (Hb) It is important that the patient is not anaemic as this will reduce the oxygen-carrying capacity of the haemoglobin molecule. This will lead to reduced O_2 uptake at cellular level.

It is important to remember that with a low Hb the patient may still have O_2 saturations of 95–100%. But it must be stressed that the O_2 content is reduced with a low Hb. Consequently, there will be an O_2 debt at cellular level.

Urea and creatinine If there is any derangement of these two electrolytes in conjunction with renal failure the outcome will be the disruption of one of the major buffering systems, resulting in an acid–base imbalance. This will lead to a metabolic acidosis or alkalosis causing a shift in the oxyhaemoglobin curve. If not corrected an O_2 debt will develop.

Phosphate Ensuring that the patient's phosphate levels are within normal limits is paramount if respiratory muscle function is to be optimised in patients who are at risk of respiratory failure. This blood test is often missed or deemed irrelevant. Reduced phosphate will cause diaphragmatic weakness and increase the risk of atelectasis, collapsed lung and respiratory failure.

Arterial blood gases (ABGs) (see Box 5.14) These will be taken as a final assessment of a patient's respiratory status once all other data have been extrapolated and analysed, and the doctor or senior nurse believes that they will add important and useful insight into the patient's condition and consequent care and treatment.

The nurse requires knowledge of normal acid–base balance and experience in analysing such results to make sense of ABGs.

The first thing to look at when analysing ABGs is the pH value. This indicates whether the patient is acidotic or alkalotic. A pH below 7.35 is indicative of acidosis and a pH above 7.45 is indicative of alkalosis. The next step is to discover

■ **BOX 5.14** Normal ABG values

pH	7.35–7.45
P aO$_2$	12–13 kPa
P aCO$_2$	4.7–6.0 kPa
HCO$_3$	22–26 mmol/l
BE	–2–+2
O$_2$ saturation	95%–100%

■ **BOX 5.15** Causes of respiratory acidosis and alkalosis

Causes of respiratory acidosis
- Oversedation
- Neuromuscular disorders
- Trauma or surgery to the chest or upper abdomen
- Obstructive lung disease
- Inappropriate mechanical ventilation
- Any condition contributing to hypoventilation

Causes of respiratory alkalosis
- Anxiety
- Hyperventilation
- Pulmonary emboli
- Pulmonary oedema
- Salicylate poisoning or overdose
- Excessive mechanical ventilation
- Congestive heart failure
- Gram-negative septicaemia – the hyperventilation may precede other evidence of septicaemia.
- Pregnancy
- Hepatic insufficiency

the primary cause of the acidosis or alkalosis, whether it is respiratory, metabolic or a mixture. Therefore, the PaO_2, PCO_2 and HCO$_3$ need to be analysed.

Once acidosis or alkalosis has been diagnosed it is important to find out the cause in order to direct appropriate nursing care and treatment.

Respiratory acidosis (see Box 5.15)

Respiratory acidosis is not a disease but an acid–base imbalance which occurs in any condition that interferes with pulmonary gas exchange and results in retention of CO_2. It may be classified as acute or chronic.

Acute respiratory acidosis is identified by sudden onset, with high $PaCO_2$ levels and a sharp decrease in serum pH that occurs before the renal system begins to compensate (this usually takes between several hours to days).

Chronic (or compensated) respiratory acidosis is identified by the body's adaptation to higher than normal CO_2 levels by the renal system, which allows retention of bicarbonate to balance the high levels of CO_2. It therefore produces a normal or near-normal serum pH.

Assessment of respiratory acidosis

Early signs and symptoms are related to central nervous system depression. They are:

- Depressed rate and depth of respirations
- Tachypnoea
- Headache
- Confusion
- Lethargy
- Arrhythmias
- Dehydration
- Slow, deep respiration or coma
- Cyanosis
- Elevated intracranial pressure (chronic)
- Dilated conjunctival and facial blood vessels for hypercapnia (chronic)
- Oedema from right ventricular failure (chronic).

CASE EXAMPLE 5.2

Miss Green, 48 years old, is admitted to the ward following a road traffic accident in which she had sustained bruising to her chest wall. Her respiratory rate is 28 breaths per minute and heart rate is 115 beats per minute. Her pattern of breathing is irregular and her breath sounds unequal. She appears distressed and agitated. Arterial blood gases are taken and pulse oximetry shows 85% saturation on air.

ABG analysis:
- *pH: 7.2*
- *PaO_2: 5.0 kPa*
- *$PaCO_2$: 8.0 kPa*
- *HCO_3: 32 mmol/l*
- *BE: −4*
- *Saturation: 85%*

The ABGs demonstrate a primary respiratory acidosis with no metabolic compensation. A chest X-ray revealed a left pneumothorax. A chest drain was inserted and supplemental oxygen given. Miss Green made a full recovery.

Respiratory alkalosis

This may result from any condition that interferes with pulmonary gas exchange and causes excessive loss of CO_2 (hyperventilation). It may be classified as acute or chronic.

Acute respiratory alkalosis is identified by a sudden onset with low $PaCO_2$ levels and a sharp increase in serum pH that occur before the renal system begins to compensate.

Chronic respiratory alkalosis is identified by the body's adaptation to lower than normal CO_2 levels by the renal system which allows excretion of bicarbonate to balance the CO_2 decrease. Consequently it produces a normal or near-normal serum pH.

Assessment of respiratory alkalosis

The early signs and symptoms are related to excitability of the peripheral and central nervous systems. Chronic respiratory alkalosis is usually asymptomatic. The following are signs and symptoms of alkalosis:

- Increased rate and depth of respirations
- Dizziness
- Numbness or tingling fingers and toes
- Sweating
- Muscle weakness
- Tetany

- Seizures
- Syncope
- Arrhythmias.

CASE EXAMPLE 5.3

A 45-year-old woman, Mrs King, is admitted to the ward following a suicide attempt – she consumed large amounts of aspirin. She is drowsy and has peripheral cyanosis. Her respiratory rate is 34 breaths per minute.
ABG analysis:
- *pH: 7.35*
- *PaO_2: 8.0 kPa*
- *$PaCO_2$: 3.5 kPa*
- *HCO_3: 15 mmol/l*
- *Saturation: 90%*

Mrs King's blood gas analysis firstly demonstrates primary respiratory alkalosis due to the effect of salicylate on the central nervous system, causing hyperventilation. Secondly it shows primary metabolic acidosis due to the production of organic acids.

The nurse's responsibility in carrying out an in-depth and meticulous respiratory assessment on a patient who has been identified as at risk of developing respiratory failure cannot be over-emphasised. A higher degree of care is required if the nurse is to observe, extrapolate and analyse such important and pertinent data and plan appropriate nursing care to optimise and maintain ventilation and perfusion.

NURSING INTERVENTIONS AND CARE

Positioning

Positioning may appear to be one of the most fundamental and essential of nursing care concepts and not, therefore, worthy of in-depth discussion here. It is, however, a particularly important area of care in relation to optimising and maintaining ventilation and perfusion. Those patients who are at risk and need a higher intensity of care are usually bedfast and will need frequent repositioning. However, those patients who have chronic lung disease need to be nursed in a position that they are used to and feel comfortable in. If they have not slept in a bed for a long time or find that their breathing is easier if they sit in a chair, then it is important to accommodate them. But it must be remembered that these patients will also need repositioning. What must be remembered is that repositioning patients not only enhances respiratory function but is part of essential nursing care in order to prevent pressure sores. This is especially significant if the patient has poor perfusion because of his condition and is therefore more likely to develop pressure sores, thus increasing risk of patient mortality.

The cardiopulmonary effects of turning or repositioning patients have been well documented (Gavigan et al 1990, Brooks-Brunn 1995). Frequent body repositioning can be effective in enhancing oxygen transport by changing the ventilation and perfusion of the lungs through gravitational effects. Changing the patient's position also enhances mobilisation of secretions. Although frequent turning is important, it is also vital to monitor the patient's response – that is, his respiratory rate, respiratory effort and pulse oximetry – to different positions. This is because repositioning patients increases their oxygen demand.

Studies by Banasik (1987) and Shively (1988) are inconclusive on the effects of repositioning on pulmonary gas exchange in the presence of atelectasis. Although a patient's FRC is reduced when he is supine this should not cause too many problems for those patients free from pulmonary abnormalities. Changing their position therefore does not significantly affect gas exchange.

There is, however, stronger evidence from the literature *for* repositioning patients and enhancing ventilation and perfusion than for not doing so. Nurses need to keep open minds and generate their own research on the positioning of patients in relation to optimising ventilation and perfusion.

Specialised kinetic therapy beds can be used to facilitate the turning process and in some studies have been found to reduce pulmonary complications in different patient groups (Gentillo et al 1988, Fink et al 1990, Hess et al 1992). These beds are usually indicated for those patients who will be bedfast for a long period of time, those with limited mobility or patients with unilateral lung disease who cannot easily be positioned on one side. Although these beds are useful in certain circumstances they are exceedingly costly and therefore not indicated for routine use or to replace quality essential nursing care and good repositioning.

Mobilisation

Mobilisation and ambulation are important aspects in the care of any patient who requires bedrest for whatever reason and who has been identified as at risk of developing respiratory failure. The physiological principles associated with early ambulation are extensions of the benefits of turning and repositioning the patient while in bed. Ambulation stimulates ventilation, increases perfusion and promotes secretion clearance and oxygenation. Further benefits of early ambulation can be seen in Box 5.16.

Deciding when and how the patient should be mobilised should be done on an individual basis in conjunction with the patient's nurse, doctor and physiotherapist. Some patients may worry about early mobilisation, becoming anxious about pain and discomfort. It is therefore of paramount importance that the nurse explains to the patient the benefits of early mobilisation. It is also important that the nurse monitors, observes and provides optimal pain management as well as comfort strategies and interventions during this period.

Physiotherapy techniques

Chest physiotherapy reduces the risk of sputum retention, chest infection and consolidation. The physiotherapist and the nurse therefore play pivotal roles in implementing specific physiotherapy interventions related to respiratory care that ensure adequate ventilation and perfusion.

It is important that the nurse whose patient requires chest physiotherapy liaises with the physiotherapist as to what interventions are suitable for a particular patient and how to safely carry them out. Care needs to be truly collaborative and will include a plan of care and assessment tailored for those patients requiring chest physiotherapy. Physiotherapy care includes:

■ **BOX 5.16** Benefits of early ambulation

- Decreased venous pooling thus reducing the risk of deep vein thrombosis and pulmonary emboli.
- Improved functional capacity.
- Decreased deconditioning related to bedrest (i.e. muscle weakness).
- Decreased psychological problems such as depression and anxiety in relation to bedrest.

- Deep breathing and coughing exercises
- Suctioning (oral and nasopharyngeal)
- Incentive spirometry
- Postural drainage
- Saline nebulisers
- Spontaneous intermittent positive pressure ventilation (SIPPV)
- Mobilisation.

It is not the intention of this chapter to explore all chest physiotherapy techniques as this is primarily the domain of the physiotherapist. Certain physiotherapy interventions may, however, be facilitated equally by both nurse and physiotherapist.

Coughing and deep breathing exercises

If the patient is to undergo surgery, instruction on deep breathing and coughing exercises should ideally be given pre-operatively. This applies to all patients who are on bedrest and identified as at risk of developing pulmonary complications. These exercises are as important as frequent repositioning, early ambulation and pain management strategies. The importance of pre-operative education for post-operative recovery and pulmonary function has been well documented in both the nursing and medical literature (Hathaway 1986, Crawford et al 1990).

The time-honoured tradition of 'cough and deep breath' is often thought of as the foundation of good pulmonary care. The concept can be attributed to Dripps and Waters (1941) who described three fundamental principles for patients who had or were at risk of developing pulmonary complications:

- The patient must be turned
- The patient must cough
- The patient must inflate his lungs adequately with deep breaths.

This should be encouraged every hour or every 30 minutes depending on the patient's physical and psychological condition. The limited human resources and complexity of today's nursing and medical care often mean a low priority for this procedure. If this essential nursing intervention is not valued, this puts patients further at risk of developing respiratory insufficiency.

Encouraging the patient to cough as a routine aspect of care is one method of facilitating clearance of airway secretions for those patients who have increased secretions or secretion management problems. Each patient must be assessed on an individual basis in relation to whether he needs to be encouraged to cough as a routine aspect of his care. The nurse must ask these questions:

- Does the patient have pre-existing lung disease?
- Does the patient have a history of secretion clearance problems?
- Is there evidence of increased secretions when listening to breath sounds?
- Will the patient benefit from coughing as an intervention?

If the nurse decides that the patient needs to be encouraged to cough it is extremely important that effective coughing is taught, primarily by the physiotherapist. Once the patient understands the procedure the nurse should continue to encourage and assist.

The patient should be placed in an optimal position to reduce tension on the abdominal muscles. If the patient has a wound site (abdominal or chest) then splinting of the wound with a pillow, rolled-up towel or crossed arms should also be encouraged.

It is important to remember that coughing is an expiratory manoeuvre that can cause pleural pressures to exceed airway pressure. This may result in alveoli collapse. Post-operative coughing is contraindicated in patients who have had ear surgery, eye surgery, neurosurgery or repair of large abdominal hernias because of this increase in pleural pressure.

Deep breathing exercises

Normal ventilation occurs through pleural pressure changes caused by the contraction and relaxation of the diaphragm. Negative pleural pressure increases during inspiration and is decreased during expiration. Therefore, any disorder that interferes with the generation and maintenance of increased negative pleural pressure on inspiration will decrease the distending forces of the lung and increase the risk of alveolar collapse and possible atelectasis.

An influential article by Bartlett Gazzanigar and Geraghti (1973) noted that if the patient had decreased tidal volume and FRC (especially post-operatively), deep and prolonged inspiratory efforts favoured reversal of atelectasis and enhanced surfactant replenishment. They went on to describe a sustained maximal inspiration (SMI) manoeuvre that was effective in increasing tidal volume and FRC. An early example of an SMI was the 'yawn' which patients were encouraged to do at least 10 times an hour in the post-operative period (Bartlett et al 1973).

In order to prevent pulmonary complications for those patients at risk of developing respiratory failure it is imperative that the nurse encourages the patient to take regular effective deep breaths. The technique is:

- Take a slow deep breath in
- Hold breath for at least 3 seconds in order to prevent alveolar collapse
- Repeat at least 3–6 times per hour.

As with coughing, patients should be assessed as to whether they are able to do deep breathing exercises. If they are, they should be placed in an optimal position that enables them to expand their lungs, and in which they feel comfortable. Success in effective deep breathing exercises relies on five strategies:

- Motivation of patient and staff
- Education of patient and staff
- Supervision of patient
- Comfort
- Assessment.

Incentive spirometry

In some areas the use of incentive spirometers (see Fig. 5.7) is advocated to help the patient take slow deep breaths and produce a voluntary sustained maximal inspiration. Spirometers measure patient effort in either flow or volume and according to some research help maintain muscle strength and promote secretion clearance. However, incentive spirometry has limited benefits for some patients and is only effective if the nurse continually supervises and encourages its proper use (Chuter et al 1989).

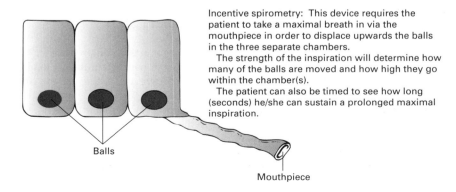

Incentive spirometry: This device requires the patient to take a maximal breath in via the mouthpiece in order to displace upwards the balls in the three separate chambers.

The strength of the inspiration will determine how many of the balls are moved and how high they go within the chamber(s).

The patient can also be timed to see how long (seconds) he/she can sustain a prolonged maximal inspiration.

Balls

Mouthpiece

Fig. 5.7 Incentive spirometry.

■ **BOX 5.17** Principles in the administration of oxygen

- Oxygen is a combustible gas and therefore a fire risk.
- Compressed oxygen is very dry and must be humidified if it is to be used for long periods – i.e. more than half an hour.
- If hypoxaemia is not accompanied with carbon dioxide retention (hypercapnia) then high concentrations of oxygen up to 60% may be given.
- In hypoxaemia associated with hypercapnia the concentration of oxygen should not be more than 30%. Serial estimates of arterial carbon dioxide should be carried out before and during oxygen therapy to ensure that ventilation is not sufficiently depressed to cause significant carbon dioxide retention.
- High concentrations of oxygen (60% or more) over prolonged periods may cause severe lung damage. High concentrations of oxygen are toxic and damage the alveolar epithelium. Therefore, inspired oxygen concentrations should always be kept to a minimum while maintaining reasonable respiratory function. Meticulous assessment of the patient is essential.

Oxygen therapy and non-invasive respiratory support

The use of supplementary oxygen is the primary treatment for patients with respiratory failure – that is, hypoxia – whether it is acute or chronic. Although giving supplementary oxygen to a patient with acute hypoxia may be of short-term benefit, it is important to find the cause of hypoxia and treat the underlying problem.

The benefits of oxygen therapy are as follows:

- It can correct hypoxaemia
- Oxygen reduces the work of breathing
- It decreases myocardial workload.

Although the administration of oxygen may appear to be straightforward the nurse needs to have a full understanding of its hazards and of respiratory physiology (see Box 5.17).

Methods of administration

Oxygen delivery systems may be high-flow or low-flow systems, with a large range of masks and nasal cannulae. Choice of system will be dictated by what type of system the ward or unit has purchased; however other factors that should be considered include the type of respiratory failure, how much inspired oxygen is required and whether the flow needs to be high or low.

The length of tubing used to deliver the inspired oxygen can have an effect on carbon dioxide retention as it increases the patient's deadspace. This increases the potential for carbon dioxide retention. For this reason, nurses should not be over-zealous with the amount of tubing used. Many companies who supply oxygen tubing have already pre-cut the tubing to a therapeutic length.

Considering patient comfort If the patient finds a mask claustrophobic, low concentrations of inspired oxygen can be given through nasal cannulae as long as the patient does not have high minute volumes. However, if the patient only mouth breathes nasal cannulae are of limited use.

Nasal cannulae can cause ulceration of the nasal and pharyngeal mucosa.

The nurse must explain what is happening to the patient at all times. She should always be available for the patient, continually assessing and evaluating the care and treatment. Pay meticulous attention to detail.

If the patient is restless the nurse may need to stay with him during the initial treatment.

The cause of hypoxia and whether or not it is accompanied by hypercapnia will direct the percentage and flow of oxygen given to the patient. Giving high concentrations of oxygen to a patient with hypercapnia will cause respiratory depression by exacerbating carbon dioxide retention.

It must be remembered that oxygen is a drug and should be prescribed by a doctor. As with any drug, the nurse must understand how to give it effectively and therapeutically and know what positive and negative effects it may have on the patient.

Patients with large minute volumes require high flow systems (unless a Venturi mask system is used – see Fig. 5.8) in order to cover the patient's own minute volume. If the flow rate is not greater than the patient's minute volume the correct concentration of inspired oxygen will not be delivered. This will cause further hypoxaemia, increase the patient's work of breathing, decrease myocardial function and lead the patient into greater respiratory distress and failure which may require further invasive support.

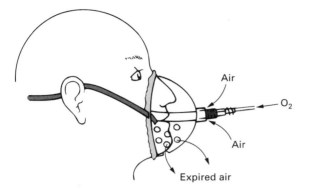

Fig. 5.8 Venturi mask. (Based on Kumar & Clark 1990 with kind permission.)

■ **BOX 5.18** Factors affecting success of CPAP and NIPPV

- The patient must be able to maintain his own airway.
- The patient must be alert.
- The patient must not have excessive bronchial secretions and be able to clear his own secretions.
- The nurse caring for patients requiring non-invasive respiratory support needs to be knowledgeable and experienced in using this type of intervention.
- There must be continuous assessment of the effectiveness of the therapy on respiratory function. Ensure meticulous attention to detail.

Non-invasive respiratory support

For a significant minority of patients supplementary oxygen is not effective in reducing hypoxaemia and further support is therefore necessary. Until recently patients with reversible respiratory failure would always have been intubated and mechanically ventilated. Alternative methods of support have now been developed which do not require endotracheal intubation. These include:

- Continuous positive airway pressure (CPAP) support
- Non-invasive intermittent positive pressure ventilation (NIPPV).

Because neither method requires endotracheal intubation, patients who receive this type of respiratory support can now be nursed within a ward environment rather than having to be moved to the unfamiliar surroundings of an intensive care unit (ICU). However, if the patient is to be nursed within a ward area higher nurse-to-patient ratios must be guaranteed as these patients require a higher level of care. It also requires the appropriate knowledge and expertise of staff to establish this type of support and care for the patient effectively throughout his treatment (see Bo 5.18).

Continuous positive airway pressure (CPAP) (see Box 5.19)

CPAP benefits three interdependent aspects of respiratory physiology:

- It increases functional residual capacity (FRC).
- It improves lung compliance. There will therefore be a decrease in the work of breathing.
- CPAP improves ventilation/perfusion ratio.

Success of CPAP can be evaluated through observing an improvement in the patient's oxygenation determined by arterial blood gas analysis and pulse oximetry. There is also a decrease in the patient's respiratory rate and an increase in tidal volume due to an improvement in lung compliance and increase in FRC.

A reduction in the patient's work of breathing will be noted, indicated by decrease in heart rate and stress response and the use of fewer accessory muscles.

Methods of delivery CPAP may be delivered by continuous flow or by demand flow.

Both methods require the patient to wear a tight-fitting mask that may be extremely uncomfortable and frightening. CPAP can be delivered through a nasal mask as opposed to a full-face mask, but mouth breathing can result in a significant loss of positive pressure in the airways.

Continuous flow Gas flows through the system continuously throughout the respiratory cycle. These systems are extremely noisy. They use large volumes of piped gases – 50–120 l/min.

Demand flow Gas is only allowed to flow when inspiration is initiated by the patient, and is stored within a reservoir in the form of suspended rubber bellows or a bladder from which the patient draws his breath. These systems are quieter and use less gas. The patient has to open the valve in order to receive gas flow. This may increase the patient's respiratory work and so he may tire more easily.

The amount of continuous positive pressure that the patient receives is determined by a valve attached to the mask (see Fig. 5.9). Patients can receive low (2.5 to 7.5 cm H_2O) or high (10 to 20 cm H_2O) values of CPAP. Valves creating lower values of CPAP are more easily tolerated by the patient but they may not increase FRC sufficiently to be effective. However, it may help the patient to get accustomed to the therapy by first starting with a low amount of CPAP and then gradually increasing the pressure once tolerated.

Valves creating higher values of CPAP are more difficult for the patient to breathe through. While the higher value valves may have better results in increasing FRC

> A patient who needs CPAP is likely to be frightened and distressed. He will already have a marked degree of dyspnoea and feel extremely tired. On top of this he is being asked to wear a tight-fitting mask and breathe out against a degree of resistance caused by the CPAP valve. Gaining the patient's trust and making him feel safe in the early stages is paramount if the treatment is to be successful.

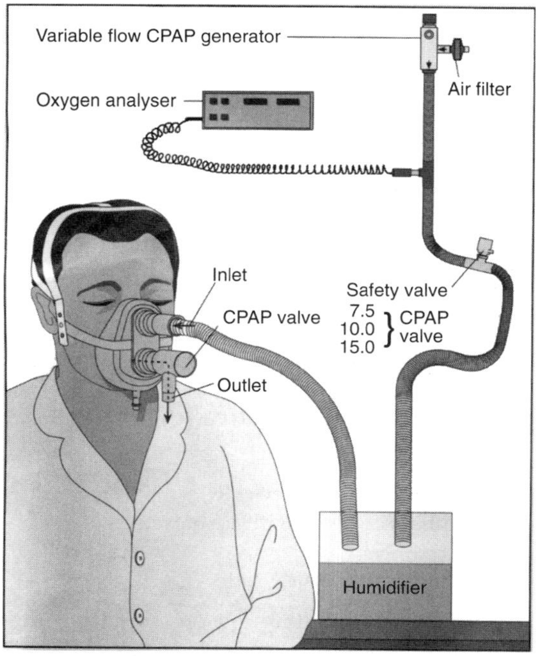

Fig. 5.9 Patient wearing a CPAP mask. (Reproduced with kind permission from Nursing Times (Place 1997).)

■ **BOX 5.19** Indications for CPAP

- Acute hypoxaemia without carbon dioxide retention, i.e. those patients having problems with oxygenation and not ventilation.
- Basal lung collapse.
- Fluid overload causing pulmonary oedema. Applying positive pressure throughout the respiratory cycle can 'squeeze' fluid out of flooded alveoli and reduce the inward flow of water into alveolar and interstitial spaces.
- Patients with COPD may also benefit from CPAP but have to be carefully selected. NIPPV is the preferred method of respiratory support for these patients.
- Weaning from mechanical ventilation.

and reducing the work of breathing these benefits may be offset because of the patient's distress and difficulty in breathing through the valve.

There has therefore to be a balance between what feels comfortable for the patient and what is therapeutic. Establishing CPAP requires time, patience, effort, motivation, knowledge, understanding, creativity and a partnership of trust and safety between nurse and patient.

Establishing CPAP

The first few hours of treatment are extremely important. If managed correctly and with sensitivity, treatment should be effective. The nurse should sit with the patient and explain the benefits of the treatment and what equipment is involved, allowing the patient to touch and feel the equipment.

Any questions should be answered honestly, and the nurse should be calm, confident, compassionate and caring. Listen to the patient. Then:

- Allow the patient to hold the mask and ask him to ensure a seal between the mask and his face.
- Once he is used to the mask, gently attach the head straps and tighten them until a satisfactory seal is obtained.
- If the seal is difficult to achieve, remove some of the air from the inflated mask flange. This may allow the mask to mould more easily to the face.
- Continually talk to the patient and explain what you are doing.
- Encourage the patient.
- Ensure that there is adequate gas flow through the circuit throughout the patient's respiratory cycle. The gas flow should be able to generate a constant airway pressure independent of the inspiratory flow generated by the patient.
- Ensure that the patient is able to see a nurse at all times and that the nurse can observe the patient continuously. Anticipation of when the patient may need a rest from the treatment is vital.
- When CPAP is removed, positive end expiratory pressure (PEEP) is lost. When CPAP is put back on again, the level of PEEP returns but its effect may take longer to be seen.

Potential dangers associated with CPAP

Valve failure or expiratory valve occlusion Inspiration will be able to occur but expiration and asphyxiation will follow quickly. A safety PEEP valve must be included within the circuit 5 cm H_2O higher than the therapeutic PEEP valve attached to the mask.

If flow coming out of the CPAP valve ceases at any stage during inspiration then the gas flow needs to be increased.

Vomiting and aspiration Because of the large flow of gas some is unavoidably swallowed. This causes gastric distension and increases the risk of vomiting. Quick-release head straps should be used which may reduce the risk of aspiration if vomiting does occur.

Hypotension can occur when CPAP is applied. CPAP raises mean intrathoracic pressure and reduces venous return. In the long term this reduced cardiac output will cause tissue hypoxia.

An oxygen analyser must always be incorporated within the system.

Patient comfort

It is essential that the nurse helping the patient establish CPAP is competent. Competency here does not just mean the ability to carry out a set of skills. The nurse must have the knowledge, skills, energy, compassion, confidence and motivation to respond effectively to the patient's needs and situation. This will lead the patient to trust the nurse, feel safe and ultimately feel comfortable in commencing the therapy.

Other factors relating to patient comfort are as follows:

- A well-fitting mask is essential.
- Adequate humidification of inspired gases is required to prevent drying and ulceration of mucosa.
- Humidification can make the mask slip from the nose and cause skin irritation. Using an adhesive gauze dressing may help to stop the mask from slipping and thus protect the skin.
- Pressure of the CPAP mask can cause nasal bridge necrosis. Constant observation of this pressure point is paramount.
- Air leaks from the mask may cause drying of the eyes. Ensuring there is an adequate seal is important.
- Abdominal discomfort from air swallowing. Encouraging the patient to breathe nasally some of the time may reduce abdominal discomfort.
- Immobility. It is important to encourage the patient to change position. This will enhance secretion clearance and reduce the risk of pressure sores. Deep breathing exercises should also be encouraged.
- Isolation and loneliness. Impaired communication as a result of the treatment as well as the patient's vulnerable physiological condition, may mean that some patients begin to feel isolated and lonely. It is important to establish other forms of communication such as writing and touch, and encourage the patient's loved ones to visit when they can. Patients need to be kept in touch as to what is going on in terms of their present condition and their social wellbeing. Actively listen to the patient.
- Sleep deprivation. Patients receiving CPAP may find sleep difficult, and sleep is vital both for the healing process and for the patient's psychological be difficult for wellbeing. Sleep may be difficult for the patient because the CPAP system is too noisy, or because of physical discomfort. It may be that he is frightened to go to sleep, afraid that he will not wake up again. It is important when caring for these patients to encourage rest and sleep: staying with them as they go to sleep may help. Other interventions may include massage, relaxation tapes and music. Organising nursing care in order to optimise the patient's rest period will also help.

> CPAP must never be used in isolation from other strategies and interventions that help to maintain respiratory function. The patient requires continuous assessment and evaluation.

Non-invasive intermittent positive pressure ventilation (NIPPV) (see Box 5.20)

There are two types of non-invasive intermittent positive pressure ventilators.

■ **BOX 5.20** Indications for NIPPV

- Type II respiratory failure that is characterised by raised carbon dioxide levels. For example: patients with acute exacerbation of chronic obstructive pulmonary disease (COPD), chest wall defects or neuromuscular disorders.
- Obstructive sleep apnoea (OSA).
- Patients recovering from critical illness or surgery.
- Patients being weaned from mechanical ventilation.
- Improvement of pre-operative cardiorespiratory function in patients with chronic ventilatory failure.

Pressure-preset machines These deliver a preset amount of positive pressure flow over a predetermined length of time. The size of each breath is determined by setting the maximum inspiratory pressure. By setting the inspiratory and expiratory time dials, the respiratory rate is determined.

Volume-preset machines These deliver a breath of a preset volume. Where carbon dioxide levels are raised and lung compliance is very poor, preset volume machines are more useful because they can generate even higher flow rates than pressure-preset machines. Both require a mask and a circuit of ventilator tubing.

Expected outcomes with NIPPV therapy

- Inspiratory muscle effort should decrease because each breath is assisted.
- The patient's tidal volume should increase because inspiratory effort is reduced for each breath.
- The patient's respiratory rate should decrease as the work of breathing is lessened.

Establishing and caring for the patient receiving NIPPV

Comments made earlier with regard to CPAP apply here. The first few hours of treatment are the most important and establishing an effective nurse–patient relationship is crucial at this stage. Ensuring that there is a nurse available for the patient at all times is also extremely important.

The machine should be set up by a doctor or an experienced senior nurse or physiotherapist.

Establishing both CPAP and NIPPV requires an intricate blend of comforting nursing strategies combined with knowledge of the complex physiological and psychological reactions the patient may manifest.

DRUG THERAPY IN RESPIRATORY FAILURE

Drug therapy (see Box 5.21) is used both in the short term and acute management of respiratory failure and for the long-term relief of symptoms in chronic respiratory disease.

■ **BOX 5.21** Common drug therapy

- Bronchodilators: salbutamol
  aminophylline
  ipratropium bromide
- Corticosteroids

- Antibiotics
- Respiratory stimulants: doxapram
- Mucolytics

This section will focus briefly on the drug therapy most commonly used in the management of patients presenting with an acute episode of respiratory failure (Fig 5.10). See Further reading for specific drug therapy texts.

Bronchodilators

These drugs are beta-adrenoceptor agonists. Salbutamol is the most commonly used, and can be given via a tablet, an inhaler, a nebuliser or intravenously. Bronchodilators are commonly used in the treatment of asthma and chronic obstructive pulmonary disease (COPD) especially during exacerbations.

Side effects

1. Increase in heart rate due to stimulation of beta-1 receptors. This will cause an increase in myocardial oxygen demand which in turn may lead to a decrease in myocardial function, decreased cardiac output and a further decrease in tissue perfusion and oxygenation to an already hypoxic patient.
2. Tremor of skeletal muscle. This can sometimes be quite marked and may stop the patient performing daily activities such as drinking and eating. It is relieved by reducing the dose.

Nursing considerations

Patients with an acute exacerbation of asthma may be prescribed 2–4 hourly nebulised bronchodilators over 24-hour periods. It is extremely important that these

Fig. 5.10 Drug therapy in respiratory failure.

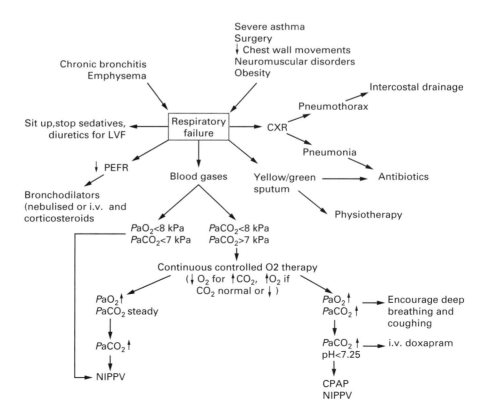

patients receive their nebuliser at the prescribed times even throughout the night. The nurse must wake the patient up at the appropriate times to administer the, therapy.

These patients have what are termed 'morning dips' when their peak expiratory flow rate (PEFR) is reduced to a critical level in the early hours of the morning. Such dips can cause severe hypoxia which may lead to respiratory arrest.

The nurse must record the patient's PEFR pre- and post-nebuliser to assess the efficacy of the treatment.

If patients are unable to produce a PEFR greater than 60 l/min then a low reading peak-flow meter should be used.

Respiratory stimulants

Intravenous doxapram has been tried as a respiratory stimulant in patients with varying degrees of respiratory failure with contrasting results (Jansen et al 1990). Doxapram may help to arouse the patient sufficiently to encourage him to cough and breathe deeply in order to remove secretions. However, its use is limited and it should only be used as a short-term measure.

Mucolytics

There is little evidence that mucolytics are of any benefit. What is essential is the nurse's role in encouraging the patient to cough and breathe deeply enough to remove any secretions. If the patient's sputum is thick and tenacious, nebulised saline or steam inhalations may help to liquefy it so that it can be more easily coughed up.

As with all treatment and interventions for respiratory failure, constant observation, assessment and evaluation of the patient's respiratory function are vital in order to ensure that the treatment is effective and that the patient is able to cope with such therapy.

CHEST DRAIN MANAGEMENT (see Box 5.22)

It is essential that the nurse caring for patients with chest drains in situ has a sound understanding of their management in order to optimise the patient's respiratory function and prevent complications.

Although there are various underwater seal drainage systems available, the basic principle remains the same: to allow air and excess fluid to escape from the pleural cavity while preventing any reflux (see Fig. 5.11). Chest drainage bottles must always be kept lower than the patient's chest to prevent water being sucked into the chest. This is due to the decrease in pressure inside the pleural cavity during inspiration, causing air to be sucked up the tube usually to height of about 10–20 cm.

■ **BOX 5.22** Indications for chest drains

- Pneumothorax
- Tension pneumothorax
- Haemothorax
- Empyema
- Thoracic or cardiac surgery

Fig. 5.11 Basic principles of chest drainage.

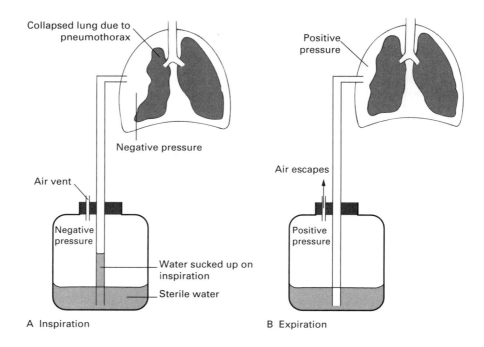

A Inspiration   B Expiration

Assessment

Fluid level and type of fluid within the chest drain bottle This should be recorded regularly. Any signs of fresh bleeding into the drain must be reported immediately. If the fluid looks cloudy or infected a specimen must be sent for culture and sensitivity.

Fluid swing There should always be a 'swing' of fluid in the tube of the chest drainage bottle during inspiration and expiration if the system is patent. This should also be recorded.

Bubble/air leak If the chest drain is in situ for the treatment of a pneumothorax then there should be a visible bubbling within the chest drain until the pneumothorax has resolved. It is important when assessing for such an air leak that the patient is sitting upright and is asked to take a deep breath in and out and to cough.

Pain and discomfort Chest drain tubes can be extremely painful and cause discomfort especially if they are not secured correctly and are accidentally pulled.

Infection The longer a chest drain is in situ the more likely the risk of infection around the site of insertion. The patient will often complain of increased pain and discomfort around this area. Careful observation of the site is needed. If the infection goes unchecked it can translocate into the pleural cavity and cause an empyema.

Respiratory function Continuous assessment of a patient's respiratory function during chest drain therapy is essential in order to prevent complications (see Box 5.23).

■ BOX 5.23 Troubleshooting

If the bubbling suddenly stops:
• Check there are no kinks in the tubing system
• Check level of fluid. Is there an adequate seal? Is the level too high and does the drainage bottle need changing?
• Ask patient to cough
• If unresolved inform medical staff
• Observe for signs of tension pneumothorax

If the drain is blocked:
• Check that there are no kinks in the tubing
• Check level of fluid is not too high as this may stop drainage
• If the drain is on low flow suction increase this slightly
• Milk the tubing (this is the only time that tubes should be milked as it may dislodge the blockage)
If unresolved inform medical staff
• Continue to observe patient's respiratory function and signs of tension pneumothorax

If there is a broken underwater seal:
• Sit the patient down
• Re-connect drain and/or re-establish underwater seal
• Ask patient to take a deep breath in and out
• Ask patient to cough
• Assess patient's respiratory function
• Inform medical staff

If there is an airleak around the insertion site:
• Assess insertion site for infection
• Does the drain site need further suturing?
• Ensure adequate dressing around site. DO NOT USE SLEEK.
• Look for signs of surgical emphysema

If the chest drain falls out:
• Put patient into bed
• Inform medical staff
• Put a gauze dressing over insertion site
• Assess patient's respiratory function

Signs of tension pneumothorax
• Bubbling ceases within chest drain
• No fluid swing
• Respiratory rate rapidly increases
• Heart rate increases
• Patient exhibits signs of shock
• Displaced mediastinum
• Respiratory arrest

Complications arising from chest drains can include:

• Infection
• Surgical emphysema
• Pain
• Blocked drain
• Broken seal
• Tension pneumothorax
• Air leak from insertion site.

Nursing considerations

Chest drains may interfere with respiration as they can be uncomfortably painful. Ensure that the patient has adequate pain control and that he feels comfortable.

This will allow him to take deep breaths, mobilise and help reduce fear and anxiety. Patients must be taught the basics of managing their own chest drain bottles. This will encourage them to mobilise.

The nurse should encourage the patient to mobilise when and where appropriate.

Ensure that the dressing around the insertion site is comfortable and not too bulky. A small keyhole dressing with gauze should be sufficient.

Secure the chest drain tubing to the patient's skin in order to stop it from pulling. Do not pin it to the patient's nightwear as this is sometimes forgotten and on removing nightwear the chest drain may become dislodged or pulled out.

Do not clamp chest drains when mobilising or moving patients as this may cause a tension pneumothorax. Clamp only briefly when changing chest drain bottles.

Do not milk chest drain tubing unless the chest drain appears blocked. Milking the tubes causes an increase in intrathoracic pressure and may cause further pneumothoraces, tension pneumothorax and a decrease in cardiac output.

There are no set rules regarding when to change chest drain bottles. What needs to be remembered is that the more they are changed the more the underwater seal is broken, increasing the risk of introducing infection. Chest drain bottles should only be changed when absolutely necessary.

CASE EXAMPLES FOR ASTHMA, PNEUMONIA AND COPD

The following section presents the reader with three case scenarios in relation to caring for and managing patients with three specific disease processes of the espiratory system:

- Asthma
- Pneumonia
- Acute exacerbation of chronic obstructive pulmonary disease (COPD)

The reader is advised to seek further information on the pathophysiology of each of the disease processes presented (see Further reading).

The asthmatic patient

Asthma is an acute reversible airways disease that occurs from a variety of causes such as allergens, infection and exercise. It results from an airway obstruction that may spontaneously reverse but usually requires pharmacological intervention to reverse the obstruction.

For many years asthma was considered to result only from airway constriction-induced bronchospasm that progresses to airway obstruction. As such, asthma therapy was based on reversing the bronchoconstriction with bronchodilator agents such as beta 2-adrenergic agonists (e.g. salbutamol) and theophylline, which relax the bronchial smooth muscle constriction and induce bronchodilation. However, it has now been established that asthma is more than just a bronchospastic event. Asthma is an inflammatory disorder. Inflammation is central to the airway hyperresponsiveness that leads to airway narrowing and obstruction (Djukanovic et el 1990, The British Guidelines on Asthma Management 1997).

The three main aims of managing an acute asthmatic event are:

- Rapid assessment and appropriate measures to treat hypoxaemia
- Relieve airflow limitation and symptoms
- Reverse airway inflammation.

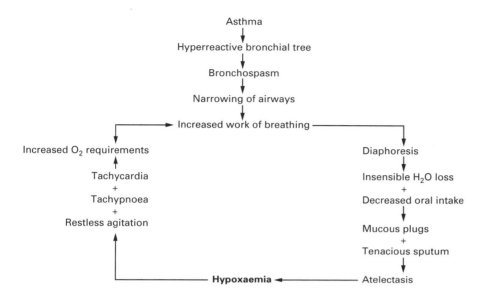

Fig. 5.12 Cycle of events leading to critical hypoxaemia.

If these three main areas are not adequately managed and controlled a cycle of events will develop leading to life-threatening status asthmaticus and critical hypoxaemia (Fig. 5.12).

Assessment, treatment, monitoring and care of a patient suffering an asthmatic event is based upon an understanding of the pathogenic mechanisms (see Box 5.24).

■ **BOX 5.24** Aspects of asthma care

- Thorough ongoing respiratory assessment
- Frequent monitoring of PEFR and/or FEV1
- Drug therapy (See Box 5.25)
- Physiotherapy strategies
- Patient teaching and education
- Humidified oxygen
- Adequate hydration
- Adequate nutrition
- Blood profiles (magnesium, phosphate, haemoglobin, calcium, potassium, white cell count)
- ABG's
- Pulse oximetry

It is of paramount importance that regularly prescribed nebulisers are given to the patient even during the night. The patient must be woken up to receive them.

Signs and symptoms of an acute event

- Increasing respiratory rate of greater than 20 breaths per minute at rest.
- Use of accessory muscles, especially the sternomastoid and shoulders, confirming respiratory distress. This may also reflect the severity of bronchospasm.
- *Breath sounds*

Expiratory wheezes, although the hallmark of asthma, are not specific for this disease. A very tight asthmatic with poor respiratory effort may have little evidence of wheezing. The patient may have a 'silent chest', indicative of insufficient air movement or mucus plugging. There may be signs of a pneumothorax due to hyperinflation of the lungs.

- Mouth breathing.
- Inability to talk in sentences. As the respiratory distress worsens the patient will not be able to speak at all.
- Tachycardia.
- *Pulsus paradoxus*
  In normal subjects the systolic pressure and the pulse pressure fall during inspiration due to the response of the right side of the heart responding to changes in intrathoracic pressure. In asthma there is an increased and sudden negative intrathoracic pressure on inspiration which will enhance the normal fall in blood pressure.

- Initial rise in blood pressure (BP) due to the sympathetic response. The patient will then manifest signs of hypotension as decompensation results and respiratory distress worsens.
- The patient will be anxious and extremely frightened.
- The patient will be restless, agitated and/or experience alteration in consciousness. These signs need to be taken extremely seriously as the patient may be hypoxic and/or hypercapnic.
- Reduced peak expiratory flow rate (PEFR) from the patient's normal. Pre- and post-treatment PEFR is essential in relation to the management and treatment of an acute asthmatic event.
- Low oxygen saturations with or without supplemental oxygen therapy will indicate critical hypoxaemia. As already discussed, pulse oximetry should be viewed as a trend and always in conjunction with a thorough respiratory assessment.
- Arterial blood gases (ABGs) should be considered if PEFR is less than 200 l/min or if there is evidence of clinical deterioration to assess gas exchange and acid–base balance.
- Raised temperature will indicate infection which may have precipitated the event.
- Diaphoresis.
- Dehydration.

■ BOX 5.25 Drug therapy

Beta 2-agonists	**Non-steroidal prophylactics**
• Salbutamol	• Sodium cromoglycate
• Terbutaline	• Nedocromil sodium
• Fenoterol	**Corticosteroids**
• Reproterol	• inhalers
• Ipratropium bromide	• Tablets
Anticholinergics	• Intravenous administration
Theophyllines	

Sedatives should *never* be administered to an asthmatic who is experiencing a mild or severe asthma event unless he is to be intubated and mechanically ventilated.

CASE EXAMPLE 5.4

A 42-year-old woman, Mrs Jenner, was admitted to a medical ward with an acute exacerbation of her asthma. This was her first hospital admission relating to her asthma, as she is usually well controlled and managed at home by her GP and practice nurse. She has suffered from asthma since the age of 16 but has no previous relevant medical history. She has stated that what appears to trigger a mild event is either stress or a cold. Her medication is then adjusted accordingly in negotiation with the practice nurse.

For the past 5 days she has been having flu-like symptoms and experiencing night sweats. She adjusted her medication as she was having increasing bronchospasm and difficulty in breathing at night. Her GP arranged for her admission to hospital. Observations and investigations on admission were:

- HR: 115 bpm sinus tachycardia
- BP: 140/90 mmHg
- MAP: 106 mmHg
- RR: 32 bpm
- Temperature: 38°C
- Using accessory muscles
- Mouth breathing
- Alert but unable to talk in sentences
- Frightened
- Breath sounds: Loud expiratory wheeze, silent bases
- PEFR: Unrecordable as patient too breathless. Her normal PEFR is around 400 l/min
- Pulse oximetry: SpO_2 88%–90% on air
- CXR: Consolidation in the right lower lobe

As a result of the above data Mrs Jenner was given a ventolin nebuliser and written up for them 4-hourly, along with i.v. hydrocortisone 100 mg bd. She was also written up to have 35% oxygen via a face mask.

After a couple of hours Mrs Jenner became more settled and her respiratory rate came down to 24 bpm and her loud expiratory wheeze had lessened. She was able to perform a PEFR which was 380 l/min. Pulse oximetry showed 98% saturation on 35% oxygen. However, it was noted that there was a significant difference between her pre-nebuliser and post-nebuliser PEFR and that Mrs Jenner's work of breathing significantly increased three-quarters of an hour prior to receiving her nebulisers. Her prescription is changed to 3-hourly nebulisers with good effect. Sputum cultures revealed a Gram-positive organism Streptococcus pneumoniae. Mrs Jenner received erythromycin.

On the basis of the data Mrs Jenner was diagnosed with an acute exacerbation of asthma secondary to bronchiole pneumonia. 48 hours after admission at 07.30 hours Mrs Jenner became restless and agitated. Her vital signs were:

- HR: 120 bpm, full and bounding pulse
- BP: 160/98 mmHg
- RR: 44 bpm
- Pulse oximetry: 82% on 35% oxygen
- Prominent sternocleidomastoid
- Silent chest on auscultation

Arterial blood gases were taken. An adrenaline nebuliser was given with little effect. ABG results:

- pH: 7.2
- PaO_2: 6.0 kPa
- $PaCO_2$: 9.0 kPa
- HCO_3: 18 mmol/l
- BE: −9
- Saturation: 80%

It was noted that Mrs Jenner had not received her 3-hourly nebulisers overnight as she had 'been asleep'.

A secondary diagnosis was made of acute respiratory failure type II. It was decided to intubate and mechanically ventilate Mrs Jenner. She was transferred to the intensive care unit (ICU).

Mrs Jenner responded well to ventilatory support, i.v. antibiotics, corticosteroids and bronchodilator therapy and made a full recovery. She was discharged home 12 days following her admission.

The patient with pneumonia

CASE EXAMPLE 5.5

Mr Cowley, a 60-year-old man, is admitted to a surgical ward for repair of his hiatus hernia. He has been a smoker for 40 years and continues to smoke 15–20 cigarettes per day. He has no other relevant past medical history.

His operation was successful and he had an uncomplicated immediate post-operative recovery. 24 hours following his surgery Mr Cowley complained of feeling very unwell and had pain in his chest on inspiration. Further observations revealed the following:

- *HR: 115 bpm*
- *BP: 155/85 mmHg*
- *RR: 26 bpm*

Respiratory rhythm demonstrated shallow, fast breathing with the right side of the chest moving less than the left.

- *Decreased breath sounds, especially to the bases. A pleuritic rub could be heard*
- *Cough with sputum production*
- *Temperature: 38.5°C*
- *Pulse oximetry: 90% on air (previously 95%)*

A sputum specimen and blood cultures were sent and supplemental oxygen was started, 35% via a face mask. Mr Cowley was rehydrated with intravenous fluid and regular analgesia was given for his pleuritic pain. He was seen by the physiotherapist and taught and encouraged to deep breathe and cough in order to expand his bases and clear secretions. Chest X-ray revealed consolidation mostly in the right lung base. Mr Cowley was commenced on i.v. ampicillin 1 g 6-hourly and erythromycin 500 mg. Sputum cultures revealed Gram-negative bacilli.

Mr Cowley responded well to antibiotic therapy and intense physiotherapy. He made a good recovery and was discharged from hospital.

Discussion

There were three factors which predisposed Mr Cowley to pneumonia:

- *He was a smoker*
- *He had had a general anaesthetic*
- *He had had upper abdominal surgery.*

All of these factors have been previously identified and discussed earlier in the chapter. Atelectasis and pneumonia still account for the most common post-operative complications. Nurses must therefore be aware of the clinical signs and symptoms of both and be able to identify those patients who are at greater risk of acquiring a pneumonia.

The most important aspects of caring for a patient who presents with pneumonia are:

- *Meticulous attention to detail of their respiratory function*
- *Adequate hydration*
- *Adequate nutrition*
- *Adequate analgesia, but opiates should be used with care because they cause respiratory depression*
- *Supplemental oxygen if there are any signs of hypoxia. (However, the hypoxia is often due to a physiological shunt, and it may make little difference to the hypoxaemia).*
- *Physiotherapy techniques – deep breathing exercisess coughing Mobilisation as soon as possible*
- *Comfort measures.*

The patient with an exacerbation of COPD

CASE EXAMPLE 5.6

Mr Reeves, a 68-year-old man, has had chronic bronchitis for the past 10 years. He recently developed a chest infection and was being treated with antibiotics at home by his GP. Unfortunately he was unresponsive to treatment and his respiratory function continued to deteriorate. He was therefore admitted to hospital. On admission his observations were:

- HR: 110 bpm
- BP: 158/98 mmHg
- RR: 34 bpm
- Temperature: 39.9°C
- WBC: 20.000/mm3
- Hct: 56%

ABG's on air:

- pH: 7.25
- PaO_2: 6.9 kPa
- $PaCO_2$: 7.2 kPa
- HCO_3: 30 mmol/l
- Saturation: 80%

Mr Reeves requested to sit out of bed as he found it much easier to breathe. He often slept in a chair at home. He was placed on 28% humidified oxygen via a facial mask. However, despite aggressive therapy (physiotherapy, bronchodilators, corticosteroids, antibiotics, controlled oxygen therapy, rehydration) he was still deteriorating at the end of the first day. His blood levels of carbon dioxide were still rising which was evident even before blood gas analysis. Mr Reeves was becoming increasingly confused and agitated; his peripheries became very warm. He developed flapping tremors, a bounding pulse, headaches and drowsiness.

It was decided that Mr Reeves would benefit from non-invasive positive pressure ventilation (NIPPV) rather than intubation and mechanical ventilation. He was put on NIPPV using a fitted mask. Within an hour he showed signs of improvement. Although his PaO_2 levels remained low, his $PaCO_2$ levels fell. Mr Reeves made an effective recovery from his chest infection and was able to go home.

Discussion

Some patients with chronic lung disease lose their ability to respond to rising $PaCO_2$. This is partly due to mechanical obstruction on breathing in and they are incapable of increasing their work of breathing any further. However, some patients have a reduced responsiveness to CO_2 and instead become dependent on the hypoxic drive to breathe. Administering high-dose oxygen to these types of patients can eliminate this drive altogether and cause total cessation of breathing. Therefore, judicious use of oxygen is warranted, and low-dose oxygen should always be given in the first instance.

As previously discussed in this chapter there are now alternative methods of non-invasive ventilation for these patients. It is extremely important that nurses, doctors and physiotherapists who are going to care for patients receiving NIPPV are confident and have a full understanding of how it works, its limitations and potential dangers. Patients need to be able to trust and feel secure about those who are caring for them so that they will co-operate with the treatment.

CONCLUSION

This chapter has given nurses a greater understanding of the concepts of patient assessment, nursing care and therapeutic interventions in order to optimise and maintain effective respiration for those patients who require high dependency care in any setting. Nurses caring for such patients must realise that they are the pivot for effective respiratory care and prevention of complications. To achieve this, the nurse caring for the high dependency patient must be knowledgeable, proactive, dynamic and creative in all aspects of nursing care and intervention.

By using their clinical wisdom and demonstrating an understanding of both the physiological and psychological response to breathing, nurses will realise that they are not just instruments of other professionals in curing the patient but rather are uniquely significant in the patient's recovery.

The definitive outcome of such good nursing care will be improvement in the quality of patient care and comfort, especially in terms of reducing patient morbidity and mortality.

REFERENCES

Banasik J L 1987 Effect of position on arterial oxygenation in postoperative coronary revascularization patients. Heart and Lung 16 November: 652–657

Bartlett R H, Gazzaniga A B, Geraghty T R 1973 Respiratory maneuvers to prevent postoperative pulmonary complications: a critical review. Journal of the American Medical Association 224: 1217–1021

Benner P 1984 From novice to expert. Addison-Wesley, London

British Guidelines on Asthma Management 1997 Thorax 52 (Suppl. 1)

Brooks-Brunn J A 1995 Postoperative atelectasis and pneumonia. Heart and Lung 24(2): 94–115

Chuter T M, Weisman C, Starker P M, Gump F E 1989 Effect of incentive spirometry on diaphragmatic dysfunction following cholecystectomy. Surgery 105: 488–493

Chuter T M, Weisman C, Starker P M 1990 The effect of coached abdominal breathing on diaphragmatic activity following cholecystectomy. Chest 97: 1230–1235

Crawford B L, Blunnie W P, Elliott A G P 1990 The value of self administered perioperative physiotherapy. Irish Journal of Medical Science 90: 51–52

Djukanovic R et al 1990 Mucosal inflammation in asthma. American Review of Respiratory Disorders 142: 434

Dripps R D, Waters R M 1941 Nursing care of surgical patients 1: the 'stir up'. American Journal of Nursing 41: 534–537

Fink M P, Helsmoortel G M, Stein K L 1990 The efficacy of an oscillating bed in the prevention of lower respiratory tract infection in the critically ill victims of blunt trauma. Chest 97: 132–137

Foyt M M 1992 Impaired gas exchange in the elderly. Geriatric Nursing September/October: 262–268

Gavigan M, Kline-O' Sullivan C, Klumpp-Lybrand B 1990 The effect of regular turning on CABG patients. Critical Care Nursing Quarterly 12: 69–76

Gentillo L, Thompson D A, Tonneson A S 1988 Effect of a rotating bed on the incidence of pulmonary complications in critically ill patients. Critical Care Medicine 16: 783–786

Giroux J M, Lewis S, Holland L G 1987 Postoperative chest physiotherapy for abdominal hysterectomy patients. Physiotherapy Canada 39: 89–93

Hathaway D 1986 Effect of preoperative instruction on postoperative outcomes: a meta-analysis. Nursing Research 35: 269–275

Hess D, Agarwal N N, Myers C L 1992 Positioning, lung function and kinetic bed therapy. Respiratory Care 37: 181–197

Hinchliff S, Montague S 1988 Physiology for nursing practice. Baillière Tindall, London

Kumar P J, Clark M L 1990 Clinical medicine, 2nd edn. Baillière-Tindall, London

McConnell E A 1991 Problems. Nursing 91 November: 35–40

Matthay M A, Wiener-Kronish J P 1989 Respiratory management after cardiac surgery. Chest 95(2): 425–434

Place B 1997 Using airway pressure. Nursing Times 93(31): 42–47

Roach S M 1985 A foundation for nursing ethics. In: Carmi A, Schneider S (eds) Nursing law and ethics. Springer-Verlag, Berlin, p 170–177

Shively M 1988 Effect of position change on mixed venous oxygen saturation in coronary artery bypass surgery patients. Heart and Lung 17: 51–59

Stoneham M D, Saville G M, Wilson I H 1994 Knowledge about pulse oximetry among medical and nursing staff. Lancet 344: 1339–1342

FURTHER READING

Pre-requisite knowledge

Cole R B 1975 Essentials of respiratory disease, 2nd edn. Pitman Medical, London

McCarthy E J 1987 Ventilation perfusion relationships. Journal of American Association of *Nurse Anaesthetists* 55(5): 437–439

Merieb E N 1995 Human anatomy and physiology, 3rd edn. Benjamin/Cummings, San Francisco

Respiratory failure

Davies J M 1991 Pre-operative respiratory evaluation and management of patients for upper abdominal surgery. Yale Journal of Biological Medicine 64: 329–349

Ephgrave K S, Kleiman-Wexler R, Pfaller M, Booth B, Werkmeister L, Young S 1993 Postoperative pneumonia: a prospective study of risk factors and morbidity. Surgery 114: 185–190

Pulse oximetry

Davidson J A H, Hosie H E 1993 Limitations of pulse oximetry: respiratory insufficiency – a failure of detection. British Medical Journal 307: 372–373

Hutton P, Clutton-Brock T 1993 The benefits and pitfalls of pulse oximetry. British Medical Journal 307: 457–458

Assessment/interventions

Anderson S 1990 Six easy steps to interpreting blood gases. American Journal of Nursing August 42–45

Dickson S 1995 Understanding the oxyhemoglobin dissociation curve. Critical Care Nurse October 54–58

Good M 1996 Effects of relaxation and music on postoperative pain: a review. Journal of Advanced Nursing 24: 905–914

Grossman R F 1998 The value of antibiotics and the outcomes of antibiotic therapy in exacerbations of COPD. Chest 113 (suppl. 4): 249S–255S

Metheny N M 1996 Fluid and electrolyte balance. J B Lippincott, Philadelphia

Pillet O, Manier G, Castaing Y 1998 Anticholinergic versus beta 2-agonist on gas exchange in COPD: a comparative study in 15 patients. Archives of Chest Diseases 53(1): 3–8

Snyder M 1992 Independent nursing interventions, 2nd edn. Delmer, USA

Non-invasive respiratory support

Place B 1997 The skill behind the mask. Nursing Times 93(26): 31–32

Romand J-A, Donald F 1995 Physiological effects of continuous positive airway pressure ventilation in the critically ill. Care of the Critically Ill 11(6): 239–243

Simonds K (ed.) 1996 Non-invasive respiratory support. Chapman and Hall Medical, London

Chest drains

Gift A G, Bogiano C S, Cunningham J 1991 Sensations during chest drain removal. Heart and Lung 20: 131–137

Kinney M R, Kirchoff K T, Puntillo K A 1995 Chest drain removal practices in critical care units in the United States. Heart and Lung 4(6): 419–424

Asthma and specific respiratory disorders

Adrogue H J, Tobin M J 1997 Respiratory failure. Blackwell, USA

British Guidelines on Asthma Management 1997 Thorax 52 suppl. 1

Kumar P J, Clark M L 1990 Clinical medicine, 2nd edn. Baillière-Tindall, London

Nunn J F 1994 Nunn's applied respiratory physiology, 4th edn. Butterworth-Heinemann, London

Cardiac care

Nigel Davies

> ### Key learning objectives
>
> - To relate the structure and function of the cardiovascular system with specific reference to the knowledge required to provide care to high dependency patients.
> - To undertake a comprehensive cardiovascular nursing assessment and plan appropriate care.
> - To make best use of monitoring equipment and other devices commonly used to assess cardiovascular status in high dependency patients.
> - To understand the rationale for care in a patient with acute circulatory failure and relate this to the concept of shock.
> - To recognise common conduction defects and care for a patient with a temporary pacing system.
> - To consider the nurse's role in advanced life support.
> - To explore advances in the care of clients with acute myocardial infarction and recognise ECG changes manifested by clients with chest pain.
> - To demonstrate a greater awareness of the cardiac drugs most commonly used for high dependency patients and the nurse's role in the maintenance of the patient's stability.

INTRODUCTION

This chapter will discuss the cardiovascular aspects of high dependency care, commonly needed either for patients with a primary cardiac condition (e.g. acute myocardial infarction or cardiac surgery) or for patients with underlying ischaemic heart disease who are admitted to hospital for other reasons (e.g. elective surgery).

Around 3% of all hospital admissions in the UK and 10% of admissions of men aged 45–64 years are due to coronary heart disease (Boaz & Rayner 1995). It is estimated that 2 million people in the UK experience angina and that 1.4 million people have experienced a heart attack at some time in their lives. Due to this high underlying prevalence of heart disease an appreciation of the principles of cardiac care is needed by nurses, not only in designated cardiac or coronary care units, but also by those caring for patients in other medical and surgical high dependency areas.

BACKGROUND PHYSIOLOGY

In this section, an overview will be given of the control mechanisms that can affect cardiac output. These may be manipulated by medical and nursing interventions for patients requiring high dependency care.

An introduction to the knowledge required by nurses caring for high dependency patients is also given. You may wish to explore cardiovascular physiology in greater depth by consulting one of the textbooks and electrocardiography (ECG) guides suggested in the Further reading list at the end of this chapter.

Cardiac output

In health, the normal cardiac output (CO) is around 5 litres per minute at rest increasing to 25 litres during exercise. It represents the amount of blood ejected by the heart in a minute and is calculated by multiplying the stroke volume (SV) by the heart rate (HR):

$$CO = SV \times HR$$

Heart rate and stroke volume are both controlled by, and dependent upon, a number of factors (summarised in Box 6.1) including the action of the conduction system, the effectiveness of the heart muscle and the peripheral vasculature.

The cardiac cycle

The cardiac cycle is the period from the end of one heartbeat to the end of the next. The heart contracts (systole) and then relaxes (diastole). At an average heart rate of 72 beats per minute, each cardiac cycle lasts 0.8 seconds with the relaxation phase (0.5 seconds) being slightly longer.

The terms systole and diastole are usually used to refer to the contraction and relaxation of the ventricles. The sequence of events happens in both the right and left sides of the heart; however, the pressure exerted by the right side is less due to the resistance to flow being less in the pulmonary circulation than in the systemic circulation. This difference is reflected in the comparative size of the muscular walls of the left and right sides of the heart. Despite the lower pressure exerted by the right side of the heart, the same amount of blood is ejected with each contraction.

In late diastole, the atria and ventricles are relaxed and blood enters the atria. When enough blood has entered the atria the pressure causes the mitral and tricuspid valves to open, for blood to pass into the ventricles. Towards the end of

■ **BOX 6.1** Factors affecting the control of heart rate	
• Conducting system	Inherent 'pacemaker' cells
• Nervous control	Sympathetic nervous system increases heart rate Parasympathetic nerves (vagus) decrease heart rate
• Hormonal control	Adrenaline from the adrenal medulla
• Stretch	Increased venous return can stretch the right atrial wall and result in an increase in heart rate by 10–15% (Bainbridge reflex)
• Temperature	Affects the SA and AV nodes. Raised temperatures increase heart rate; low temperatures decrease heart rate, e.g. in hypothermia and following cardiac surgery
• Drugs	Drugs that affect heart rate are known as chronotropes. Examples of positive chronotropes which increase heart rate are isoprenaline and adrenaline; negative chronotropes include beta adrenergic blocking agents
• Other factors	Electrolyte concentration Hormones (other than adrenaline)
Factors affecting stroke volume	
• Preload	Volume of blood returning to the heart
• Contractility	'Stretchability' of the myocardium
• Afterload	Resistance to ventricular ejection, e.g. aortic valve, peripheral vascular resistance

diastole, the atria contract and pump some more blood into the ventricles. The ventricles receive 80% of their blood passively before the atria contract; the last 20% is sometimes referred to as the 'atrial kick' and its absence (e.g. in people with atrial fibrillation) can sometimes lead to symptoms of dyspnoea, confusion and 'light-headedness'. The amount of blood remaining in the ventricles at the end of diastole is called the ventricular end-diastolic volume (EDV).

As the ventricles begin to contract the pressure in them begins to rise. This causes the mitral and tricuspid valves to close and so prevent backflow of blood into the atria. This can be heard as the first heart sound. When the pressure in the ventricles exceeds the pressure in the great arteries the aortic and pulmonary valves open causing, at first, rapid ejection of blood. The amount of blood ejected is called the stroke volume. The ejection fraction is the ratio between stroke volume and end-diastolic volume and is normally between 60% and 70%.

Almost as soon as the ventricular muscle relaxes the pulmonary and aortic valves close. This can be heard as the second heart sound. As ventricular pressure falls below atrial pressure the mitral and tricuspid valves open and ventricular filling occurs fairly rapidly.

The conduction system and the normal ECG

The conduction system within the heart consists of the sinoatrial (SA) node, the atrioventricular (AV) node, the atrioventricular bundle (also known as the bundle of His), the left and right bundle branches and the Purkinje fibres (see Fig. 6.1). The electrical activity that occurs when an impulse passes along this system can be observed on an electrocardiogram (ECG). Figure 6.2 shows a normal ECG complex.

The impulse is initiated in the SA node, which has the ability to self-generate an impulse (automaticity). The impulse spreads through the atria and is represented on the ECG by the P wave. The SA node controls the pace of the heart and is known as the heart's normal pacemaker. Although its inherent rate is about 100 per minute, the actual heart rate is slowed to an average of 70–80 per minute by the effects of the parasympathetic nervous system, exerted through the vagus nerve. Other parts of the conducting system also have a 'pacemaker' ability, though at slower rates. For example, the AV node has an inherent rate of 40–60 per minute, and the Purkinje fibres about 20–40 per minute.

The atria and ventricles are separated by connective tissue, which does not permit the spread of impulses. Therefore, the AV node and AV bundle provide the only connection. Conduction through the AV node is delayed for approximately 0.1 seconds, which allows the atria to contract and empty into the ventricles before the ventricles are depolarised and subsequently contract. This pause can be seen on the ECG during the PR interval, when the wave returns to the isoelectric (zero amplitude) line for a short period.

When the impulse leaves the AV node it is conducted rapidly which results in the entire ventricles contracting more or less simultaneously. The speed of depolarisation through the ventricles is shown by the narrow QRS complex.

An impulse generated by the conduction system leads to depolarisation (or electrical activity) in the heart, which then causes the heart muscle to contract. The ECG waveform is, therefore, a representation of the electrical activity of the heart rather than actual contraction.

Effectiveness of the heart muscle

The Frank-Starling mechanism (Guyton & Hall 1996, pp 115–116) explains that the greater the amount of stretch of the myocardial fibres at the end of diastole, the greater the force of the ensuing contraction. Up to a certain point, with healthy myocardium, the more filling that takes place, the greater the contractility and the

Fig. 6.1 Conduction system. (From Jowett & Thompson 1995, p 22. Reproduced by kind permission of Baillière Tindall.)

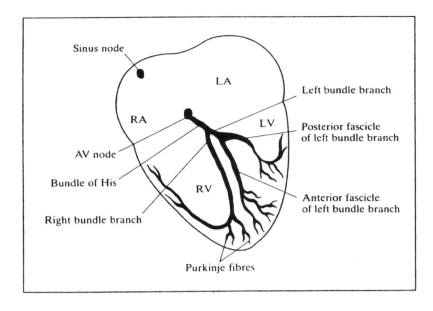

Fig. 6.2 The normal ECG. (Based on Hinchliff et al Montague & Watson 1996, p 399. Reproduced by kind permission of Baillière Tindall.)

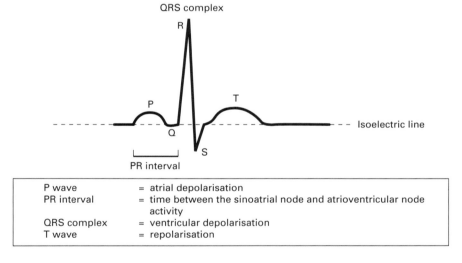

P wave	= atrial depolarisation
PR interval	= time between the sinoatrial node and atrioventricular node activity
QRS complex	= ventricular depolarisation
T wave	= repolarisation

greater the stroke volume (i.e. more fluid entering is followed by more fluid being pumped out).

In practice, with patients who have 'unhealthy' myocardial tissue (poor ventricular function or heart failure), cardiac output becomes compromised when preload is increased. This can occur, for example, following a blood transfusion or fluid administration where the heart muscle does not have the capacity (or stretchability) to increase stroke volume. More fluid enters the circulation but is not pumped adequately resulting in pooling in the pulmonary or peripheral vasculature, leading to oedema.

Positive inotropes are frequently administered in acute settings to patients with the aim of improving the effectiveness of the heart muscle's action. An inotrope is a substance that affects the contractility of the heart. The term is often incorrectly used in practice to refer only to positive inotropic drugs that increase contractility (see Box 6.2). Strictly speaking positive inotropes increase contractility – for example, adrenaline, dopamine – whereas negative inotropes decrease contractility – calcium antagonists (nifedipine, verapamil) and beta-adrenergic blocking agents (atenolol, propranolol).

■ **BOX 6.2** Positive inotropes

- Dopamine
- Noradrenaline (Norepinephrine) } naturally occurring catecholamines
- Adrenaline (Epinephrine)

- Dobutamine } synthetic substances
- Isoprenaline

All act directly on adrenergic receptors:
- **Alpha-1** effects: vasoconstriction of most peripheral vessels. Some increased myocardial contractility
- **Beta-1** effects: increased heart rate, rate of AV conduction, and myocardial contractility
- **Beta-2** effects: peripheral vasodilatation of some vascular beds, e.g. some skeletal muscle, bronchodilatation.

Adrenaline (Epinephrine)
Has beta effects at lower doses. At higher doses, e.g. during resuscitation, alpha effects produce a higher blood pressure leading to increased coronary and cerebral perfusion.

Dose	1–12 mcg/min as continuous infusion 1 mg every 2–3 minutes during CPR
Administration	1:1000 ampoules (1 mg/ml) to be diluted in 5% glucose 1:10 000 (1 mg/10 ml) recommended for use during CPR

Dopamine
Increases stroke volume but little effect on heart rate. Causes peripheral vasoconstriction but has a selective renal arterial vasodilatation effect which is most marked at low doses. Can cause localised peripheral tissue ischaemia and should therefore always be given via a central line.

Dose	1–5 mcg/kg/min	Renal effects leading to increased urine output
	5–10 mcg/kg/min	Inotropic effect. Increases cardiac output and heart rate. Doses above 10 mcg are likely to cause arrhythmias
	> 15 mcg/kg/min	Alpha receptors activated. Vasoconstriction doses of dopamine are not beneficial
Administration	Continuous infusion in 5% glucose or 0.9% sodium chloride Dilute to maximum concentration of 1.6 mg/ml	

Dobutamine
Increases force of myocardial contraction with only a small increase in heart rate. Used predominantly for cardiogenic shock and heart failure. Often given in combination with low (renal) dose of dopamine.

Dose	2.5–15 mcg/kg/min
Administration	Continuous infusion in 5% glucose or 0.9% sodium chloride Maximum concentration 5 mg/ml via syringe driver, i.e. 20 ml vial diluted to 50 ml. May be diluted further

(Cont'd.)

(Box 6.2 cont'd)

Isoprenaline

Used mainly for its chronotropic effect (increasing heart rate) rather than its inotropic (contractility) effect. Useful following MI or cardiac surgery for patients showing signs of sinus or junctional bradycardia or transient second degree AV block which is unresponsive to atropine.

Dose	1–10 mcg/min
Administration	Continuous infusion in 5% glucose or dextrose saline. Large volume dilution, e.g. 500 ml suggested (BNF); however many units dilute to much smaller quantities, e.g. 50 ml

Noradrenaline (Norepinephrime)

Generally only given under full monitoring conditions in intensive care environments. Useful in septic shock.

All catecholamines have very short biological half-lives (1–2 min) due largely to reuptake into tissues and to degradation in the liver and lungs. A steady state plasma concentration is achieved within 5–10 min after the start of a continuous infusion.

Adrenaline (epinephrine), noradrenaline (norepinephrine) and isoprenaline have 100 times greater potency than dopamine and dobutamine. Note that the dosages of the former (mcg/min) are much smaller than the latter (mcg/kg/min). As the effects may vary greatly, patients must be continuously monitored and the dose of the drug titrated as necessary.

ASSESSMENT

In order to make a comprehensive assessment of a patient's cardiovascular status, the following approaches may be adopted:

- Interpretation of vital signs
- Physical examination
- Interview with patient and any close family/friend
- Review of previous health information
- Analysis of laboratory findings.

> The stress caused to the patient by multiple assessments should be avoided. In evaluating the patient's condition, the multidisciplinary team should work as a whole.

For patients needing high dependency care, this assessment needs to be undertaken collaboratively with other members of the healthcare team, including doctors, physiotherapists, cardiac technicians and support workers. Repeated assessments by these different health professionals should be avoided, particularly in acutely ill patients, and assessment should be ongoing and synonymous with evaluation. Communication and co-ordination of activities between the different members of the healthcare team are vital to reduce the amount of disruption and disturbance for the patient.

Interpretation of vital signs

Observation of a patient's vital signs often constitutes a large proportion of a high dependency nurse's time. The interpretation of alterations in vital signs gives an insight into changes occurring within the patient's internal environment and the homeostatic mechanisms being used to counter any problems. Changes can act as triggers to other aspects of the patient's care. For example, an increase in heart rate and blood pressure may be a result of pain, while emotions such as anxiety can also affect vital signs. It is important that vital signs are interpreted correctly therefore, and not in isolation from other factors and the patient as a whole. Furthermore, baseline observations, preferably obtained before the acute event, can provide important points for comparison.

Pulse and heart rate

Arterial pulses should be examined for rate, rhythm and volume. The radial artery is usually used but may be difficult to palpate if there is peripheral shutdown, in which case the femoral or carotid arteries should be palpated. The pulse should be counted for 1 minute to assess heart rate and rhythm; however, it is more usual in high dependency or cardiac units to rely upon continuous ECG monitoring to obtain these details. In this case care should be taken to assess whether there is a peripheral pulse deficit by recording any difference between the apical rate and the peripheral pulse. Normal heart rate in the resting adult is around 70 beats per minute but can be between 60 and 100 per minute and should be regular.

The volume of the pulse depends on the pulse pressure, which is the difference between the systolic and diastolic blood pressure. A small volume pulse is often seen following a myocardial infarction whereas large volumes can be found in patients with anaemia or aortic regurgitation.

ECG monitoring

Monitoring the ECG gives a continuous picture of the heart's electrical activity, which includes the heart rate. There are different situations in which continuous ECG monitoring may be performed (see Box 6.3) but the overall aim is to identify or anticipate potentially life-threatening disturbances as early as possible. However, it should be borne in mind that the monitor trace is just an additional tool for assessment and sight should not be lost of the patient's general condition and status.

The reason for continuous ECG monitoring needs to be explained to the patient and family together with the explanation that being attached to the monitor does not necessarily imply that he is critically ill. Patients generally do not mind being attached to a monitor and a significant proportion find its presence reassuring (Thompson et al 1986).

Many monitors enable the nurse to place the electrodes on a patient in a 'colour co-ordinated' manner with the lead view then being selected at the press of a button. However, this facility is not always available and knowledge of lead

> The ECG monitor trace is just an additional tool for assessment. Don't lose sight of the patient and what *all* the vital signs are telling you.

■ BOX 6.3 Indications for continuous cardiac monitoring

- Surveillance of heart rate and rhythm
- Dysrhythmia identification and evaluation
- Acute myocardial infarction
- Undiagnosed chest pain
- Unstable angina. Monitoring may be discontinued if pain free for period of time (usually at least 24 hours) or if extent of coronary artery disease is known, e.g. following cardiac catheterisation
- Atrial–ventricular block (third degree/complete heart block and some patients with second degree depending on symptoms)
- Evaluation of temporary pacing
- Evaluation of response to drug therapy
- Peri- and post-operatively (length of time will depend on procedure and other factors, e.g. effect of drug therapy)
- Emergency and life-threatening conditions, e.g. trauma, overdose, poisoning

placement may be useful when older equipment or smaller portable monitors are used to transfer patients between units (see Fig. 6.3).

The ECG tracing should be observed for the following features:

- Rate
- Rhythm
- PR interval
- Ectopic beats.

A regular heart rate between 60 and 100 per minute is known as sinus rhythm. (A slight slowing and quickening with respiration, known as sinus arrhythmia, is quite normal). Slower rates, less than 60 per minute, are referred to as sinus bradycardia. Rates faster than 100 are known as sinus tachycardia, if the rhythm remains regular and controlled by the sino-atrial node (see Fig. 6.4 and Box 6.4).

■ **BOX 6.4** ECG electrode skin preparation

Although self-adhesive ECG electrodes usually require minimal or no skin preparation the following steps can help if the signal is poor:
- Rub the skin lightly with dry gauze or a proprietary 'skin prep' tape to remove loose dry skin
- Shave the skin if the patient is particularly hirsute to improve electrode contact (and make removal painless)
- Excess body oil and perspiration should be removed by washing with soap and water. Wiping the skin with alcohol-impregnated swabs is no longer recommended as the alcohol dries the skin excessively
- The electrode site should be observed daily for allergic reaction.

Fig. 6.3 Electrode positions for cardiac monitoring. (a) Lead II. This is the lead most commonly used by nurses (Drew & Sparacino, 1991). The QRS has the greatest amplitude in people with a normal electrical axis.
Suitable if reason for monitoring is heart rate surveillance and detection of life threatening arrhythmias.

- Positive electrode (+): lower left abdomen below the rib cage
- Negative electrode (-): right infra-clavicular space
- Ground electrode (G): left infra-clavicular space

(b) MCL1 (Modified chest lead 1)
This is a dipolar equivalent of V1 and is best for recognising arrhythmias and bundle branch block.

- Positive electrode (+): V1 position, 4th intercostal space, right sternal border
- Negative electrode (-): left infra-clavicular space
- Ground electrode (G): right infra-clavicular space

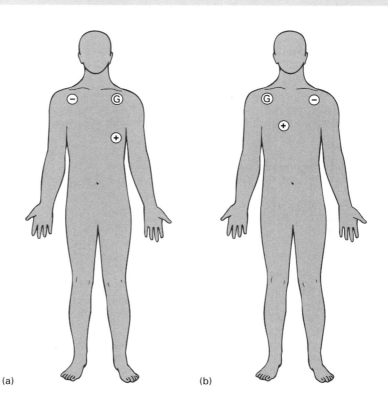

(a)　　　　　(b)

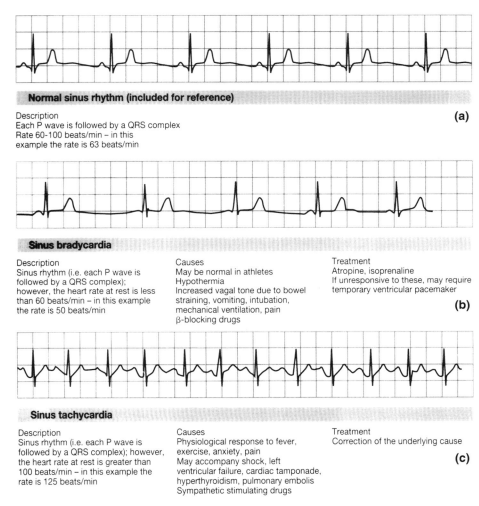

Normal sinus rhythm (included for reference)

Description **(a)**
Each P wave is followed by a QRS complex
Rate 60-100 beats/min – in this
example the rate is 63 beats/min

Sinus bradycardia

Description	Causes	Treatment
Sinus rhythm (i.e. each P wave is followed by a QRS complex); however, the heart rate at rest is less than 60 beats/min – in this example the rate is 50 beats/min	May be normal in athletes Hypothermia Increased vagal tone due to bowel straining, vomiting, intubation, mechanical ventilation, pain β-blocking drugs	Atropine, isoprenaline If unresponsive to these, may require temporary ventricular pacemaker **(b)**

Sinus tachycardia

Description	Causes	Treatment
Sinus rhythm (i.e. each P wave is followed by a QRS complex); however, the heart rate at rest is greater than 100 beats/min – in this example the rate is 125 beats/min	Physiological response to fever, exercise, anxiety, pain May accompany shock, left ventricular failure, cardiac tamponade, hyperthyroidism, pulmonary embolis Sympathetic stimulating drugs	Correction of the underlying cause **(c)**

Fig. 6.4 ECG tracings. (a) Sinus rhythm, (b) sinus bradycardia, (c) sinus tachycardia. (From Hinchliff et al 1996. Reproduced by kind permission of Baillière Tindall.)

Nurses working in areas where ECG monitoring takes places should be familiar with the operation of the monitor, including setting alarm limits appropriately and dealing with common problems (see Box 6.5 on p. 120).

Blood pressure

Arterial blood pressure is an important clinical observation that is used extensively to assess and monitor patient progress. For high dependency patients it may be recorded in three ways:

- Using a stethoscope and sphygmomanometer
- Using an automatic device with cuff that measures non-invasively
- Direct and continuous intra-arterial measurement following the insertion of a catheter into (usually) the radial artery which is then connected to a transducer (see Fig. 6.5 on p. 121).

The decision concerning which method is to be adopted will depend on the acuity of the patient, the resources available in the ward or unit and whether rapid

■ **BOX 6.5** Troubleshooting ECG monitors (adapted from Nurse's Ready Reference 1992, pp 199–200)

Problem	Possible causes	Solutions
False high-rate alarm	• Monitor interpreting large T waves as QRS complexes and doubling the rate • Skeletal muscle activity	• Reposition electrodes to lead where QRS complexes are taller than T waves • Place electrodes away from major muscle masses
False low-rate alarm	• Patient movement causing change in axis making complexes too small • Low amplitude of QRS • Poor contact between electrode and skin	• Reapply electrodes, increase size/gain control • Increase size/gain control • Reapply electrodes, wash skin
Low amplitude or no waveform	• Size/gain control set too low • Poor contact between skin and electrode; dried out gel • Broken or loose lead wires, poor connections, malfunctioning monitor	• Increase size/gain • Reapply electrodes • Check connections on all leads, wires and cables
Wandering baseline	• Poor position or contact between electrodes and skin • Chest movement	• Reposition or replace electrodes • Reposition electrodes
Artefact (interference)	• Patient anxious, shivering, rigors or seizures • Patient movement • Electrodes applied incorrectly • Electrical short circuit in leads or cables	• Treat as appropriate, keep the patient warm, reassure • Help patient relax • Check and reposition Replace broken equipment
Skin excoriation under electrode	• Patient allergic to electrode adhesive • Electrode left on skin too long	• Remove and apply with non-allergenic tape • Inspect site daily

changes in blood pressure are likely to occur. The advantages of having an arterial line measuring blood pressure (i.e. continuous measurement and observation of a wave form) need to be weighed against the potential disadvantages (e.g. risk of accidental dislodgement and subsequent bleeding; potential infection; peripheral artery damage; and embolism).

When using a traditional sphygmomanometer or non-invasive device the cuff should be an appropriate size for the patient, otherwise an inaccurate recording can be made. The bladder of the cuff should be at least 80% of the arm circumference in length and 40% of the arm circumference in width.

Central venous pressure

The central venous pressure (CVP) is measured following insertion of a line into either the subclavian or internal jugular vein, which is then advanced along the vein until its tip is near the right atrium. The CVP is therefore reflective of the pressure in the right atrium.

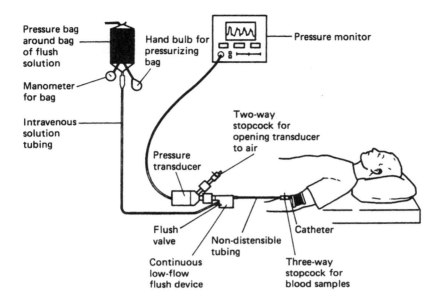

Fig. 6.5 Arterial pressure monitoring. (From Thompson & Webster 1992. Reproduced by kind permission of Butterworth-Heinemann.)

Measurement of the CVP will:

- Assist with establishing the pressure in the right atrium (filling pressure or preload)
- Help establish blood volume deficits
- Assist the evaluation of circulatory failure
- Act as a guide in fluid replacement
- Reflect response to treatment.

The normal CVP range is 3–10 mmHg (5–12 cmH₂O) although considerable variation exists in what is considered a normal value. The trend of the readings is considered more important in its association with other signs. For example, if the CVP begins to rise while urine output drops a decreased cardiac output may be indicated with circulatory overload.

The CVP can be measured either:

- Electronically using a transducer system similar to that used for measuring arterial blood pressure (see Fig. 6.5). Continuous measurements can then be obtained.
- Manually using a hard plastic water manometer that is placed on an intravenous infusion set. Measurements are obtained intermittently (see Fig. 6.6 on p. 122).

The recording should be made with the patient in the same 'baseline' position with the zero point of the manometer level with the patient's right atrium.

Manual methods measure the pressure in centimetres of water (cm H_2O) whereas electronic systems usually use millimetres of mercury (mmHg), although most new monitors can be programmed for either unit of measurement. Care should be taken when interpreting changes in CVP to check if the method used has been changed: for example, soon after a patient has been transferred from a ward, where the CVP has been recorded manually, to a high dependency area where the pressure is transduced or if the patient's position has changed. 1 mmHg is equal to 1.36 cmH₂O. Situations that commonly produce an elevated CVP include congestive heart failure; cardiac tamponade; vasoconstrictive states where the blood volume has remained the same but the vascular bed has become smaller; and

Fig. 6.6 Measuring central venous pressure (CVP) using a fluid manometer. (Based on Hinchliff 1996 et al, reproduced by kind permission of Baillière Tindall.)

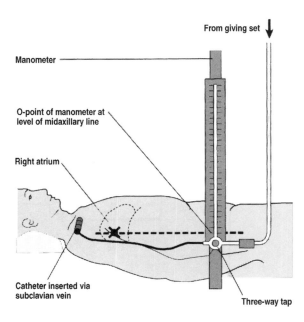

Fig. 6.7 Pressure in the heart and great vessels.

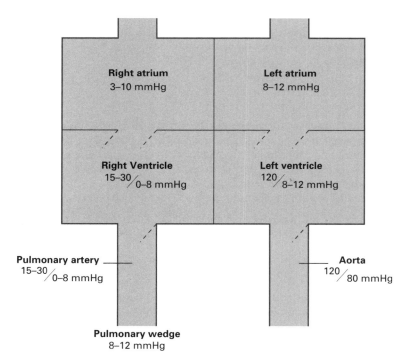

increased blood volume as a result, for example, of over transfusion. A low CVP is usually seen with hypovolaemia due to blood or fluid loss or through drug induced vasodilatation.

The pressures in the heart and main blood vessels (see Fig. 6.7) are most frequently assessed by measuring the arterial blood pressure and central venous pressure. However, in some high dependency areas it may also be possible to measure pressures in the heart and pulmonary artery together with the cardiac output using a pulmonary artery flotation catheter (Swan et al 1970). Cardiac output is measured by thermodilution. Typically, this involves a bolus of cold saline being injected into the right atrium with the cardiac output then being calculated electronically by measuring the change in temperature of the blood in the pulmonary artery. The technique and care required are explained fully in many intensive care manuals (e.g. Adam & Osborne 1997).

Measuring cardiac output indirectly is often adequate for many clinical situations. This can be done by reviewing blood pressure, heart rate and CVP measurements and relating this to information obtained during a physical examination of the patient, e.g. skin colour, peripheral temperature and changes in urine output.

> Indirect measurement of cardiac output may be adequate for most clinical situations. Review blood pressure, heart rate and CVP. Relate this to skin colour, urine output and peripheral temperature in the patient.

Physical examination

Observation of a patient's physical state can greatly aid the assessment of his cardiovascular status. Physical examination has traditionally been completed by medical staff. However, nurses undertaking specialist or expanded roles are increasingly developing the skills required to perform a comprehensive physical assessment.

Aspects of a physical examination particularly pertinent to the cardiovascular assessment include:

- Skin colour and temperature, noting any pallor, cyanosis, signs of hypo- or hyperthermia and of peripheral 'shutdown'
- Level of consciousness
- Urine output and fluid balance
- Peripheral abnormalities such as claudication.

Interview

Nurses can gain a wealth of information from the patient and any accompanying family or close friend, which may be pertinent to the cardiovascular assessment. The information may be collected in a structured interview or over a period of time. In acute situations, information may be obtained from the patient about his experience of the situation. For example, does he have a sensation of palpitations to accompany the tachycardia noted on the ECG monitor? Alternatively, is the pain he is experiencing associated with inspiration or is it continuous? Other activities of living (Roper et al 1996) which may need to be considered are summarised in Box 6.6.

Review of previous information

Valuable details that may contribute to the current assessment of the patient may be culled from previous information recorded about him. Information that may be readily available can be found in 'old' notes relating to previous hospital admissions, recent notes recorded before the current acute episode or from 'patient-held' details (e.g. current medications or anticoagulation clinic results). Medical notes may contain information about longstanding conditions (e.g. hypertension) or previous treatments (e.g. the response to nitrates). Nursing notes may give an indication of the patient's perception of his illness or his social situation, which the patient may not be able to communicate because of his current acuity. Furthermore, they may contain information relating to the patient's normal coping strategies and previous experiences of aspects of high dependency care. Charts (e.g. vital signs, fluid balance), previous ECGs and laboratory results will provide 'baseline' information to compare with current assessments.

■ **BOX 6.6** Factors to consider when undertaking a cardiovascular assessment (Based on the Activities of Living Model (Roper et al 1996))

Maintaining a safe environment
Pain:
• Do they suffer with chest pain?
• Has the pain become worse recently?
• Does it occur at rest as well as on exertion?
• What type of pain is it and where? (back, left arm, jaw, neck, chest)
• What do they usually do to relieve the pain?
• Do they know what causes it? Is it angina? Do they know what angina is?
• Do they have any other pain from any other condition?
• Do they ever suffer from dizzy spells, fainting, sweating, nausea?
Medication:
• How long have they been taking these drugs?
• Do they know what the tablets are for?
• Do they cause any side effects?
• Are the medications limiting in any way?

Communicating
• Anxiety – now and normally?
• Stressful events recently?

Breathing
• Are they breathless; were they on admission?
• Do they suffer from breathlessness with chest pain?
• Is breathlessness ever a problem? If so, does it restrict them in any way?
• Do they smoke? Have they ever? When did they give up? How much did/do they smoke per day?

Eating and drinking
• When did they last eat/drink?
• Do they normally have a good appetite?
• Do they usually eat a well balanced diet?

Eliminating
• Do they take diuretics? If so, do they cause problems?
• What time of day do they normally take them?
• Urinary catheter? Does this cause any distress? Do they understand reason for catheter?
• Are bowels regular? Constipation – do they need aperient while in hospital?

Personal cleansing and dressing
• Condition of skin

Controlling body temperature
• Any fevers, temperature, night sweats recently, possibly indicating infective endocarditis?
• Cold hands/feet? – poor circulation or drug side effects, e.g. beta blockers
• Does cold weather aggravate angina?

Mobilising
• Does any chest pain or breathlessness restrict mobility?
• How far can they normally walk without getting symptoms?
• Have they had an exercise tolerance test?

Working and playing
• What type of work do they do?

(Cont'd)

(Box 6.6 cont'd)

- Do they consider their work to be stressful?
- If retired – what did they used to do? Do they enjoy retirement?
- Do they still keep active?
- Have any activities been given up due to illness?

Expressing sexuality
- Relationships? Any stressful changes recently, e.g. separation, divorce, children

Sleeping
- Does angina or breathlessness wake them at night or in the morning?
- How many hours, sleep do they normally have?
- How many pillows do they need to sleep?

Dying
- How do they feel about being in hospital?
- How well do they think their family/friends are coping with their illness?
- Do they wish to see a religious representative while in hospital?

Analysis of laboratory findings

Results obtained primarily from blood samples will aid the assessment. This will include the interpretation of results obtained from equipment located within many high dependency units. Information that is frequently of use in acute settings to the cardiovascular assessment includes:

- Serum potassium (K^+) levels. In healthy individuals the normal level is 3.6–4.6 mmol/l, however, a higher level (4.5–5.0 mmol/l) may need to be maintained in some cases where the cardiac muscle is particularly irritable (e.g. after cardiac surgery). Variation from the norm (both higher and lower levels) can lead to cardiac arrest.
- Coagulation times will be needed for both hypovolaemic patients and those with a primary cardiac condition requiring anticoagulation. Activated clotting times (ACT) may be assessed easily on the ward while laboratory analysis will enable activated partial thromboplastin time (APTT) and the international normalised ratio (INR) for prothrombin time to be assessed for patients who have been anticoagulated with heparin or warfarin respectively.
- Haemoglobin and haematocrit or packed cell volume (PCV) will be needed for hypovolaemic patients or those where fluid replacement is anticipated.
- The metabolic status derived from the partial pressures of oxygen and carbon dioxide (see Ch. 5 for a full account of the interpretation of arterial blood gases).

Typical normal values are shown in Box 6.7

■ BOX 6.7 Typical normal values	
Hb	13.5–17.5 g/dl (M)
	11.5–15.5 g/dl (F)
Hct/PCV	0.4–0.45 (M)
	0.36–0.44 (F)
Platelet count	150–400 × 10⁹l)
APTT	25–37 sec
ACT	<150 sec
K⁺	3.6–4.6 mmol/l

LOW CARDIAC OUTPUT

The distinctions between the terms low cardiac output state, acute circulatory collapse and the various types of 'shock' are, largely, arbitrary. The terms can be used to denote a clinical picture in which there is inadequate perfusion of oxygen and other essential substances in the tissues caused by:

- Heart muscle pump failure
- Hypovolaemia
- Abnormalities in peripheral resistance
- A combination of one or more of the above.

The different types and typical manifestations of shock are listed in Boxes 6.8 and 6.9.

Pathophysiological changes

Cardiac changes Cardiac output may be either absent or reduced due to disruption of electrical activity, impaired contractility or inadequate filling. In the early stages, as shock begins to develop, there is more sympathetic activity, which increases the heart rate and force of contraction. This is accompanied by vasoconstriction, increasing the venous return to the heart. This compensatory mechanism ceases to work when the circulating volume is reduced by more than 15%.

■ **BOX 6.8** Types of shock

Hypovolaemic
- Haemorrhage
- Dehydration
- Burns
- (Not manifested until between 15% and 25% of circulating volume lost)

Cardiogenic
- Acute myocardial infarction
- Arrhythmias
- Tamponade
- Pulmonary embolism (caused by an inadequate cardiac output)

Neurogenic
- Spinal cord injury
- Spinal analgesia
- Severe pain
- Extreme fright (autonomic nervous system activity causes reflex vasodilatation and loss of arteriolar tone resulting in pooling of blood and loss of venous return)

Septic
- Older patients in hospital
- Following invasive procedure particularly genitourinary instrumentation
- Where there is an underlying disease which limits the use of compensatory mechanisms (caused by an overwhelming infection that results in peripheral vasodilatation leading to inadequate circulating volume)

Anaphylactic
- Antigen–antibody reaction (The release of toxic substances (e.g. histamine) produces vasodilatation and pooling of blood)

■ **BOX 6.9** Typical manifestations of shock

• Systolic BP less than 90 mmHg or reduction of more than 25% of its normal reading
• Weak, rapid and thready pulse
• Cold and clammy skin
• Oliguria – urine output less than 0.5 ml/kg body weight per hour
• Mental confusion or other signs of altered orientation such as agitation

The classic picture may show some variations, e.g. in septic shock the patient's skin may be warm and dry and the pulse bounding.

The increased heart rate causes a decreased diastolic filling time that reduces coronary perfusion. Dysrhythmias can further reduce the diastolic filling time and also lead to inefficient ventricular contractions, decreasing cardiac output.

Bleeding into the pericardial sac (cardiac tamponade) can precipitate cardiogenic shock, particularly following cardiac surgery or chest injuries. This impairs effective emptying or filling of the heart.

In the later stages of shock a number of vasoactive kinins (e.g. bradykinin, histamine) are released which have potent vasodilator effects further decreasing the circulating volume.

Peripheral vessel changes Initially, vasoconstriction diverts blood to the vital organs and blood pressure, particularly diastolic pressure, may be maintained. Blood flow to the skin and renal circulation are reduced. Prolonged vasoconstriction causes tissue hypoxia and acidosis, which eventually leads to microcirculatory failure, if not reversed or treated. Accumulating metabolites and the local acidosis cause relaxation of the precapillary sphincters, which results in the pooling of blood.

Fluid shifts Early in hypovolaemic and cardiogenic shock, fluid moves from the interstitial spaces into capillaries thus increasing the circulating volume. However, this fluid shift is later reversed and fluid leaves the vascular space. This reversal is caused by the effects of hypoxia on cellular metabolism. Ion pumping mechanisms fail due to lack of 'energy', potassium leaves the cell and sodium enters. Water follows sodium, leaving the vasculature and extending the hypovolaemia.

In septic shock, toxins result in increased permeability of capillaries with small proteins and fluid leaving the circulation. Fluid can leave the circulation at a rate of 200 ml per hour with the patient developing severe oedema and hypovolaemia.

Renal changes In the initial stages of shock the kidneys promote conservation of water through activation of anti-diuretic hormone (ADH) from the posterior pituitary gland, and through the renin–angiotensin–aldosterone response (Guyton & Hall 1996, :pp 227–229). Prolonged renal ischaemia may lead to acute renal failure with the onset of oliguria or anuria.

Coagulation changes Microcirculatory changes can lead to pooling and stasis of blood that predisposes to platelet aggregation. Disseminated intravascular coagulation is often seen in patients with septic shock with very rapid consumption of clotting factors leading to bleeding, particularly from mucosal surfaces.

Acid–base disequilibrium Initially, due to hyperventilation, respiratory alkalosis can develop. However, once tissue hypoxia occurs, anaerobic metabolism is induced and lactic acid accumulates, producing a metabolic acidosis (see Ch. 5).

Intestine and liver Prolonged vasoconstriction is thought to cause intestinal ischaemia and necrosis which permits intestinal bacteria to gain access to the blood-stream leading to sepsis. If the liver has sustained ischaemic damage, it is unable to undertake its metabolic and detoxification functions or produce clotting factors.

Pulmonary changes Extensive left ventricular damage (in cardiogenic shock) will result in vascular congestion and pulmonary oedema. Ventilation : perfusion ratios are disturbed and hypoxaemia results.

CARE OF THE PATIENT WITH A LOW
CARDIAC OUTPUT

The aim of nursing and medical interventions is to preserve oxygen and nutrient transport to the vital organs and to elicit the cause (if not known) of the low output state. Aspects of the initial management of a patient displaying signs of shock are shown in Figure 6.8. Depending on the response to initial treatment, the patient may be stabilised quickly and able to remain in a lower dependency care setting, or may require transfer to another critical care or intensive therapy unit where more comprehensive care is available. Advanced life support may be necessary (see below).

With all patients, continuous monitoring of heart rate and blood pressure is necessary. Oxygen should generally be administered as appropriate in relation to assessment of oxygen saturation or blood gas analysis. Pulse oximetry may only be useful if the patient is not peripherally 'shut down'. Skin colour and temperature, together with an assessment of the patient's conscious level, also need to be considered. The insertion of a urinary catheter and houry measurements will give some indication of renal perfusion and, hence, cardiac output. An adequate cardiac output should support renal perfusion sufficiently to produce a urine output greater than 0.5 ml per kg of body weight per hour.

Other treatments and interventions that are likely to occur will depend on the cause of the low cardiac output.

Cardiogenic shock or heart muscle pump failure is usually treated with positive inotropic drugs, generally dobutamine in conjunction with dopamine at a low dose which may improve renal perfusion (see Box 6.2). These drugs need to be titrated to the individual's response and changing condition. ECG monitoring is essential. The patient needs to be assessed (CVP, urine output) to ensure he is adequately 'filled' before inotropes are started. Diuretics, often at high intravenous doses, may be needed to reverse or prevent pulmonary oedema. If the cause is well established, then the medical team may decide that the placement of a pulmonary artery flotation catheter is not warranted.

Hypovolaemia Replacement fluid will be the first-line therapy. Colloid is given rapidly in the form of either blood or plasma expander substances (e.g. gelofusin, elohes, haemacell). Generally the packed cell volume (PCV) or haematocrit is used as a guide to choice, although some units use haemoglobin (Hb) measurement. Blood should be given if the PCV is less than 30% or the Hb less than 10 g/dl. If large replacement volumes are needed, then blood products will also be required to prevent coagulation problems.

If possible, the amount of fluid that is lost should be measured to aid in the calculation of replacement fluid e.g. fluid, loss via post-operative drainage tubes or as a result of diarrhoea.

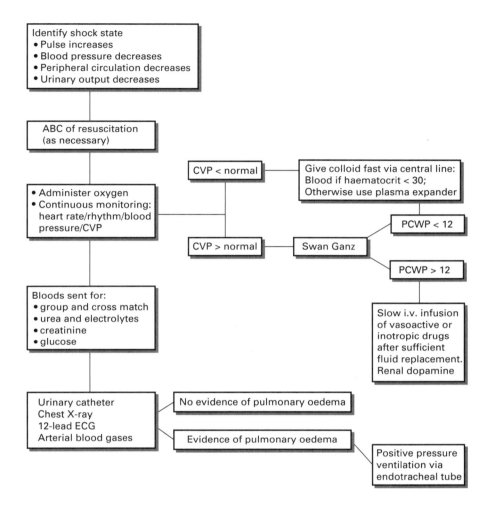

Fig. 6.8 The management of shock.

Dysrhythmias A variety of causes may precipitate dysrhythmias that compromise cardiac output. The loss of an adequate circulating volume may be as a result of either an abnormally fast or slow heart rate. Excessively fast rates are seen, for example, with ventricular tachycardia, fast atrial fibrillation or flutter and with re-entrant tachycardias. These are usually treated initially with antiarrhythmic agents such as lignocaine or amiodarone (see Box 6.11, p. 134).

Slow heart rates may be associated with parasympathetic (vagal) effects on the sinoatrial or atrioventricular nodes or with varying degrees of atrioventricular block ('heart block'). This can be the result of myocardial infarction, fibrosis of the conducting system associated with old age or cardiac surgery. Drugs with positive chronotropic (rate enhancing) effects may be used; for example, atropine, which blocks parasympathetic activity, or isoprenaline (see Box 6.2, p 115–116). Temporary pacing may also need be initiated.

TEMPORARY PACING

Artificial cardiac pacing is likely to be used for any condition resulting in failure of the heart to initiate or conduct an intrinsic electrical impulse at a rate adequate to maintain tissue perfusion throughout the body. Pacing is the repetitive delivery of very low electrical energies to the heart, thus initiating and maintaining the cardiac rhythm.

There are four main ways in which pacing may be undertaken as a temporary measure.

Transvenous (endocardial) A pacing lead is passed via a vein to the endocardial surface of the heart, most commonly the right ventricle. The wire is inserted in a similar way to a 'central line' via the subclavian vein. This is usually done under X-ray imaging guidance, many CCUs having an adjacent room set aside for pacing. Very occasionally and in emergency conditions it may be inserted 'blindly'.

Epicardial Following cardiac surgery conduction disturbances may arise due to oedema and manipulation of the conducting system. Temporary epicardial wires are frequently inserted during surgery: attached to the outer surface of the heart (epicardium) they are then brought out through the skin at the base of the sternotomy wound. They are usually removed 4 or 5 days after surgery.

Transcutaneous (external transthoracic) First introduced by Zoll in the 1950s, this method is now used in emergency situations as a rapid, simple and safe method of maintaining cardiac output. It is non-invasive and relatively simple to commence following minimal training. With modern units, which use a longer pulse duration (and thus lower amplitude), pacing is usually well tolerated, with little more than slight discomfort such as tingling or tapping (Zoll & Zoll 1985). If the patient does find the experience painful, however, analgesia (e.g. 2.5–5 mg diamorphine given intravenously) should be administered. Despite advances in technology it remains a temporary measure until appropriate transvenous pacing can be undertaken.

Transoesophageal This technique involves an electrode being inserted, in a manner rather like a nasogastric tube. Although originally described in the late 1960s, it is used infrequently and is not very reliable (Jowett & Thompson 1995).

A summary of the nursing care required for a patient with a temporary pacing system and actions that may need to be taken if problems arise are given in Box 6.10 on page 132. These aspects are discussed further in Thompson and Webster (1992, pp 194–198).

ADVANCED LIFE SUPPORT

In the event of a cardiac arrest, it is the nurse's first priority to commence basic life support (BLS) measures. Increasingly, nurses in both ward and high dependency areas are enhancing their skills to include advanced life support (ALS) techniques. Evidence suggests that the chances of a patient surviving are increased when defibrillation is implemented promptly (Advanced Life Support Working Group 1998). It is now recommended that rapid defibrillation should take precedence over basic life support measures.

The majority of sudden deaths result from arrhythmias associated with acute myocardial infarction or chronic ischaemic heart disease. However, a significant number of 'arrests' also occur after medical interventions such as line insertions or secondary to bleeding as a result of trauma or surgery. The heart usually arrests in one of three rhythms (Handley & Swain 1996) – see Figure 6.9.

- Ventricular fibrillation (VF) or pulseless ventricular tachycardia (VT)
- Asystole or extreme bradycardia

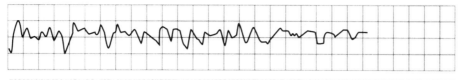

Fig. 6.9 ECG tracings during a cardiac arrest. (Reproduced by kind permission of Bailliere Tindill.)

Ventricular fibrillation

Description	Causes	Treatment
Ventricular rhythm is rapid and chaotic QRS complexes are wide and irregular No visible P waves	Myocardial ischaemia or infarction, hypo- or hyperkalaemia, congestive cardiac failure, untreated ventricular tachycardia, drug toxicity (e.g. digitalis), electrocution, hypothermia	Cardiopulmonary resuscitation Direct current shock 200-400 joules Sodium bicarbonate Antiarrhythmic drugs after resuscitation **(a)**

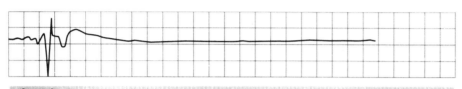

Asystole

Description	Causes	Treatment
Ventricular standstill No QRS complexes	Myocardial ischaemia or infarction, acute respiratory failure, aortic valve disease, hyperkalaemia	Cardiopulmonary resuscitation Calcium chloride Isoprenaline Adrenaline **(b)**

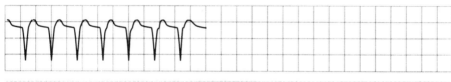

Ventricular tachycardia

Description	Causes	Treatment
QRS complexes are wide and bizarre No visible P waves Ventricular rate 140-220 beats/min – in this example ventricular rate is 166 beats/min	Myocardial infarction, drug toxicity (e.g. digitalis, quinidine), hypokalaemia, hypercalcaemia	Lignocaine If no effect, direct current cardioversion **(c)**

• Electromechanical dissociation (EMD) – the presence of an electrical rhythm compatible with circulation but with no detectable cardiac output.

Successful resuscitation after cardiopulmonary arrest is most likely when the rhythm is VF or pulseless VT.

A cardiac arrest is usually unexpected and the ensuing events may easily become very chaotic. However, with high dependency patients in both ward and specialist units, the level of monitoring may forewarn the nurse of changes to the patient's condition, enabling a potential arrest to be prevented or anticipated. The successful management of the situation requires an effective leader, and team members who are well-rehearsed in basic and advanced life support skills. Nurses taking on expanded roles need first to be competent in BLS and have a good knowledge of arrhythmias associated with cardiac arrests (Inwood 1996). As studies have shown that the resuscitation skills of healthcare professionals are poor and that ability diminishes quickly over time (Wynne et al 1987) regular retraining and competence assessment are necessary.

■ **BOX 6.10** Nursing care for the patient with temporary pacing. (Adapted from Nurse's Ready Reference 1992)

Care of the patient includes:
- Assessing pacemaker function
- Ensuring the system is intact and working
- Maintaining patient comfort and safety
- Preventing and dealing with complications
- Teaching the patient about his condition

Rhythm strip showing normal paced beat and two pacing problems

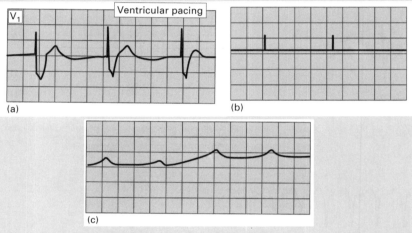

ECG	Action
(a) Ventricular paced beat Note 'pacing spike' followed by broad QRS complex	
(b) Failure to pace: P waves are not followed by a pacing stimulus or QRS complex	• Check connections • Increase voltage **NB** May be caused by 'oversensing' of electrical impulses from pectoral muscles
(c) Failure to capture: pacing spike seen but not causing depolarisation of the ventricles (no QRS)	• Move patient on to his left side • Check connections • Increase voltage

In the emergency of a cardiac arrest nurses should not forget to be sensitive to the patient's family while being professional in a high-risk scenario.

During a cardiac arrest nurses also need to be aware of their responsibility to the patient's family. Relatives may need to be telephoned and informed of the deterioration in the patient's condition. This should be done with sensitivity and a decision made about the exact extent of the information to be given based on the nurse's knowledge of the family. Relatives should be given realistic and honest information that enables them to decide how quickly and with whom to come to the hospital. If relatives are present when the patient arrests they should not automatically be excluded from the ward or unit. There is increasing evidence, mainly from research carried out in accident and emergency departments, that many relatives find it beneficial to remain and witness the resuscitation (Barratt & Wallis 1998).

The UK and European Resuscitation Councils have produced standard guidelines for the management of a cardiac arrest (Advanced Life Support

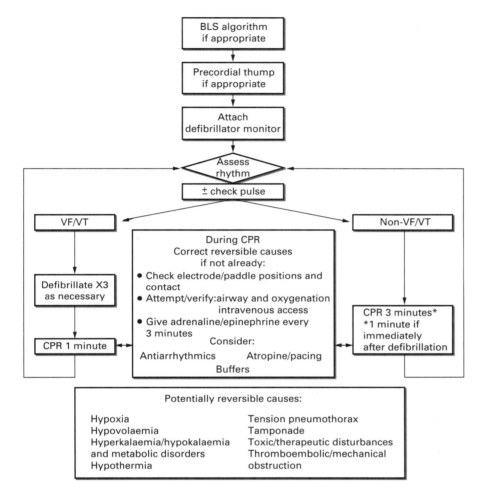

Fig. 6.10 Advanced life support algorithm. (Reproduced by kind permission of the European Resuscitation Council, from Robertson C Steen P, Adgey J et al.)

BLS algorithm
if appropriate

Precordial thump
if appropriate

Attach
defibrillator monitor

Assess
rhythm

± check pulse

VF/VT

Non-VF/VT

Defibrillate X3
as necessary

During CPR
Correct reversible causes
if not already:
• Check electrode/paddle positions and contact
• Attempt/verify: airway and oxygenation
   intravenous access
• Give adrenaline/epinephrine every 3 minutes
Consider:
Antiarrhythmics   Atropine/pacing
         Buffers

CPR 3 minutes*
*1 minute if
immediately
after defibrillation

CPR 1 minute

Potentially reversible causes:

Hypoxia
Hypovolaemia
Hyperkalaemia/hypokalaemia
and metabolic disorders
Hypothermia

Tension pneumothorax
Tamponade
Toxic/therapeutic disturbances
Thromboembolic/mechanical
obstruction

Working Group 1998) including an algorithm to assist health professionals (see Fig. 6. 10).

Although the initial drugs and dosages given during a cardiac arrest have been standardised, in a prolonged arrest different inotropic and antiarrhythmic agents may be used (see Boxes 6.2 on page 115 and 6.11 on page 134).

> Remember drugs that treat arrythmias can also cause arrythmias.

CARING FOR THE PATIENT WITH CHEST PAIN

An estimated 1.4 million people in the UK have experienced a 'heart attack' at some time in their lives. The annual incidence is 330 000 (Boaz & Rayner 1995). Although nurses working in coronary care units have specialist knowledge of the care required for patients experiencing a myocardial infarction (MI), nurses in other areas caring for highly dependent patients need to be aware of the presentation and evolution of angina and an MI. This necessitates an understanding of the ECG changes manifest during chest pain and the immediate care required.

■ **BOX 6.11** Antiarrhythmics

Most arrhythmias arise from an alteration in impulse generation, or from an abnormality in impulse conduction. Antiarrhythmic drugs can be classified according to their main effects on the action potential:

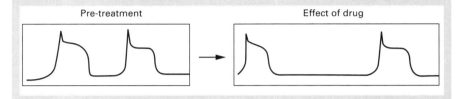

| Pre-treatment | Effect of drug |

Depolarisation occurs every 500 msec or 120 beats/min

Depolarisation is slowed or the threshold increased so that depolarisation occurs every 750 msec or 80 beats/min

Examples of antiarrhythmic drugs

CLASS I (Na⁺ channel blockers)
- Disopyramide
- Lignocaine
- Flecainide

CLASS II (Beta-adrenergic receptor blockers)
- Propranolol
- Atenolol

CLASS III (K⁺ channel blockers)
- Amiodarone
- Bretylium

CLASS IV (Ca⁺⁺ channel blockers)
- Verapamil
- Diltiazem

OTHER ANTIARRHYTHMICS
- Digoxin

Pathophysiology

The buildup of fatty deposits in the coronary arteries (atherosclerosis) leads to obstruction of blood flow and therefore a reduction of oxygen supply to the heart muscle. This imbalance between oxygen supply and demand causes pain known as angina. This usually occurs during exertion but other factors that increase the physiological stress placed upon the body, e.g. surgery or anxiety, may also precipitate chest pain. Angina that is related to exercise is generally referred to as 'stable'. In contrast, 'unstable angina' refers to chest pain that also occurs at rest. It usually implies serious coronary disease.

An acute myocardial infarction is, most commonly, the result of a rupture of part of the atheromatous plaque that has built up in the coronary arteries. This causes a clot (thrombus) to be formed, at the site of lipid accumulation, that results in total (or near total) blockage of the affected artery. The blood supply to this part of the heart is then reduced and tissue damage occurs. There are three levels of damage to the affected tissues (see Fig. 6.11)

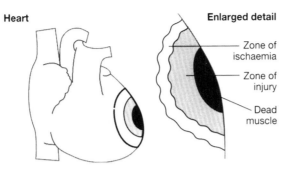

Heart

Enlarged detail

Zone of ischaemia

Zone of injury

Dead muscle

Fig. 6.11 Zones of ischaemia, injury and infarction. (Reproduced by kind permission of Bailliere Tindall.)

- *Ischaemia:* tissue damaged by lack of oxygen but potentially salvageable with an oxygen supply
- *Injury:* more jeopardised tissue but still potentially reversible
- *Infarction:* irreversible cell death.

Prompt intervention, with the administration of thrombolytics (see below), can help save myocardium.

Distinguishing between angina and myocardial infarction

The symptoms people experience when having chest pain can often be similar with angina or with an MI.

Chest pain   This is often referred to as being 'gripping' or 'vice-like' in nature and radiates to the arms, neck and jaw. Some patients (the elderly and those with diabetic neuropathy) may feel no pain and other symptoms have to be relied upon. This can lead to what is known as a 'silent infarction'. The chest pain usually comes on gradually (truly sudden onset chest pain is more often associated with dissection of the aorta).

Breathlessness   This may occur as a result of exertion or at rest.

Light-headedness or syncope   This is a result of the reduction in cardiac output brought about by the inability of the heart to pump effectively without adequate oxygen supply. Some patients have reported these symptoms in the minutes leading up to a cardiac arrest.

Nausea   This is caused by congestion in the gastrointestinal tract following the diversion of blood to the vital structures.

> Even if a myocardial infarction is excluded, the patient may still be seriously at risk from unstable angina.

Patients with these symptoms are said to be having a suspected MI until other measures are undertaken to rule this out. If an MI is excluded, this does not mean the patient is not still at risk of developing further complications or death from unstable angina. To confirm a diagnosis of myocardial infarction a 12-lead ECG needs to be interpreted and cardiac enzymes evaluated.

ECG changes in patients with chest pain

A 12-lead ECG recording is necessary for all patients experiencing chest pain. Sufficient information cannot be obtained from single monitoring leads. The ECG will need to be performed promptly as part of the initial assessment of the patient's chest pain and may need to be repeated every few minutes. Therefore, it is important that nurses have the skills and ability to perform and accurately interpret the ECG (Quinn 1996).

Fig. 6.12 The sequence of ECG changes in myocardial infarction. (From Jowett & Thompson 1995, p 139. Reproduced by kind permission of Bailliere Tindall.)

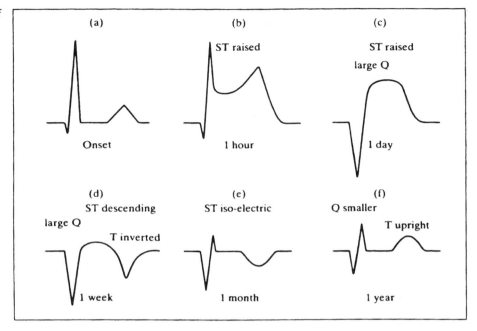

Typical ECG features that should be observed are:

- *ST segment:* either elevation or depression
- *T waves:* inversion or flattening
- *Q waves:* at least 25% of the size of the R wave.

Generally speaking, ST segment depression suggests that there is ischaemia, whereas ST segment elevation is regarded as being an indication of an emerging myocardial infarction. Correctly speaking, the only definitive diagnostic changes with myocardial infarction are changes in the QRS complexes (Rowlands 1991, p 168), i.e. reduction in R wave height and appearance of Q waves. T wave changes are seen in ischaemia (flattening or inversion) and also within days of an MI. Figure 6.12 shows the typical sequence of changes in acute MI. However, individual patients differ and any part or this entire spectrum may not be seen. Changes can occur over short periods of time, and highlight the dynamic and unstable nature of the patient.

The 12-lead ECG gives a global picture of the electrical activity of the heart. From this, it is possible to note in which area of the heart the infarction or ischaemia is occurring. Box 6.12 indicates which leads correspond to specific areas of the heart. A full explanation of the ECG manifestations found in ischaemia and infarction can be found in the many texts focussing primarily on ECG interpretation (see Further Reading suggestions at the end of this chapter).

Treatment for angina

For patients with angina the aim of care is to minimise the mismatch between the heart's oxygen demand and supply. In health extra oxygen demands (e.g. as a result of exercise or anxiety) can be met by an increased supply of oxygen to the heart tissue. in angina, however, due to the atherosclerotic changes (described above) causing narrowing or obstruction of coronary blood vessels the blood supply and therefore oxygen transport are reduced. Sufficient supply of oxygen to the heart tissue is thus not achieved. Attempts are made to address the imbalance by

■ **BOX 6.12** Identifying the area of infarction from the ECG

ECG changes indicating infarction will be seen in the leads lying over the area of damage.

Other leads may show mirror images or 'reciprocal changes' of these features (e.g. ST depression may be seen in the lead opposite to the area of infarction, where ST elevation is present).

Location of infarction	Leads showing changes
Anterior infarction	Some of the group V_{1-3} plus some of the group V_{4-6}
Inferior infarction	II, III, aVF
Posterior infarction	V_1, V_2 but inverse of the usual changes. The images in V_1 and V_2 are reciprocal changes

(An in-depth classification including more extensive MIs may be found in Rowlands 1991, p 180.)

■ **BOX 6.13** Vasodilators

Nitrates

Nitrates have been the mainstay in the treatment of angina for many years. Many different preparations have been developed to enable them to be used for treatment and prophylaxis, in oral, sublingual, transdermal and intravenous forms. They are also used intravenously in acute care settings to counteract hypertension and promote vasodilatation, e.g. after cardiac surgery.

Nitrates relax vascular smooth muscle mainly in the venous system and thus reduce preload to the heart. Coronary dilatation probably occurs although this is not a main action.

Intravenous glyceryl trinitrate (GTN) or isosorbide dinitrate
Dose : 1–10 mg/h
Administration:
- Continuous infusion in 5% glucose or 0.9% sodium chloride
- Not compatible with PVC containers but is stable with polyethylene therefore recommended that given via syringe pump (i.e. rigid plastic container)
- Usual dilution: 50 mg in 50 ml

Sodium nitroprusside (nipride)
Sodium nitroprusside is a potent intravenous vasodilator used in hypertensive emergencies and severe left ventricular failure. It relaxes both arteriolar and venous smooth muscle. It is light sensitive degrading to cyanide. Arterial blood pressure monitoring required.
Dose : 0.5–8 mcg/kg/min
Administration:
- Continuous infusion in 5% glucose or 0.9% sodium chloride.
- Cover infusion set with foil

encouraging the patient to rest, giving oxygen and by the administration of a combination of medications. Typically, patients will have one or more of the following groups of drugs:

- Vasodilators (see Box 6.13), e.g. nitrates in intravenous, sublingual or sustained release tablet or patch form
- Beta-adrenergic blocking agents e.g. atenolol

- Calcium-channel blockers, e.g. nifedipine
- Opiate analgesia, e.g. diamorphine.

Cardiac enzymes

Many biochemicals are released from dead and dying cells. In cardiac muscle three enzymes are routinely measured to diagnose myocardial infarction:

- Creatine phosphokinase (CPK or CK)
- Lactic dehydrogenase (LDH)
- Serum glutamic oxaloacetic transaminase (SGOT), also known as aspartate transaminase (AST).

None of these enzymes is cardiac specific. However, an isoenzyme of creatine kinase (CK-MB) has been developed which is virtually only found in the heart.

Within cells, each of these enzymes catalyses a specific biochemical reaction. Under normal circumstances they are only present in serum at low concentrations but this rises rapidly following cell death. The levels of these enzymes, which peak at different times between 6 hours and 5 days (Swanton 1994) after the heart attack, can be assessed to give an indication of the extent of the myocardial damage (see Fig. 6.13).

CK-MB is currently the most widely available blood test for early diagnosis of acute MI, although alternatives are currently being developed to enable earlier and rapid assessment. It is likely that in the not-too-distant future blood testing for

Fig. 6.13 Changes to enzyme levels after myocardial infarction. (From Jowett & Thompson 1995. Reproduced by kind permission of Bailliere Tindall.)

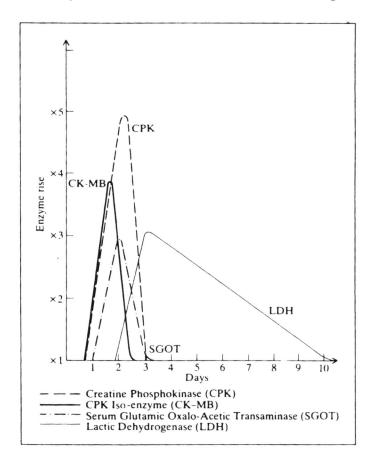

early diagnosis of MI may be as common as ward-based testing of blood glucose levels (Higgins 1996).

Care needs to be taken when interpreting these enzyme results if the patient has had external chest compression (during CPR), if intramuscular injections have been given, and after surgery.

Immediate treatment in hospital for a patient with an MI

It is important that patients with a suspected myocardial infarction receive immediate treatment with a 'fast track' system to enable them to receive thrombolytics, if appropriate, as soon as possible. The immediate measures and nursing care that need to be addressed are summarised in Box 6.14.

Medical staff originally undertook many of these measures, but nurses are increasingly taking responsibility for initiating and carrying them out. Cannulation, venepuncture, the administration of oxygen and ECG recording are now undertaken by a wide number of nurses in a variety of high dependency areas, while in some cardiac care units protocols have been established to enable nurses to commence certain drug regimens including thrombolytic therapy. In a small study, Quinn (1995) found that with clear protocols governing selection of patients, nurses' ability to assess patients for thrombolytics matched that of preregistration house physicians and middle-grade medical staff. It is important that thrombolytic therapy (see Box 6.15) is not delayed because of the logistics of the patient's location or the availability of a junior doctor. The benefits of thrombolytics in acute MI have been shown by a number of large multicentre trials (e.g. ISIS-2 1988, ISIS-3 1992, Rawles 1996).

> Thrombolytic therapy should never be delayed because of where the patient is or because a doctor cannot be found. Nurses with the relevant skills and training can and do save lives by acting quickly and appropriately.

CONCLUSION

The high prevalence of cardiovascular disease in the UK is likely to continue for a number of years. Despite public health measures to encourage healthier lifestyles that will hopefully reduce the extent of ischaemic heart disease, the manifestations of the disease are likely to be seen for some time. Demographic predictions show

---

■ **BOX 6.14** Immediate measures and nursing care in the treatment of an MI

- Rapid assessment of the patient, e.g. shock, hypotension, signs of heart failure
- Establishment of i.v. access
- Continuous ECG monitoring
- 12-lead ECG recording
- Oxygen at 40% concentration if no history of chronic airway limitation
- Medications:
  — Aspirin 150 mg orally, if no contraindications
  — Diamorphine 2.5–5 mg i.v. and repeated as necessary to control pain
  — Metoclopramide 10 mg i.v.
  — GTN spray × 2 if not hypotensive
- Portable chest X-ray
- Bloods for urgent urea and electrolytes, glucose, creatinine kinase and full blood count
- Thrombolytic therapy (see Box 6.16).
- Calm and quiet environment
- Comfort and minimal exertion

■ **BOX 6.15** Thrombolytics: dose and administration

	Streptokinase	rt-PA	APSAC
Dose	1 500 000 units	a) 15 mg i.v. bolus then b) 0.75 mg/kg over 30 min (max. 50 mg) then c) 0.5 mg/kg over 60 min (max. 35 mg)	30 mg
Diluent	100 ml 5% glucose	Supplied	
Infusion time	60 min	90 min	5 min
Half-life	30 min	4 min	90 min
Storage	Room temperature	Room temperature	Refrigerator
Source	Bacterial	Recombinant human protein	Bacterial and human plasma
Anaphylaxis	0.1%	Nil	0.1%
Allergic reaction	2–3%	Nil	2–3%
Supplemental medication	Hydrocortisone 100 mg i.v. Chlorpheniramine 10 mg i.v. (Prophylactic regime– need debated)	Heparin 5000 u bolus then 1000 u/h commencing 4 h after initiation of tPA	
Cost	£80	£750	£495

Indications for use and choice of agent
Indications
- Myocardial infarction beginning in the past 12 hours
- Patients with pain of 12–24 hours' duration should only receive thrombolysis if they are in continuing pain or if their general condition is worsening (Swanton 1994, p 218)

Special benefit:
The following patient groups particularly benefit from thrombolysis:
- Patients with anterior infarction
- Pronounced ST elevation
- The elderly over 75 years
- Patients with poor LV function
- Those receiving early administration within the first hour of symptoms

Contraindications
- Trauma, major surgery or invasive procedure (e.g. liver biopsy, lumbar puncture) in recent weeks
- Cerebrovascular accident in the last 6 months
- Gastrointestinal bleeding in recent months
- Systolic BP > 200 mmHg
- Prolonged cardiopulmonary resuscitation
- Recent (within hours) central venous or arterial line insertion

Contraindications specific to streptokinase
- Streptokinase given previously from 5 days to 4 years
- Systolic BP < 90 mmHg
- Anticipated central access (cardiac catheter, temporary pacing) in next 24 hours
- Recent (within past month) streptococal infection

(Cont'd)

(Box 6.15 cont'd)

Choice of agent

1) Streptokinase
2) rt-PA (recombinant tissue plasminogen activator) – Alteplase
3) APSAC (anisoylated plasminogen streptokinase activator complex) – anistreplase

rt-PA and APSAC are much more expensive than streptokinase with no clear benefit in uncomplicated cases (Swanton 1994, ISIS-3 1992), therefore streptokinase remains the first line agent of choice in most centres.

Complications

- Haemorrhage. Seen in up to 10% of patients, as bleeding from cannulae and i.m. injection sites. More seriously, occasional haematemesis and melaena from occult peptic ulcers.
- Allergic reactions. A low grade fever and rash are common with streptokinase. A vasculitis and bronchospasm have been reported with APSAC.
- Systemic emboli. If pre-existing thrombus, e.g. with abdominal aneurysm or enlarged left atrium with atrial fibrillation.
- Cerebrovasular bleed. Risk is between 0.3% and 0.7%.
- 'Early hazard' (Swanton 1994, p 224). Refers to the slight increase in mortality in the first day after receiving thrombolysis probably due to cardiac rupture causing EMD.

a vast increase in the numbers of elderly people in society in the future, and a large proportion of these older adults are likely to have a degree of cardiovascular disease underlying other illnesses for which they might be admitted to hospital. Nurses working in all acute care settings will need to be able to give skilful and knowledgeable cardiovascular care not only to patients admitted with a primary cardiac condition but also to those clients admitted to other specialties who happen to have underlying heart disease.

REFERENCES

Adam S K, Osborne S 1997 Critical care nursing. Science and practice. Oxford University Press, Oxford

Advanced Life Support Working Group, The European Resuscitation Council 1998 The 1998 European Resuscitation Council guidelines for adult advanced life support. British Medical Journal 316: 1863–1869

Barratt F, Wallis D N 1998 Relatives in the resuscitation room: their point of view. Journal of Accident and Emergency Medicine 15(2): 109–111

Boaz A, Rayner M 1995 Coronary heart disease statistics. British Heart Foundation/Coronary Prevention Group, London

Drew B J, Sparacino P S 1991 Accuracy of bedside electrocardiographic monitoring: a report on current practices of critical care nurses Heart and Lung. 20(6): 597–609

Guyton A C, Hall J E 1996 Textbook of medical physiology, 9th edn. W B Saunders, Philadelphia

Handley A, Swain A 1996 Advanced life support manual, 2nd edn. Resuscitation Council (UK), London

Higgins C 1996 Laboratory diagnosis of acute myocardial infarction. Nursing Times 92(3): 36–37

Hinchliff S M, Montague S E, Watson R 1996 Physiology for nursing practice, 2nd edn. Baillière Tindall, London

Inwood H 1996 Knowledge of resuscitation. Intensive and Critical Care Nursing 12: 33–39

ISIS-2 1988 Randomised trial of intravenous streptokinase, oral aspirin, both or neither among 17 187 cases of suspected acute myocardial infarction (Second International Study of Infarct Survival Collaborative Group). Lancet ii: 349–360

ISIS-3 1992 ISIS-3: a randomised comparison of streptokinase vs tissue plasminogen activator vs anistreplase and of aspirin plus heparin vs aspirin alone among 41 299 cases of suspected acute myocardial infarction (Third International Study of Infarct Survival Collaborative Group). Lancet 339: 753–770

Jowett N I, Thompson D R 1995 Comprehensive coronary care, 2nd edn. Scutari Press, London

Nurse's Ready Reference 1992 Quick ECG interpretation. Springhouse Corporation, Pennsylvania

Quinn T 1995 Can nurses safely assess suitability for thrombolytic therapy? A pilot study. Intensive and Critical Care Nursing 11: 126–129

Quinn T 1996 Myocardial infarction: the role of the nurse. Nursing Times 92(6): Supplement 5–8

Rawles J 1996 Magnitude of benefit from earlier thrombolytic treatment in acute myocardial infarction: new evidence from Grampian region early anistreplase trial (GREAT). British Medical Journal 312: 212–216

Robertson C, Steen P, Adgey J et al 1998 The 1998 European Resuscitation Council guidelines for adult advanced life support. Resuscitation 37: 81–90

Roper N, Logan W W, Tierney A J 1996 The elements of nursing, 4th edn. Churchill Livingstone, Edinburgh

Rowlands D J 1991 Clinical electrocardiography. Gower Medical, London

Swanton R H 1994 Cardiology: pocket consultant, 3rd edn. Blackwell Scientific Publications, Oxford

Swan H J C, Ganz W, Forrester J S et al 1970 Catheterisation of the heart in man with the use of a flow-directed balloon catheter. New England Journal of Medicine 283: 447–451

Thompson D R, Webster R A 1992 Caring for the coronary patient. Butterworth-Heinemann, Oxford

Thompson D, Bailey S, Webster R 1986 Patients' views about cardiac monitoring. Nursing Times (occasional paper) 82(25): 54–55

Wynne G, Marteau T M, Johnston M et al 1987 Inability of trained nurses to perform basic life support. British Medical Journal 294: 1198–1199

Zoll P M, Zoll R H 1985 Non-invasive temporary cardiac stimulation. Critical Care Medicine 13: 925–926

FURTHER READING

Physiology
The following suggestions of general textbooks have comprehensive chapters exploring cardiovascular physiology which you might wish to consult.

Brooker C G 1998 Human structure and function: nursing applications in clinical practice, 2nd edn. Mosby, London
This textbook is aimed primarily at Dip H E (Project 2000) students. However, it is also useful for nurses who have not studied recently or as a relatively quick and straightforward revision text.

Hinchliff S M, Montague S E, Watson R 1996 Physiology for nursing practice, 2nd edn. Baillière Tindall, London
Marieb E 1998 Human anatomy and physiology, 4th edn. Addison Wesley Longman, California
Both these textbooks are very popular especially among nurses studying aspects of biological sciences at degree level, for example, as part of a post-registration clinical course. Marieb (1998) is a North American publication whereas Hinchliff et al (1996) has been written by experienced British nurse educationalists.

Specialist cardiac nursing texts
These books contain comprehensive specialist nursing knowledge related to cardiac care. They will be particularly useful for nurses working in designated cardiac units.

Shuldham C 1998 Cardiorespiratory nursing. Stanley Thornes, Cheltenham
The chapters in this book are written almost entirely by nurses working in clinical practice at the Royal Brompton Hospital.

Jowett N I, Thompson D R 1995 Comprehensive coronary care, 2nd edn. Scutari Press, London
Thompson D R, Webster R A 1992 Caring for the coronary patient. Butterworth-Heinemann, Oxford
There are, as might be expected, many similar features in both these books. They are both extremely useful for nurses working in CCUs and cardiology/medical wards.

Canobbio M M 1990 Cardiovascular disorders. Mosby Clinical Nursing Series, St Louis
Although originating from the US, this book has a wealth of high quality photographs, diagrams, care plans and suggested patient information 'handouts'.

Underhill S 1982 Cardiac nursing Lippincott, Philadelphia
This is a comprehensive US text covering all aspects of cardiac disease and care.
ECG guidebooks
These books are useful for nurses who want to increase their knowledge relating to ECG interpretation.

Gardiner J 1981 The ECG – what does it tell? Stanley Thornes, Cheltenham
Although this book is now relatively old (published in 1981), its slim pocket size nature and easy to understand explanations continue to make it popular as an initial read.

Hampton J R 1986 The ECG made easy, 3rd edn. Churchill Livingstone, Edinburgh
Hampton J R 1986 The ECG in practice. Churchill Livingstone, Edinburgh
The series of pocket ECG books by Hampton are popular with most nurses. They contain relatively comprehensive information for their size but do not provide any links to nursing practice.

Paul S, Hebra J 1998 The nurse's guide to cardiac rhythm interpretation – implications for patient care. W B Saunders, Philadelphia
This is a very comprehensive and well-presented new ECG guide. It has a more 'textbook' feel (and size) than the ECG books above. Its introductory section reviews basics and then the three subsequent sections (and numerous chapters) address basic cardiac rhythms, paediatric ECGs and advanced concepts. It contains information about related care, drug therapy and patient teaching.

Critical care
Adam S K, Osborne S 1997 Critical care nursing: science and practice. Oxford University Press, Oxford
This book is aimed primarily at intensive care nurses but contains information that is useful to those in high dependency units as well. Its strong points are that it is a recent British publication with an emphasis on the practical aspects of critical care.

The following texts may be useful, especially as some aspects of cardiac care undertaken in 'critical' or 'intensive' care units in other countries would fall within the remit of lower dependency areas in Britain.
Bongard F S, Sue D Y 1994 Current critical care diagnosis and treatment. Appleton & Lange, Norwalk
Hudak C M, Gallo B M 1994 Critical care nursing: a holistic approach, 6th edn. J B Lippincott, Philadelphia
Oh T E 1990 Intensive care manual, 3rd edn. Butterworths, Sydney
Swearingen P L, Hicks-Keen J 1991 Manual of critical care, 2nd edn. Mosby, St Louis

Pocket guides
The following are examples of 'pocket' books containing factual information related to the cardiovascular system which are useful for quick reference.
Parr M, Craft T 1992 Resuscitation: key data. Quick reference guide. BIOS Scientific, Oxford
Pepper J, Millner R 1990 A manual of cardiac surgical intensive care. Edward Arnold, London
Tinker J, Jones S N 1986 A pocket book for intensive care. Data drugs and procedures. Edward Arnold, London

OTHER RESOURCES

There are an increasing number of useful computer-based resources which you may wish to consult rather than the traditional texts suggested above.

Two examples of multi-media physiology on CD-ROM include:
• ADAM Software Incorporated 1995 Interactive human anatomy series (5 CDs). Details on www.adam.com
• Marieb E, Branstrom 1996 Interactive physiology – cardiovascular system. Churchill Livingstone, Edinburgh

Additionally if you have access to the Internet (either at home or through your local library or university) the following world wide web (www) sites may have useful information:
Association of Resuscitation Training Officers. *http://www.arto.org*
Personal site with many links maintained by an American resuscitation enthuiast. *http://www.defib.net*
Details of resuscitation simulation interactive program. *http://www.resussim.com*
Hewlett Packard's cardiology page provides information about their products together with other links and resources. *http://www.hp.com/go/heart*
American Heart Association. *http://www.amhrt.org*

Neurological care

Deborah Dawson

INTRODUCTION

The human brain is by far the most complex structure in the known universe
(Thompson 1993)

This quotation could be extended to include the whole nervous system, and it is that element of the unknown that ensures that the study and care of patients with neurological problems are both challenging and rewarding. The challenge includes the quick recognition of acute events and the unravelling of information to uncover the chronic condition. The patient with a head injury for overnight observation and the surgical patient with a history of seizures who requires post-operative care – both these patients will be admitted into the high dependency unit. This chapter explores the care of patients who might require high dependency care, and this includes patients who may have head injury, seizures, Guillain–Barré syndrome, meningitis or CVAs. It describes the assessment of these patients and the medicines they may require. In order to care for them it is important to have an understanding of the anatomy and physiology of the nervous system, so this is where we start.

ORGANISATION OF THE NERVOUS SYSTEM

Prerequisite anatomy and physiology

- The neuron
- The nerve impulse including saltatory conduction
- Electrical and chemical synapses
- Neurotransmitters
- The skull and facial bones
- The peripheral nervous system

The nervous system is generally divided into two main functional units, the central nervous system (CNS) and the peripheral nervous system (PNS). The central

■ **BOX 7.1** The major structures of the brain

Cerebrum	Cerebellum	Brainstem
• Cerebral hemispheres		• Midbrain
• Corpus callosum		• Pons
• Basal ganglia		• Medulla
• Diencephalon		
• Hypophysis		

nervous system consists of the brain and the spinal cord: these process new sensory information and combine that information with previous experience to provide appropriate motor responses. The peripheral nervous system consists of the spinal and cranial nerves which convey nerve impulses to and from the brain and the spinal cord.

THE BRAIN (ENCEPHALON)

The brain consists of three main areas: the cerebrum, the cerebellum and the brainstem. The major structures within these divisions are summarised in Box 7.1.

The cerebrum

The cerebrum consists of two cerebral hemispheres, which are partially separated by the longitudinal fissure, and connected at the bottom by the corpus callosum. It is generally accepted that one hemisphere is more highly developed than the other and this is usually the left: only a small proportion of left-handed people have right hemisphere dominance. The left side of the brain has been shown to control the right side of the body: spoken and written language and scientific, reasoning and numerical skills, whereas the right side is more concerned with emotion and artistic and creative skills. However, at birth the hemispheres are of equal ability and very early injury to one side or another usually results in skills being acquired by the opposite side of the brain. Each cerebral hemisphere has an area of grey matter called the basal ganglia, which assists in the motor control of fine body movements.

The surface area of the brain, the cerebral cortex (grey matter), is much increased by the presence of gyri (folds) and sulci (dips) (Fig. 7.1), resulting in a 3 : 1 proportion of grey to white matter. Below the cortex is the white matter. The cerebral hemispheres are composed of four lobes, the frontal, parietal, temporal and occipital lobes. Box 7.2 summarises the main functions of the lobes.

The diencephalon is located deep into the cerebrum and consists of the thalamus, hypothalamus, subthalamus and epithalamus. It connects the midbrain to the cerebral hemispheres. The thalamus is the relay and processing centre for all sensory information except smell. The basal ganglia are a collection of motor nucleii which help to co-ordinate muscle movement by relaying information via the thalamus to the motor cortex in the cerebrum. Parkinson's disease is a disorder associated with the basal ganglia. The hypothalamus is responsible for autonomic regulation and endocrine control through the pituitary gland (hypophysis), and is the point where the two optic tracts cross (optic chiasma).

The cerebellum

The cerebellum is situated behind the pons and attached to the midbrain, pons and medulla by three paired cerebellar peduncles. It consists of three main parts:

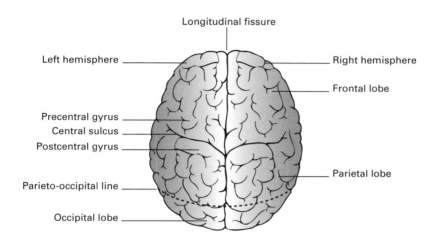

Fig. 7.1 The surface area of the brain, showing the gyri, sulci and fissures of the cerebral hemispheres. (From Carola, et al 1990, p 378.)

Longitudinal fissure

Left hemisphere

Right hemisphere

Frontal lobe

Precentral gyrus
Central sulcus
Postcentral gyrus

Parietal lobe

Parieto-occipital line

Occipital lobe

■ **BOX 7.2** The functions of the cerebral cortex by lobe

Frontal	Parietal	Temporal	Occipital
• Motor	• Sensation	• Auditory	• Visual
• Expression	• Spatial	• Equilibrium	
• Moral		• Interpretive	
		• Intellectual	

How might the symptoms of cerebellar dysfunction affect normal life?

---

the cortex; the white matter, which forms the connecting pathways for impulses joining the cerebellum with other parts of the central nervous system; and four pairs of deep cerebellar nuclei. The cerebellum is the processing centre for co-ordination of muscular movements, balance, precision, timing and body positions. It does not initiate any movements and is not involved with the conscious perception of sensations. Disorders of the cerebellum such as tumours or CVAs may result in jerky movement, diminished reflexes, ataxia and tremors – symptoms of cerebellar dysfunction can be seen following an overindulgence in alcohol! The symptoms occur on the same side as the lesion due to impulses crossing in both the midbrain and lower medulla.

Fig. 7.2 Brainstem, dorsal view. (From Carola, et al 1990, p 369.)

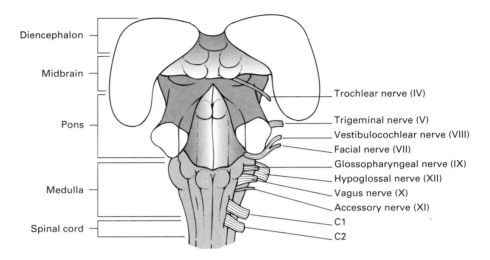

Diencephalon

Midbrain

Pons

Medulla

Spinal cord

Trochlear nerve (IV)

Trigeminal nerve (V)

Vestibulocochlear nerve (VIII)

Facial nerve (VII)

Glossopharyngeal nerve (IX)

Hypoglossal nerve (XII)

Vagus nerve (X)

Accessory nerve (XI)

C1

C2

The brainstem

The brainstem is the connection between the brain and the spinal cord, and is continuous with the diencephalon above and the spinal cord below. Within the brainstem are ascending and descending pathways between the spinal cord and parts of the brain. All cranial nerves, except the olfactory and optic, emerge from the brainstem (Fig. 7.2). It is formed from three main structures, the midbrain, pons and medulla.

The midbrain connects the pons and cerebellum to the cerebrum. It is involved with visual reflexes, the movement of the eyes, focussing and the dilation of the pupils. Contained within the midbrain and upper pons is the reticular activating system, which is responsible for the 'awake' state. The pons is located between the midbrain and the medulla and serves as a relay station from the medulla to higher structures in the brain. It is involved with the control of respiratory function. The lowermost portion of the brainstem is the medulla. This connects the pons and the spinal cord; motor fibres cross from one side of the medulla to the other and this is known as the point of decussation of the pyramidal tract. In the deeper structures of the medulla are found the vital centres associated with autonomic reflex activity. These are the cardiac, respiratory and vasomotor centres and the reflex centres of coughing, swallowing, vomiting and sneezing.

To further increase the understanding of the structures and function of the brain it is worthwhile discovering more about the limbic system, the pituitary gland (hypophysis) and the reticular activating system.

ASSOCIATED STRUCTURES

The meninges

The brain and the spinal cord are encased by three layers of membrane, the dura mater, the arachnoid mater and the pia mater, known collectively as the meninges (Fig. 7.3).

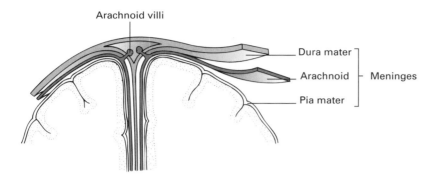

Arachnoid villi

Dura mater ⎤
Arachnoid ⎦ Meninges
Pia mater ⎦

Fig. 7.3 The cranial meninges. (From Hickey 1992, p 19.)

The dura mater consists of two layers, the outer being the periosteal layer of the skull which terminates at the foramen magnum; and the inner, a strong, thick membrane that is continuous with the spinal dura mater. There is only a potential space between the two dura, except at the falx cerebri, which divides the left and right hemispheres of the cerebrum; the tentorium cerebelli, which divides the cerebrum and cerebellum; the falx cerebelli, which divides the lateral lobes of the cerebellum; and the diaphragma sellae, creating a roof for the sella turcica (which houses the pituitary gland). These compartments provide support and protection for the brain and form the sinuses which drain venous blood from the brain.

The arachnoid mater In total contrast to the dura mater the arachnoid mater is fine serous membrane that loosely covers the brain. There is a potential space between this and the inner dura mater, known as the subdural space. Between the arachnoid mater and the pia mater is an actual space, known as the subarachnoid space; this contains the arachnoid villi, cerebrospinal fluid (CSF) and small arterial blood vessels.

The pia mater follows the convolutions and is attached to the surface of the brain. It consists of fine connective tissue, housing the majority of the blood supply to the brain.

■ BOX 7.3 The blood–brain barrier

The blood–brain barrier protects the brain and maintains homeostasis. It is a diffusion barrier between the brain and vasculature and the substance of the brain formed by tight junctions between capillary endothelial cells (Purves et al 1997). The brain is further protected by an alliance between astrocytes and the capillary endothelial cells. This ensures that only certain substances can enter the brain.

Water, carbon dioxide and oxygen pass readily through the blood–brain barrier, whereas glucose, which is the primary source of metabolic energy for nervous tissue, requires a lipid transporter. This can be a problem for clinicians attempting to deliver drugs to the brain.

The ventricles and cerebrospinal fluid

Within the brain there are four connected cavities called ventricles which contain cerebrospinal fluid (CSF). These are the left and right lateral ventricles, the third ventricle and the fourth ventricle. The lateral ventricles lie in the cerebral hemispheres, the third in the diencephalon and the fourth in the brainstem. The lateral ventricles are connected to the third ventricle by the interventricular foramen, sometimes

Fig. 7.4 Ventricles of the brain, and circulatory path of cerebrospinal fluid through the cranial pathways, (From Carola. et al 1990, p 368.)

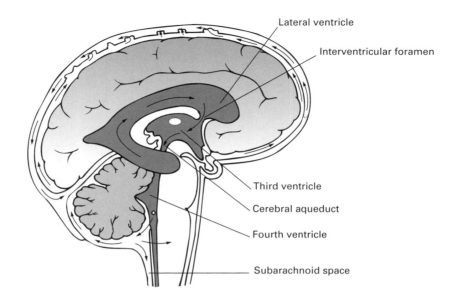

Lateral ventricle

Interventricular foramen

Third ventricle

Cerebral aqueduct

Fourth ventricle

Subarachnoid space

known as the foramen of Munro, and the third ventricle is connected to the fourth by the cerebral aqueduct, sometimes known as the aqueduct of Sylvius (Fig. 7.4).

CSF is a clear, colourless fluid composed of water, some protein, oxygen, carbon dioxide, sodium, potassium, chloride and glucose. Its purpose is to protect the brain from injury by providing a cushioning effect. The major source of CSF is from the secretions of the choroid plexus, found in the ventricles. The choroid plexus produces approximately 500 ml of CSF daily, although the average adult brain only holds between 125 and 150 ml. CSF is renewed and replaced approximately three times daily, being reabsorbed through the arachnoid villi, which drain into the superior saggital sinus, when the CSF pressure exceeds the venous pressure. Normal CSF pressure is 60–180 mm water in the lumbar puncture position (lateral recumbant) and 200–350 mm water in the sitting position.

Cerebral circulation

The brain is supplied with blood by four major arteries: two internal carotid, which supply most of the cerebrum and both eyes, and two vertebral, which supply the cerebellum, brainstem and the posterior part of the cerebrum (Fig. 7.5). Before the blood enters the cerebrum it passes through the circle of Willis, which is a circular shunt at the base of the brain consisting of the posterior cerebral, the posterior communicating, the internal carotid, the anterior cerebral, and the anterior communicating arteries. These vessels are frequently anomalous – however they allow for an adequate blood supply to all parts of the brain, even if one or more is ineffective (Fig. 7.6).

The venous drainage from the brain does not follow a similar pathway. Cerebral veins empty into large venous sinuses located in the folds of the dura mater: bridging veins connect the brain and the dural sinuses and are often the cause of subdural haematomas. These sinuses empty into the internal jugular veins which sit on either side of the neck, which return the blood to the heart via the brachiocephalic veins (Fig. 7.7).

The brain – especially the grey matter – has an extensive capillary bed, requiring approximately 15–20% of the total resting cardiac output, about 750 ml/min.

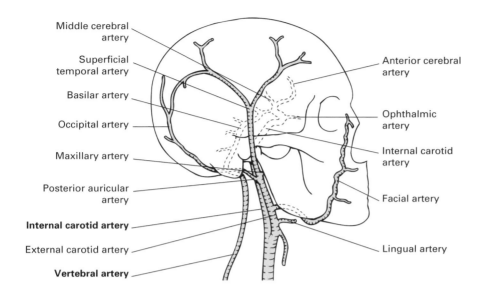

Middle cerebral artery

Superficial temporal artery

Basilar artery

Occipital artery

Maxillary artery

Posterior auricular artery

Internal carotid artery

External carotid artery

Vertebral artery

Anterior cerebral artery

Ophthalmic artery

Internal carotid artery

Facial artery

Lingual artery

Fig. 7.5 Major arteries of the head and neck: lateral view. (From Carola et al 1990, p 368.)

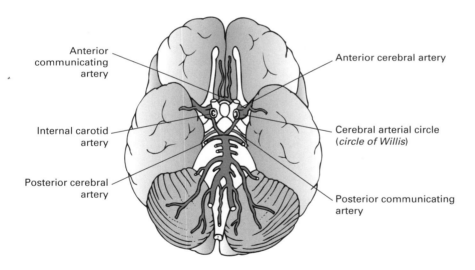

Anterior communicating artery

Internal carotid artery

Posterior cerebral artery

Anterior cerebral artery

Cerebral arterial circle (*circle of Willis*)

Posterior communicating artery

Fig. 7.6 Major arteries of the head and neck: ventral view. (From Carola, et al 1990, p 587.)

Glucose, required for metabolism in the brain, requires about 20% of the total oxygen consumed in the body for its oxidation. Blood flow to specific areas of the brain correlates directly to the metabolism of the cerebral tissue.

Spinal cord

The spinal cord is continuous with the medulla oblongata: it extends from the superior border of the first cervical vertebra (atlas) to the upper border of the second lumbar vertebra. The cone-shaped lower end of the spinal cord becomes the conus terminalis, located at the first lumbar vertebra (L1), which in turn becomes the filum terminale consisting mainly of fibrous connective tissue. The cord is about 1 cm in diameter, except for two areas, the cervical and lumbosacral

Fig. 7.7 Major veins of the head and neck. (From Carola, et al 1990, p 591.)

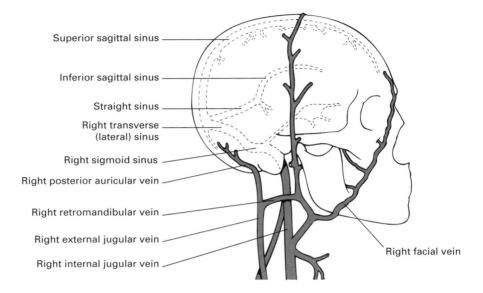

Superior sagittal sinus

Inferior sagittal sinus

Straight sinus

Right transverse (lateral) sinus

Right sigmoid sinus

Right posterior auricular vein

Right retromandibular vein

Right external jugular vein

Right internal jugular vein

Right facial vein

Fig. 7.8 The spinal cord and spinal nerves, and their relation to the vertebral column. (From Carola, et al 1990, p 337.)

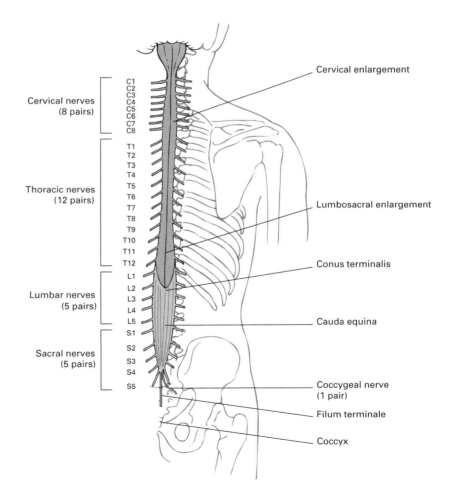

Cervical nerves (8 pairs)
C1
C2
C3
C4
C5
C6
C7
C8

Thoracic nerves (12 pairs)
T1
T2
T3
T4
T5
T6
T7
T8
T9
T10
T11
T12

Lumbar nerves (5 pairs)
L1
L2
L3
L4
L5

Sacral nerves (5 pairs)
S1
S2
S3
S4
S5

Cervical enlargement

Lumbosacral enlargement

Conus terminalis

Cauda equina

Coccygeal nerve (1 pair)

Filum terminale

Coccyx

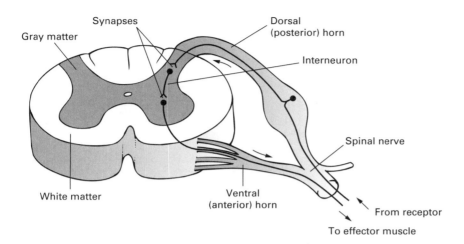

Fig. 7.9 A cross section of the spinal cord.

enlargements, from which the 31 pairs of spinal nerves emerge. The spinal nerves that emerge below the conus terminalis (L1) are known as the cauda equina. Figure 7.8 shows the spinal cord and nerves in relation to the vertebral column.

The cord is surrounded by the three layers of the meninges, pia, arachnoid and dura. Cerebrospinal fluid flows through the central canal – this is continuous with the fourth ventricle. The spinal cord has two functions. Firstly, it acts as a relay station between the peripheral nervous system and the brain, and secondly, as an activating centre in its own right, taking incoming sensory impulses and initiating outgoing motor signals, as in the reflex arc.

The spinal cord is composed of two layers, the outer white matter and the inner grey matter (this is the opposite to the brain where the grey matter is outermost).

The white matter consists of mainly myelinated axons, and the cell body of these fibres can be in either the brain or the spinal cord. The grey matter consists of neurons and synapses. It is shaped like a letter 'H', which can be divided into three functional areas. The dorsal (posterior) horns carry sensory impulses, the ventral (anterior) horns carry motor impulses, and the middle zone which undertakes association functions between the dorsal and ventral horns of the same and opposite sides (see Fig. 7.9).

> Think about the physiological effects of a whiplash injury which normally affects the high cervical area.

The spinal cord is protected by the spinal column. This is composed of 33 vertebrae, seven cervical, 12 thoracic, five lumbar, five sacral and the four fused bones of the coccyx. Table 7.1 on p. 154 describes the various effects of the autonomic nervous system.

Cranial nerves

There are 12 pairs of cranial nerves, three sensory, five motor and four mixed. They are named according to their function and numbered in the order they emerge from the brain. Table 7.2 on p. 154 describes their diverse functions.

NEUROLOGICAL ASSESSMENT

Neurological assessment provides both the basic tool for diagnosis of neurological deficit and the means for measuring progress. It also provides a common language for clinicians to communicate symptoms and changes in condition. It is therefore essential that it is completed accurately, with any uncertainties communicated.

Table 7.1 The effects of the autonomic nervous system

Activity	Sympathetic	Parasympathetic
Heart rate	Increased	Decreased
Blood pressure	Increased	Decreased
Cardiac output	Increased	Decreased
Blood vessels in cardiac muscles	Dilated	Constricted
Blood vessels in abdomen and skin	Constricted	No effect
Blood vessels in skeletal muscles	Dilated	No effect
Respiratory rate	Increased	Decreased
Bronchioles	Dilated	Constricted
Blood sugar	Increased	No effect
Peristalsis (GI)	Decreased	Increased
Bladder	Contracted	Relaxed
Sphincters Sweat	Increased	No effect
Adrenals	Adrenaline and nor-adrenaline secretion	No effect
Pupils	Dilated	Constricted

Table 7.2 Functions of cranial nerves

Number	Name	Type	Function
I	Olfactory	Sensory	Smell
II	Optic	Sensory	Vision
III	Oculomotor	Motor	Movement of eyeball, elevation of upper eyelid, constriction of pupil, focussing of lens
IV	Trochlear	Motor	Downward and outward eye movements
V	Trigeminal	Mixed	Mastication, sensory regulation of ophthalmic, maxillary and mandibular areas
VI	Abducens	Motor	Abduction of eye
VII	Facial	Mixed	Taste, salivation, lacrimation, movement of facial muscles
VIII	Acoustic	Sensory	Hearing, equilibrium
IX	Glossopharyngeal	Mixed	Taste, secretion of saliva, swallowing
X	Vagus	Mixed	Swallowing, monitors blood levels of O_2 and CO_2, blood pressure regulation
XI	Accessory	Motor	Voice production, movement of head and shoulders
XII	Hypoglossal	Motor	Movement of tongue during speech, swallowing

This will ensure timely and appropriate patient care. A complete neurological assessment (Hickey 1992) should include:

- Level of consciousness
- Cranial nerves
- Motor function
- Sensory function
- Cerebellar function
- Vital signs.

This assessment should be completed on admission and thereafter at regular intervals to determine the patient's condition, although it may not be appropriate in an emergency situation. This type of full assessment would usually be performed by a clinician with neurological experience. Commonly, a reduced assessment is performed which includes:

- Level of consciousness
- Motor function
- Pupillary signs
- Vital signs.

In practice this requires an assessment of the Glasgow Coma Score (motor and level of consciousness), a limb assessment (motor) and pupil assessment.

Glasgow Coma Scale

The Glasgow Coma Scale (GCS) was developed in 1974 by Teasdale and Jennett (Box 7.3 on page 156). It forms a quick, objective and easily interpreted mode of neurological assessment, avoiding subjective terminology such as 'stupor', 'semi-coma' and 'deep coma'. The GCS records what you see, measuring arousal, awareness and activity, by assessing eye opening, verbal response and motor ability. Each activity is allocated a score, therefore enabling objectivity, ease of recording and comparison between recordings. It also provides useful information for patient outcome prediction. The score is from 15 (fully conscious) to 3 (no response).

As a stimulus is applied, it is good practice to commence with light pressure and increase to elicit a response. There is debate as to whether it is better to use a peripheral stimulus, for example a pen pressed into the side of a finger near the nail (never press into the nailbed as this can cause the nails to die) or whether to apply central pressure. This is usually done by pressing into the trapezius muscle unless there is local injury in which case use a sternal rub. The nurse must decide the most appropriate stimulus for the situation. Applying central stimuli will always provide the most accurate response and should be used at all times when there is uncertainty, but a mildly drowsy patient will not thank you for waking him up with a sternal rub! Always record the best arm response. There is no need to record left and right differences – the GCS is not aiming to measure focal deficit, as this should be completed in the limb assessment. There is no reason to measure leg response as this may be measuring a spinal rather than a brain-initiated response.

When recording the GCS it is important to record the individual scores as well as the total score, i.e., E2 V3 M4 GCS = 9, the motor response being the most reflective for determining prognosis.

The GCS may be misleading in patients who have a high cervical injury, or brainstem lesion, or who are hypoxic, haemodynamically shocked, fitting or post-ictal. These patients may be unable to move their limbs, or show no responses at all. It is important to attempt to assess the spinal patient using facial movements, being aware of the possibility of a combined head and neck injury. Patients who

What different challenges would be encountered in making a neurological assessment of
- a sedated patient?
- an unco-operative patient?
- a patient who had suffered multiple trauma?

■ **BOX 7.3** Glasgow Coma Scale

EYE OPENING

4 Spontaneously This is when the patient's eyes open without stimulation of any sort.

3 To speech The patient's eyes open to verbal stimulation which may need to be repeated, but no physical stimulation is required.

2 To pain The patient's eyes open either to vigorous shaking or following the application of a painful stimulus.

1 None The patient's eyes do not open even with persistent verbal or adequate painful stimuli.

VERBAL RESPONSE

5 Orientated The patient is able to tell the assessor with complete accuracy the date, where he is and who he is.

4 Sentences The patient is not orientated, but formulates a full sentence or sentences. These may be inappropriate.

3 Words The response from the patient is restricted to words which are comprehensible, but may be inappropriate.

2 Sounds The patient makes sounds that are not recognisable as words.

1 None No sound is made by the patient in response to either verbal or painful stimuli.

The patient may have difficulty in speaking (dysphasia). If so, the letter D should be put in the 'none' column. If the patient is intubated then the letter T should be put in the 'none' column.

MOTOR RESPONSE

6 Obeys commands The patient follows simple instructions, such as 'hold up your arms' or 'squeeze *and* release my hands'.

5 Localising The patient raises his hands at least to chin level, in response to a stimulus applied above that level.

4 Normal flexion The patient's arms bend at the elbow in response to a painful stimulus, without rotation at the wrist.

3 Abnormal flexion The patient's arms bend at the elbow, the forearm rotates and the wrist is flexed, in response to a painful stimulus.

2 Extension The patient's arm straightens at the elbow and rotates towards the body, while the wrist flexes, in response to a painful stimulus.

1 None There is no response following the application of a deeply painful stimulus.

If the patient is receiving medicines to maintain muscle paralysis, record the letter P in the 'none' column.

show no response should be re-evaluated following correction of any shock or hypoxia (Atkinson Morley Hospital Neurosurgical Guidelines).

Limb assessment

A limb assessment is useful to assess for focal damage; however, although it is usual for a hemiparesis or hemiplegia to occur on the opposite (contralateral) side to the lesion, it may occur on the same (ipsilateral) side. This is due to indentation of the contralateral cerebral peduncle and is known as a false localising. Spontaneous movements are observed for equality: if there is little or no spontaneous movement, then painful stimuli must be applied to each limb in turn comparing the result. It is most appropriate to complete this while assessing the motor component of the GCS.

Pupil assessment

Pupils are assessed for their reaction to light, size and shape, cranial nerves II (optic) and III (oculomotor). Each pupil needs to be assessed and recorded individually. Pupils are measured in millimetres – normal range 2–6 mm in diameter – and are normally round in shape. Abnormalities are described as ovoid, keyhole or irregular (Hickey 1992). A bright light, preferably a bright pen torch, is shone into the side of each eye to assess the pupil's reaction to light: this should produce a constriction in both pupils, the consensual light reflex. Pupil response should be recorded as brisk, sluggish or fixed. The reaction in the non-stimulated pupil may be less brisk than in the stimulated side.

A common abnormality is a 'blown' pupil, where the pupil is large and usually unreactive to light. This follows herniation of part of the temporal lobe through the small space in the tentorium which directly damages the oculomotor (third) nerve. Following damage to the pons, with the use of some eye drops (especially those for glaucoma) and during opiate administration the pupils become pinpoint and unreactive.

Neurological assessments are usually recorded on a chart such that in Figure 7.10. It is important to record the GCS alongside vital signs as this will graphically display events. For example, pressure on the brainstem will cause not only neurological changes but changes in cardiac and respiratory patterns. Important points to remember (American College of Surgeons 1997) are:

> Record vital signs alongside GCS to gain the fullest picture of events.

- Hypotension is only of neurological origin in extremely dire circumstances: signs of hypovolaemia (or other causes of hypotension) should always be looked for in the hypotensive neurological patient.
- Hypertension, bradycardia and decreased respirations (Cushing's triad) are specific responses to a potentially lethal rise in ICP.
- Hypertension +/− hyperpyrexia may indicate autonomic dysfunction.

A CT scan should be ordered for any of the following reasons:

- GCS < 15 + skull fracture
- Abnormal neurology + skull fracture
- Seizure + skull fracture
- GCS < 15 for > 8 hours
- Developing neurological signs without coma
- Fall in GCS with normal blood pressure and PO_2
- Persistent vomiting with no other obvious cause.

Patients with any of the following should receive an urgent neurosurgical consultation:

- GCS < 8
- Rising BP and falling pulse
- Depressed skull fracture
- Otorrhoea or rhinorrhoea
- GCS < 15 for > 8 hours
- Fall in GCS with normal blood pressure and pO_2
- Abnormal CT scan.

In patients with trauma, either as a precipitating event for example in head injury, or as a sequela possibly following a cerebrovascular accident, it is important to examine the patient physically, looking for signs of laceration or bruising. Deep lacerations could conceal evidence of depressed skull fracture; however as it is easy to confuse the firm edges of a scalp haematoma with a fracture, a skull X-ray should be performed if there is doubt. Always ensure the neck is fully examined

Fig. 7.10 Observation chart.

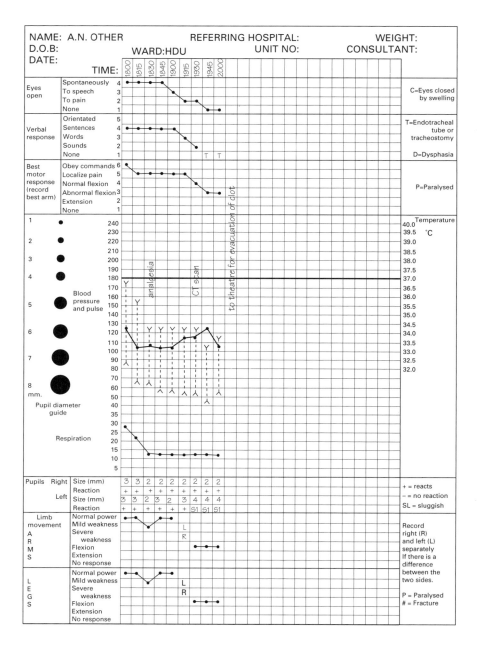

and a collar applied if there is any uncertainty regarding the integrity of the spine. Basal skull fractures are diagnosed clinically. Box 7.4 describes the clinical signs.

THE PHYSIOLOGY OF RAISED INTRACRANIAL PRESSURE (ICP)

Intracranial pressure is the pressure exerted by the cerebrospinal fluid within the ventricles of the brain (Hickey 1992). Normal ICP is 0–15 mmHg, with an average

■ BOX 7.4 Clinical signs of a basal skull fracture

- Rhinorrhoea
- Otorrhoea
- Bilateral periorbital haematoma (raccoon eyes)
- Subconjunctival haemorrhage
- Battle's sign (bruising over the mastoid)

range of 0–10 mmHg, when measured from the foramen of Munro. Intracranial pressure varies with daily activities such as coughing, sneezing and straining. To understand the physiology of raised intracranial pressure it is useful to consider the modified Munro–Kellie hypothesis (Hickey 1992) which states:

> *The skull, a rigid compartment, is filled to capacity with essentially non-compressible contents; brain matter (80%), intravascular blood (10%) and CSF (10%). The volume of these three components remains nearly constant in a state of dynamic equilibrium. If any one component increases in overall volume, another component must decrease for the overall volume and dynamic equilibrium to remain constant; otherwise, ICP will rise.*

There are limited ways for the brain to maintain normal ICP, by altering one or other component:

- Increased CSF absorption
- Decreased CSF production
- Shunting of CSF to the spinal subarachnoid space
- Vasoconstriction, reduction in cerebral blood volume (CBV).

In the healthy brain, autoregulation and chemoregulation maintain a cerebral blood flow (CBF) sufficient to maintain the energy requirements of the brain tissue, while maintaining ICP (Fig. 7.11)

The cerebral perfusion pressure (CPP) is the pressure required to maintain cerebral blood flow (CBF). Cerebral perfusion pressure needs to be above 60 mmHg to maintain CBF; autoregulation fails below this point or above 160 mmHg (Lindsay et al 1991). Following head injury autoregulation is impaired and it is vital to maintain cerebral perfusion pressure to ensure adequate oxygen to the brain tissue. To calculate cerebral perfusion pressure, the ICP needs to be subtracted from the mean arterial pressure.

$$CPP = ICP - MAP$$

In head injury, ICP rises globally due to cerebral oedema, with or without haematoma formation, and latterly a breakdown of autoregulation and chemoregulation. Figure 7.12 shows the cyclical nature of progressive brain swelling.

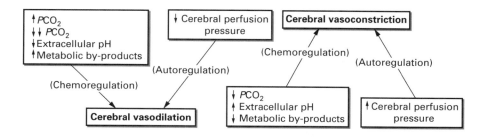

Fig. 7.11 Vasodilatation and vasoconstriction. (Based on Lindsay, et al 1991.)

Fig. 7.12 Cycle for malignant progressive brain swelling. (Based on Hudak & Gallo 1994, p 677.)

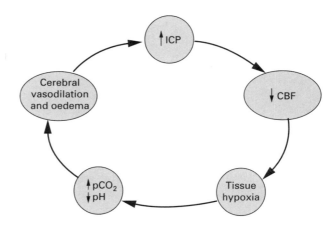

Fig. 7.13 Volume pressure curve. (Based on Lindsay et al 1991, p 75.)

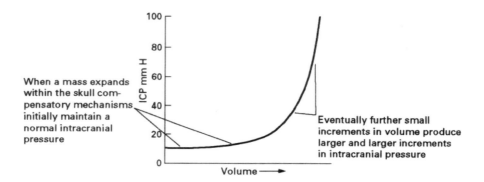

When a mass expands within the skull compensatory mechanisms initially maintain a normal intracranial pressure

Eventually further small increments in volume produce larger and larger increments in intracranial pressure

Once the compensatory mechanisms have been exhausted, a small additional change in volume results in a large pressure rise, as shown in Figure 7.13. It is therefore important to monitor for signs of rising ICP in the unresponsive patient.

Definitive management of an increased ICP requires monitoring of arterial, central venous and intracranial pressures, under neurosurgical direction (American College of Surgeons 1997).

THE MANAGEMENT OF NEUROLOGICAL CONDITIONS

The nursing management of neurological patients requires an understanding of the pathophysiology to ensure appropriate management. Many areas of care apply to all conditions, however. Box 7.6 on page 162 describes the management of the unconscious patient, and is intended to be read in conjunction with the subsequent sections describing the management of specific conditions.

Think about the care of patients with problems in addition to neurological trauma.

HEAD INJURIES

Head injuries fall into two categories. Acceleration injuries occur when a moving object strikes a stationary head: for example, a gunshot wound or a blow from a blunt object. Deceleration injuries occur when the head hits a solid object, for example a windscreen or the ground. These injuries can also occur at the same time: during an assault, for instance, a patient might be hit over the head and then fall to the ground. During the injury the head may also be subjected to rotational forces, causing stretching and shearing of the white matter and brainstem.

■ **BOX 7.5** Lumbar puncture

A sample of cerebrospinal fluid can be tested for many factors to assist in the diagnosis of many neurological diseases. The standard tests would be bacteriology (WBC < 5 mm³) and biochemical, usually protein (normal value 0.15–0.45 g/l) and glucose (normal value 0.45–0.70 g/l). However there are many other tests that can be performed: cytology, virology, fungal and parasitic tests, gamma globulin, HIV, cryptococcus and VDRL. A sample can be immediately observed for blood (normal CSF is crystal clear) – three consecutive samples are required to avoid contamination from the puncture site – and for pressure by connecting a manometer (normal pressure 100–150 mm CSF).

To avoid injury a lumbar puncture is performed below the second lumbar vertebrae, usually between L3 and L4. The spinal cord ends at about L1–L2. The patient lies on his side in the fetal position, with his knees drawn up to the chest and the neck flexed, as in Figure 7.14. This ensures the spine is flexed, separating the spinous processes.

If there is any suspicion of raised intracranial pressure or a space occupying lesion, then a lumbar puncture should not be attempted. These circumstances could precipitate tentorial herniation and consequently death.

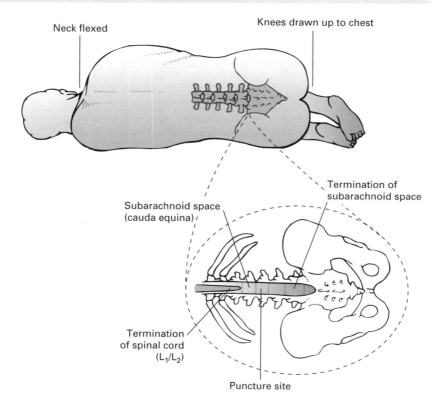

Neck flexed

Knees drawn up to chest

Subarachnoid space (cauda equina)

Termination of subarachnoid space

Termination of spinal cord (L_1/L_2)

Puncture site

Fig. 7.14 Position for lumbar puncture. (Based on Carola et al 1990, p 339.)

■ **BOX 7.6** The nursing management of the unconscious patient

Problem	Nursing intervention
Inadequate airway/poor gag reflex	Ensure clear airway through positioning patient on side with neck in neutral position, or if appropriate use of nasal or oral airway. Elevate head of bed to 30°. Care of tracheostomy/endotracheal tube.
Ineffective clearance of secretions/poor cough reflex	Assess patient's requirement for suctioning, pre-oxygenate if appropriate, limit active suctioning to 15 seconds, observe patient throughout suctioning for eteriorating cardiovascular signs, ensure recovery from suctioning.
Poor respiratory pattern/deteriorating gas exchange	Observe rate, depth and regularity of respirations. Listen to chest sounds, monitor tidal volumes and arterial blood gases. Position patient appropriately, avoiding the use of prone positioning. Chest physiotherapy to reduce secretions and improve gas exchange. Administer oxygen as required. Monitor CO_2, via either arterial blood gases or end tidal CO_2 (see Box 7.7)
Potential for alteration in normal cardiac status	Observe pulse rate, rhythm and regularity; blood pressure, where appropriate CVP and skin colour of patient, including peripheries. Maintain normal temperature. Observe for signs of infection.
Immobility	Reposition patient regularly, ensuring neck in neutral position, avoiding positions that may cause a rise in intracranial pressure, i.e., hip flexion. 6-hourly passive movements. Assess Waterlow score, using the appropriate tools to prevent and treat pressure/skin damage. Use thigh-length pressure stockings/subcutaneous heparin (contraindicated in patients with cerebral bleeds) and monitor for signs of deep vein thrombosis.
Neurological impairment	Regular Glasgow Coma Scale, pupil and limb assessments, increasing frequency if any deterioration noted. Avoid sensory deprivation/overload, planning workload to avoid clustering of activities, promote social interaction encouraging appropriate visitors to assist with care. Consider patient's potential for pain, assessing any other injuries and managing appropriately.
Maintenance of hydration and nutritional status	Monitor input and output of fluids – a catheter is usually passed in the unconscious patient, especially if he is receiving diuretics. (A high ICP can cause inappropriate ADH production and urinary retention will increase ICP). Assess skin turgor, urine specific gravity, urine and serum osmolarity. Administer fluids and nutrition enterally where possible to maintain gut integrity. Fluid infusion should be isotonic and any electrolyte imbalance corrected. (Hypernatraemia promotes cerebral oedema.)

(Cont'd)

(Box 7.6 cont'd)	
Potential for seizure activity	Observe for origin, sequence of events and start/finish time. The patient should be placed in the left lateral position, when the seizure is over, and observation should continue. The GCS is affected by the post-ictal state, and should be completed regularly, until the pre-seizure status is regained. Anti-convulsants should be administered, in an attempt to stop the seizure, and subsequently administered regularly to inhibit seizure activity. Seizures will increase the ICP, and if continuous, i.e., status epilepticus, can cause severe cerebral oedema, occasionally causing brainstem death.
Maintenance of hygiene requirements Rehabilitation	Regular care of skin, ensuring particular care for mouth, eyes and areas around invasive catheters. Support and preparation of longer term carers, making discharge plans.

The injuries may be classified in many ways. The terms 'open' (a penetrating injury) and 'closed' (a non-penetrating injury) are commonly used, although there is no common agreement on the definition of these terms. An open head injury may describe both a bullet lodged in the brain and a scalp laceration, thus it does not convey a degree of severity. 'Coup' (injury directly below the site of impact) and 'contracoup' (injury opposite the original site) are also common terms, but again describe location rather than severity of injury (see Fig. 7.15).

Gennarelli et al 1982 described the terms focal and diffuse, in an attempt to relate outcome to location. These are very useful terms, especially if used in conjunction with the Glasgow Coma Score (GCS). The GCS is commonly used in association with the terms mild, moderate and severe, mild being a score of GCS 13–15, moderate GCS 9–12 and severe GCS 3–8.

Head injuries may be described as belonging to three anatomical sites: the scalp, the skull and the brain.

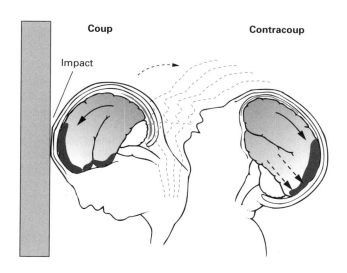

Coup   Contracoup

Impact

Fig. 7.15 Coup and contracoup injury. (Based on Hudak & Gallo 1994.)

SCALP INJURIES

There are four types of injury to the scalp:

- **Abrasions** Minor injuries that may cause a small amount of bleeding.
- **Contusions** There is no break in the skin, but bruising to the scalp may cause blood to leak into the subcutaneous layer.
- **Laceration** A cut or tear of the skin and subcutaneous fascia that tends to bleed profusely.
- **Subgaleal haematoma** A haematoma below the galea which is a tough layer of tissue under the subcutaneous fascia and over the skull. The veins here empty into the venous sinus, thus any infection can spread easily to the brain, despite the skull remaining intact.

Abrasions may not require any treatment, but ice applied to the area may reduce any haematoma formation (Hickey 1992). Lacerations can bleed extensively, however, although bleeding from the scalp alone is unlikely to cause shock in an adult. In small children, a scalp laceration may be sufficient to cause hypovolaemia. Scalp lesions should be explored under local anaesthetic for foreign bodies, or skull fracture, with an X-ray examination if there is any doubt in diagnosis, and any wound sutured or glued according to depth and position. There is controversy surrounding the treatment of subgaleal haematomas because of the risks of infection. Some doctors therefore argue that it is best to evacuate the haematoma, while others argue that it is best to let it reabsorb. If the scalp injuries are only part of other injuries, it is important that they are documented to allow further investigation at a more appropriate time. They may need to be cleaned and dressed or temporarily sutured.

SKULL INJURIES

Only 2% of head injury casualty attendees will have a skull fracture; however, the majority of the complications will occur within this 2% (Atkinson Morley Hospital Neurosurgical Guidelines). A skull X-ray should be performed with any of the following:

- Loss of consciousness
- Post-traumatic amnesia
- Scalp damage
- GCS < 15
- Abnormal neurological signs
- Vomiting.

Skull fractures are usually classified in four groups: linear, depressed, basal and comminuted. Linear are the most commonly occurring fractures. They are diagnosed following skull X-rays and will probably need no specific management unless they accompany other injuries (Hickey 1992).

Depressed skull fractures may be very evident clinically, but will require X-ray examination to discover the full extent of damage. They are managed according to their severity and whether there are any accompanying injuries. If there are no other injuries requiring surgical management, they may not be surgically elevated, due to the risks of infection. However, if there is debris disturbing the brain tissue then surgery will be required.

Basal skull fractures are often difficult to visualise on an X-ray and are usually diagnosed clinically (see Box 7.4). If there is any suspicion of a basal skull fracture and the patient requires stomach aspiration, then an orogastric tube must be

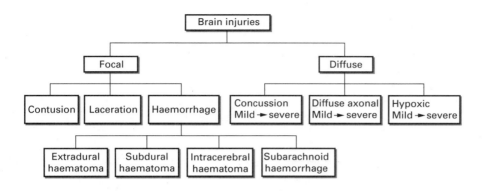

Fig. 7.16 Types of brain injury. (Adapted from Hickey 1992, p 361.)

passed, to avoid any risk of a nasogastric tube entering the cranium. When caring for head injured patients, it wise to have a policy of only passing orogastric tubes routinely for these patients.

BRAIN INJURIES

These may be focal or diffuse as shown in Figure 7.16.

Focal brain injuries

Contusion

Cerebral contusions are bruises of the surface of the brain, most commonly the frontal and temporal lobes, diagnosed by CT scan. Bleeding may occur into contusions, and it is this that would cause an early decrease in the conscious level (Lindsay et al 1991). Unfortunately, the brain will swell around the sites of contusion and if the contusions are large or widespread, the swelling may cause the ICP to rise, raising the mortality rate for this type of injury to 45% (Hudak & Gallo 1994). Lacerations are tears of the cortical surface and occur in similar locations to contusions.

Haemorrhage

There are four types of traumatic bleed, extradural (EDH), subdural (SDH), intra-cerebral (ICH) and subarachnoid (SAH). Subarachnoid bleeds are usually not traumatic in origin; however, they may be seen on CT scan following trauma. This is for one of two reasons. Either the patient has suffered an SAH prior to an incident (possibly the cause of the incident) (Sakas et al 1995), or the vessels in the subarachnoid space have been damaged by shearing forces.

> How might a blockage by a tumour or a haemorrhage affect correct drainage?

Extradural haematomas These are situated between the periosteum and the dura mater (see Fig. 7.17). They are usually caused by a laceration to the middle meningeal artery or vein or less commonly the dural venous sinus, following a blow to the temporal–parietal region. EDHs make up 16% of all haematomas (Lindsay et al 1991), and in 85% of patients the EDH will be accompanied by a skull fracture (Hickey 1993, Hudak & Gallo 1994).

Patients with extradural haematomas present with a history of transient loss of consciousness. If the EDH is not diagnosed they will then be lucid for a period of time – hours to days, dependent on the rate of the bleed. They will then rapidly

Fig. 7.17 Extradural haematoma. (From Hickey 1992, p 364.)

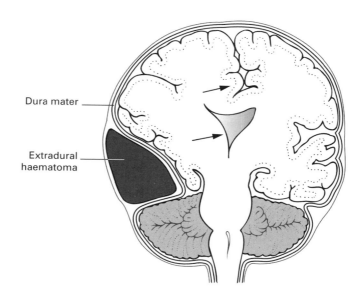

Fig. 7.18 Subdural haematoma. (From Hickey 1992, p 365.)

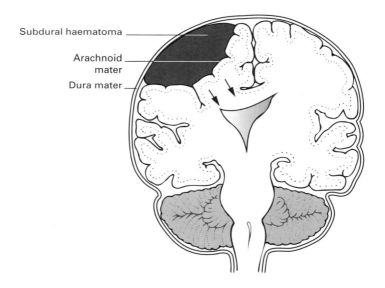

lose consciousness and deteriorate very quickly. A common presentation is the patient who falls, gets up after a short period of time, then goes home to bed; the next morning his family or friends are unable to rouse him and he is taken to A&E. Surgical treatment is to evacuate the haematoma and ligate the damaged blood vessel. Early signs of deterioration are irritation and headache, and later signs include seizures, ipsilateral pupil dilation, reduced level of consciousness and contralateral hemiplegia (Sherman 1990). Relatives or friends of these patients require a great deal of reassurance, as they often feel responsible for not bringing the patient to hospital earlier.

Subdural haematomas are situated between the dura mater and arachnoid mater and make up 22% of all haematomas (Lindsay et al 1991) (see Fig. 7.18).

These haematomas are caused by the rupture of bridging veins from the cortical surfaces to the venous sinuses. SDHs can be seen in isolation, but are more commonly associated with cerebral contusions and intracerebral haematomas – this group totals 54% of all haematomas. SDHs are classified into acute, subacute and chronic. Acute refers to symptoms which manifest within 48 hours after injury, while chronic symptoms emerge after 2 weeks and subacute between 48 hours and 2 weeks. Subacute and chronic SDHs are often seen in the elderly and in alcoholics as both groups can suffer regular falls, and have a degree of cerebral atrophy which puts strain on the bridging veins. Acute SDHs are associated with major cerebral trauma: the onset of symptoms such as headache, drowsiness, slow cerebration and confusion is slower than in EDH, but is often associated with other injuries and therefore the symptoms can become confused within a general head injury picture. Small SDHs may be treated conservatively, as they will reabsorb over time. Larger SDHs will require evacuation, because of the secondary damage they will cause.

Intracerebral haematomas are found deep within the brain parenchyma. As mentioned before they are related to contusions and are therefore usually found in the frontal and parietal lobes. Other causes include penetrating/missile injuries and a shearing of blood vessels deep within the brain following acceleration/deceleration injuries. They are caused by bleeding within the substance of the brain (see Fig. 7.19). Symptoms include headache, contralateral hemiplegia, ipsilateral dilated/fixed pupil and a deteriorating level of consciousness, progressing to deep coma (GCS < 8).

Treatment tends to be conservative because of the associated injuries and the difficulty of evacuating a haematoma that is situated so deeply within the brain. Not surprisingly, mortality is high within this group of patients.

Diffuse brain injuries

Concussion

This is a mild form of diffuse injury, involving disorientation, headache, dizziness, inability to concentrate and irritability. This may be with or without a loss of consciousness and/or memory for a short period of time. Recovery is usually within minutes to hours. Concussion is usually clinically diagnosed, but if performed, a negative CT scan would be produced. It is caused by shearing injuries from acceleration/deceleration forces.

Acute axonal injury

This occurs as a result of high speed acceleration/deceleration injuries, typically road traffic accidents, causing a mechanical shearing of axons in the white matter.

Initially there may be very little obvious injury on the CT scan. The patient is deeply unconscious, however, and with repeated scanning small diffuse haemorrhagic lesions appear, commonly in the corpus callosum, midbrain and pons, accompanied by generalised cerebral oedema (see Fig. 7.20). Patients with this type of injury have high mortality or morbidity rates, the survivors requiring long-term care.

Hypoxic injury

This occurs when the brain is deprived of adequate oxygen, for example in cardiac or respiratory arrest which may or may not be associated with head injury. Injury can be of varying degrees according to the length of the hypoxic event, from mild cognitive deficits to death. The hypoxic tissue becomes oedematous and this compounds the brain injury.

Fig. 7.19 Intracerebral haematoma. (Based on Hickey 1992, p 366.)

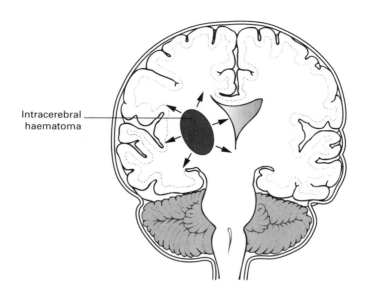

Intracerebral haematoma

Fig. 7.20 Diffuse axonal injury. (From Hickey 1992, p 366.)

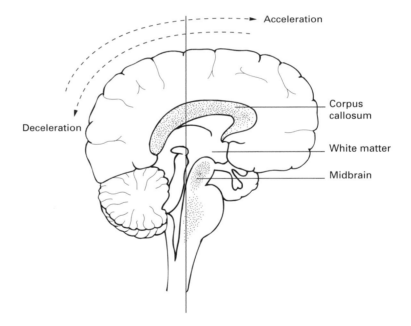

Acceleration

Deceleration

Corpus callosum

White matter

Midbrain

Management of the head injured patient is aimed at preventing or limiting secondary damage, as a result of oedema, haematoma, ischaemia and infection. Thorough assessment is essential, to gather as much early information as possible, followed by continuous assessment of the patient's neurological state.

Nursing management in the high dependency unit includes regular assessment of neurological signs (as described in the section on assessment), vital signs, recognition of the signs of rising ICP, seizure control, management of fluid input and output, management of associated injuries and accurate documentation of events.

Type	Respiratory pattern	Neuroanatomical lesion
Cheyne–Stokes respiration		Usually bilateral in cerebral hemispheres Cerebellar sometimes Midbrain Upper pons
Central neurogenic hyperventilation		Low midbrain Upper pons
Apneustic breathing		Mid pons Low pons
Cluster breathing		Low pons High medulla
Ataxic breathing		Medulla

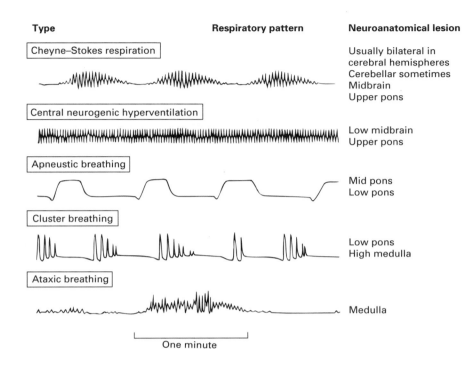

One minute

Fig. 7.21 Respiratory patterns in neurological dysfunctions. (Based on Hudak & Gallo 1994.)

Nursing management

Respiratory Observation of the patient's respiratory pattern is a particularly useful tool when caring for the head–injured patient. The neurophysiology of respiration is complex and involves many areas of the brain, therefore early observation of altered breathing patterns can assist in determining the area of neurological insult (see Fig. 7.21).

Occasionally a patient may develop neurogenic pulmonary oedema, best described by Theodore and Robin (1975). The raised ICP causes a massive adrenergic (sympathetic) discharge; the systemic vascular resistance (SVR) is increased resulting in a shift of blood from the systemic circulation to the pulmonary circulation with resultant damage to the pulmonary capillaries. Treatment is with diuretics, positioning (sitting upright if possible) and ventilation, with positive end expiratory pressure (PEEP) if the condition continues. Suctioning is not particularly helpful, but may be unavoidable. It should, however, be kept to a minimum as the distress caused by the trauma and change in gaseous exchange will cause the ICP to increase. The patient should be sedated to tolerate the endotracheal tube and may need a bolus of sedation to reduce the undesirable effects. Arterial blood gases should be taken from any patient with a sustained deterioration in their GCS, or who is respiratory or cardiovascularly unstable. If mechanical hyperventilation is required to reduce hyperaemia and therefore ICP, then a $PaCO_2$ between 3.5 and 4.5 kPa should be maintained. Mechanical ventilation should be instituted in any patient who has one or more of the following:

- $pO_2 < 10$ kPa on maximal oxygen therapy
- Hyperventilation causing $pCO_2 < 3.5$ kPa
- Hypoventilation causing $pCO_2 > 6.0$ kPa
- Spontaneous extensor posturing

■ **BOX 7.7** The role of carbon dioxide

Carbon dioxide (CO_2) in the blood causes dilatation of blood vessels. In brain injury this can result in an increased cerebral blood flow (CBF) and therefore an increased cerebral blood volume (CBV) (hyperaemia) which in turn causes a rise in intracranial pressure (ICP). CO_2 rises due to inadequate respiratory function are a major indication for mechanical ventilation.

There has been much debate regarding the use of hyperventilation to reduce CO_2 levels to below normal. Most units will hyperventilate to control ICP (Waldmann & Thyveetil 1998). There is, however, a danger of reducing CBF too far and so causing cerebral ischaemia.

■ **BOX 7.8** Brainstem death

Unfortunately – and despite appropriate management – it is sometimes impossible to reduce the ICP sufficiently and maintain cerebral blood flow. The brainstem becomes starved of oxygen following herniation of the temporal lobe through the tentorium and consequent cerebellar tonsillar herniation through the foramen magnum.

The diagnosis of brainstem death is usually made in the intensive care unit, although in some cases this may occur in the high dependency unit. Certain initial preconditions must be fulfilled: these are that a known cause of irremediable structural brain damage exists, and that any reversible causes of apnoeic coma have been excluded. These are:

• Metabolic or endocrine disturbances
• Hypothermia
• Presence of CNS depressant drugs or neuromuscular blockade.

Having satisfied the preconditions the patient is tested to ensure the absence of brainstem reflexes and apnoea:

• The pupils are fixed and dilated, not responding to sharp changes in the intensity of light.
• There is no corneal reflex when a piece of gauze or cotton wool is brushed across the cornea.
• There are no vestibular–ocular reflexes. When 20 ml of ice cold water is irrigated across the tympanic membrane the eyes do not deviate (ensuring that the tympanic membrane is clear of debris and not ruptured).
• There is no gag or cough reflex.
• There is no motor response.
• There is no respiratory effort, despite allowing the $P\,CO_2$ to rise above the threshold for stimulus of respiration.

Two senior doctors must perform these tests on two occasions. These may be documented on a pre-printed form, but must also be documented in the medical notes, the date and time of death being recorded when the second set of tests is completed. At this point the patient may be disconnected from, or not reconnected to, mechanical ventilation. Also at this time the procedure for donating solid organs may be initiated if wished.

The nurse is responsible for ensuring a clear communication of events to the patient's relatives during these procedures, and for providing appropriate reassurance and support.

- Hyperpyrexia
- Flail chest
- GCS < 8
- Marked oedema on CT scan.

Cardiovascular Assess vital signs: hypotension is rarely neurological in origin, but it is important to assess for any internal bleeding. If the patient remains hypotensive, and his ICP is higher than normal, the patient may suffer tissue hypoxia due to a poor resulting cerebral perfusion pressure (CPP). (See section regarding the physiology of raised intracranial pressure p. 158.) Cardiac arrhythmias may be due to brainstem irritation. Late signs of a very high intracranial pressure include a change in respiratory pattern, raised blood pressure and bradycardia, known as Cushing's triad.

Intracranial pressure Disorientation, irritation, headache, seizures, nausea and vomiting are also signs of raised intracranial pressure. Various measures can be taken to reduce ICP, including:

- Maintain head and neck in a neutral position
- 30° head elevation
- Mechanical hyperventilation to no lower than 3.5 kPa
- Fluid restriction to 70% of normal maintenance
- Diuresis usually with 20% mannitol +/− frusemide (frusemide decreases CSF production and increases its absorption)
- Treatment of pyrexia.

Hydration An orogastric tube should be passed to reduce the chance of aspiration; a nasogastric tube should only be passed if there is absolutely no possibility of a basal skull fracture. Always pass an og/ng tube in patients with an endotracheal tube. Fluid infusion should be isotonic, and any electrolyte imbalance should be corrected.

CEREBROVASCULAR ACCIDENTS (CVAs)

A CVA or stroke occurs when there is either a blockage (ischaemic stroke) or bursting (haemorrhagic stroke) of a cerebral artery. It is characterised by either sudden or slow onset of a wide range of neurological deficits, which may vary in severity and permanence. It is the third largest killer in affluent countries, behind heart disease and cancer, and in the UK 150–200 per 100 000 population will suffer stroke annually, of which approximately one-third will be fatal (Lindsay et al 1991).

Ischaemic stroke

Ischaemic strokes make up about 85% of all strokes but carry a lesser mortality rate (about 25%) than haemorrhagic strokes. They may be embolic or thrombotic in origin, with thrombosis carrying the higher mortality. The embolus or thrombus causes ischaemia and latterly infarction and necrosis to the part of the brain supplied by that vessel. Thrombus formation in the cerebral arteries is the cause of transient ischaemic attacks (TIAs), and should be seen as a warning sign of a stroke. The signs and symptoms of a thrombotic stroke usually develop over a period of hours. Embolic strokes are usually secondary to atrial fibrillation, mitral stenosis or a mural thrombosis. These strokes are usually rapid in onset and may resolve quickly if the embolus disperses.

Clinical presentation

The presentation will vary according to the area of brain involved and the severity of the stroke, but may however include:

- Reduced level of consciousness (the lower the GCS the higher the mortality and morbidity)
- Hemiparesis or hemiplegia
- Either left or right hemianopia (blindness of one side of both eyes)
- Deviation of the head and eyes to one side (the same side as the stroke, the opposite to the hemiparesis or hemiplegia)
- Receptive and/or expressive aphasia (dominant hemisphere stroke)
- Inattention to one side of the body (the opposite side to the stroke).

The patient's clinical history will commonly include TIAs, hypertension, cardiac disease, arteriosclerosis, diabetes mellitus or a family history of vascular disease.

Haemorrhagic stroke

These account for approximately 15% of all strokes; however, the mortality rate is high at 70% (Lindsay et al 1991). These haemorrhages can be *intracerebral* as a result of the rupture of a small, deep artery bleeding into the brain substance; *subarachnoid* as a result of the rupture of an aneurysm causing bleeding into the subarachnoid space; or the result of a rupture of an *arteriovenous malformation* causing either an intracerebral bleed or an intraventricular bleed. Onset of symptoms is usually rapid, with further progression over the next few hours.

Clinical presentation

This is often similar to that of ischaemic stroke; however, typical presentation includes:

- Sudden, severe headache
- A period of decreasing consciousness
- Nausea or vomiting
- Possibly seizures
- Hemiparesis or hemiplegia.

Diagnosis is based on clinical presentation and history. CT scanning may be useful to determine the area of stroke as might MRI, in suspected subarachnoid haemorrhage. In the absence of raised intracranial pressure, a lumbar puncture will be performed. Management is according to symptoms and aimed at reducing ischaemic damage and complications. The patient would be admitted to a high dependency unit to manage the airway and prevent aspiration, to manage hypertension while maintaining the cerebral circulation and for observation of neurological status.

Nursing management

Respiratory function Violent coughing may precipitate a re-bleed in the patient with a ruptured aneurysm. Ventilation or a tracheostomy may be required if severely compromised.

Cardiovascular function Monitor blood pressure, administering anti-hypertensives as prescribed in the ischaemic stroke and maintaining pressure in the haemorrhagic stroke to prevent vasospasm.

Neurological function Observe deficits, and assist with their management, i.e., communication aids, promoting use and knowledge of affected limbs, encouraging the patient to assist in his own care as much as possible.

Hydration promote fluid intake in the patient following SAH to prevent vasospasm.

Immobility Position limbs, involving physiotherapist to advise on the use of splints and passive movements.

BACTERIAL MENINGITIS

This acute inflammation of the meninges and subarachnoid space has three main causative organisms.

- *Neisseria meningitidis* Usually occurs in children and young adults. Symptoms may include purpuric skin rash, a severity related to sudden onset, septicaemia, DIC, and circulatory collapse. These symptoms indicate a poor prognosis.
- *Streptococcus pneumoniae* Usually occurs in adults; associated with sickle-cell disease, pneumonia, alcoholism, splenectomy and ear infections. A poor prognosis is seen with sudden onset.
- *Haemophilus influenzae* Usually seen in small children; associated with upper respiratory tract and ear infections. Generally, a good prognosis.

Meningitis occurs when the causative organisms, which are commonly found in the nasopharynx, enter the blood stream. It may also occur as a complication of sinus infection or head injury. Purulent exudate forms in the subarachnoid space causing inflammation of the meninges. The infection is quickly spread by the CSF around the brain and spinal cord. Intracranial pressure may rise as exudate inhibits the flow of CSF causing hydrocephalus and irritates the vasculature causing a cerebral vasculitis, thrombosis with resultant necrosis and haemorrhage.

Clinical presentation

- Headache; often frontal or occipital and usually the first sign. This will be described as very severe.
- Fever.
- Meningeal irritation including neck stiffness, photophobia (cranial nerve V), Kernig's sign (see Fig. 7.22).
- Reduced level of consciousness; initially loss of concentration, leading to disorientation and an inability to obey commands. Latterly the patient is drowsy or unresponsive.
- Skin rash in meningococcal varieties.
- Seizure activity; may be general or focal, and indicates irritation of cerebral cortex.
- Increased ICP; often indicated by the onset of vomiting. If severe may lead to tentorial herniation.
- Cranial nerve dysfunction; II, III, IV and VI – difficulty moving the eye, ptosis (drooping upper eyelid), unequal pupils and diplopia; VII – facial paralysis; and VIII – tinnitus, vertigo and deafness.
- Endocrine disorders; increased antidiuretic hormone; hyponatraemia.
- Waterhouse–Friderichsen syndrome; adrenal insufficiency following infarction of the adrenal glands.

Fig. 7.22 Kernig's sign.
(From Hickey 1992, p 609.)

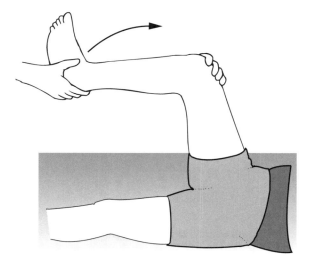

Kernig's sign is elicited by flexing the knee to 90°, bringing it up toward the body and then attempting to straighten the leg. This stretches the inflamed lumbar nerve roots causing pain.

The disease is diagnosed from clinical signs and confirmed by lumbar puncture. The earlier appropriate antibiotics can be commenced the better the outcome for the patient, reducing the risk of the more severe complications. Further treatment is supportive and particular to the symptoms being displayed.

Nursing management

Control of pyrexia Regular assessment and recording of temperature; antipyretics; patient-cooling measures such as removing excess bed linen, cooling the environment and cool washes.

Pain control Reduce environmental stimuli. Patients may be hypersensitive to touch, sound and light; analgesia, measuring degree of pain and monitoring response.

Respiratory function The patient may deteriorate to require mechanical ventilation in the ICU.

Hydration The patient may be nauseous and require parenteral hydration.

Nutrition Assess requirements according to level of consciousness.

SEIZURES

Seizures describe intermittent abnormal neural activity in the brain, characterised by a number of stages including predrome, aura, ictal (including tonic, clonic, unconscious), and post-ictal. (Lindsay et al 1991, Worthley 1994). When seizures are chronic they are usually known as epilepsy; however this term still carries a stigma and should be used with caution (Hudak & Gallo 994).

Seizures fall into three major categories: partial, generalised and unclassified. Partial seizures describe abnormal neuronal discharge localised to one area of the cortex. This discharge may remain localised or progress to a generalised seizure. A patient suffering a partial seizure may have a warning (predrome and/or

---

■ **BOX 7.9** Causes of seizures (from Worthley 1994, p 694)

- Idiopathic
- Multiple sclerosis
- Alzheimer's disease
- Febrile convulsion
- Electrocution, electroconvulsive therapy
- Eclampsia
- Pancreatitis
- Cerebrovascular diseases
  — Hypertensive encephalopathy
  — Embolism, infarction, atrioventricular malformation
  — Subarachnoid haemorrhage
  — Cerebral arterial or venous thrombosis, systemic lupus erythematosus, thrombotic thrombocytopenic purpura
- Structural cerebral defect
  — Trauma, neoplasm, abscess, infarct
  — Meningitis, encephalitis (particularly herpes simplex)
- Metabolic abnormality
  — Hypo: capnoea, glycaemia, natraemia, calcaemia, magnesaemia, phosphataemia
  — Uraemia, dialysis disequilibrium, hepatic failure, pyridoxine deficiency
- Drug withdrawal
  — Antiepileptics, alcohol, barbiturates, benzodiazepines, opiates, corticosteroids
- Drug toxicity
  — Aminophylline, lignocaine, phenothiazines, tricyclics, lithium
  — Penicillin (CSF penicillin > 10 u/ml, 6 μg/ml), imipenem
  — Isoniazid (due to pyridoxine deficiency)
  — Insulin (due to hypoglycaemia)

---

aura). Generalised seizures can also be a primary event, and are commonly known as a grand mal seizure. According to the area of the brain affected, different manifestations will occur; these can be motor, psychic, sensory or autonomic.

The most commonly recognised seizure is the convulsive generalised. Here the patient will go through all the stages described above. Without warning, he will lose consciousness and fall to the ground – this is the tonic phase and the body becomes rigid. Following this he exhibits clonic movements – rhythmic jerking of the body – and then he will become flaccid, often being incontinent. The patient then enters the post-ictal phase: his GCS may be below his normal and he may be confused, gradually returning to normal. Generalised seizures can also be non-convulsive. Occasionally the seizure activity, either clinically or on EEG, will continue for 30 minutes or more. This is known as status epilepticus and is a medical emergency (Hudak & Gallo 1994). Seizures are associated with many causes as shown in Box 7.9.

Nursing management

During seizure Maintain airway, observe respirations, observe type of seizure, duration and recovery; ensure patient safety. During status epilepticus diazepam, thiopentone, phenytoin or muscle relaxants may be administered. These require documentation for effect.

Table 7.3 Investigations

Investigation	Rationale
Serum biochemistry – glucose, sodium, calcium, magnesium, phosphate, acid–base balance, PCO_2	To ensure within normal limits
Drug levels	To establish cause
ECG, echocardiography	To assess for cardiac origin, such as cardiac syncopal, embolus
EEG	To establish a focus
CT scan/MRI scan	To identify structural brain disorders

■ **BOX 7.10** The electroencephalogram (EEG)

The EEG records the amplified electrical potential of the brain through approximately 20 electrodes placed across the patient's scalp. The first EEG was recorded by Berger in 1929, and the use of the EEG has greatly increased the understanding of seizure activity and its source (Lindsay et al 1991). It is recorded to show the location and type of cerebral disturbance and is used as a diagnostic tool in conjunction with patient history, clinical examination and biochemical results.

The normal EEG shows alpha and beta waves. Alpha waves are recorded at rest from the parietal and occipital regions and may be slowed by hypoglycaemia, hypercapnoea and hypothermia. When an individual is concentrating, with the eyes open, there is more beta activity recorded from the anterior region of the brain. Alpha and beta waves are normally bilaterally symmetrical. The abnormal EEG displays delta and theta waves and spikes, with asymmetry (Hickey 1992; Worthley 1994). Figure 7.23 contrasts the normal EEG with an EEG during a convulsive seizure.

The EEG is of reduced diagnostic value in the patient who is heavily sedated, which may be the case in the HDU. It can however be of help in distinguishing between metabolic and hypoxic encephalopathies (Bion & Oh 1997).

Following seizure Reassure patient, check for any injuries, record event; if regular record on a seizure chart to allow comparison and evaluation of any drug therapy.

Ongoing care Ensure patient is complying with the drug regimen, educate to any new regimen and give information regarding the seizures and any investigations that may be required as in Table 7.3. Address patient's pyschosocial concerns.

GUILLAIN–BARRÉ SYNDROME (GBS)

This is an acute inflammatory polyneuropathy, and is thought to be an autoimmune response to a viral infection with an incidence of 1–2 per 100 000 population. It affects slightly more males than females, occurring in all age groups, although peaks have been noted in young adults and those in their 40s–70s (McMahon-Parkes & Cornock 1997). The disease usually proceeds rapidly, primarily affecting the motor component of the peripheral nerves. Most patients survive and recover completely; those who deteriorate so as to require ventilatory support are more likely to have residual disabilities. Death may occur due to cardiac or respiratory arrest.

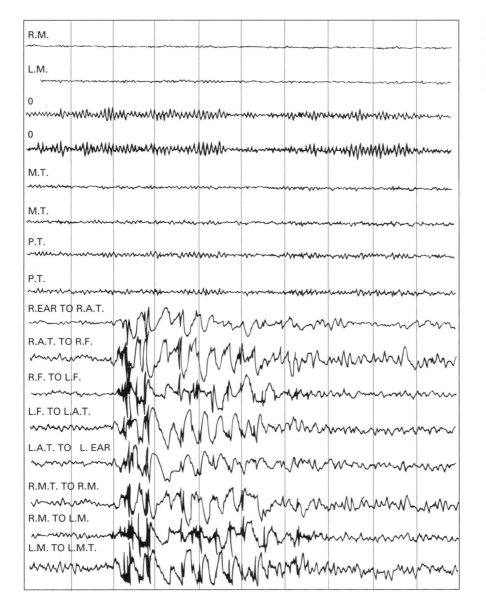

Fig. 7.23 Comparison of a normal EEG (top) with that of an epileptic patient during a tonic–clonic seizure (bottom). (Based on Hickey 1992, p 584.)

GBS is though to be caused by an immune-mediated response to a viral illness. This causes destruction of the myelin sheath, in both the spinal and cranial nerves, causing a loss of saltatory conduction and a resultant slowing of nerve impulses. The peripheral nerves become oedematous and inflamed causing varying degrees of axonal damage. The greater the damage the less the recovery.

Clinical presentation

There are four variants of Guillain–Barré syndrome: ascending, descending, Miller Fisher variant and pure motor GBS. The most common presentation is the ascending variety:

- Ascending, symmetrical weakness and numbness commencing in the lower limbs and progressing upward to the arms, trunk and cranial nerves
- Dysphagia
- Reduced vital capacity
- Hyperalgesia.

In 65% of patients these symptoms occur 2–3 weeks following a viral illness or an immunisation.

Management is generally symptomatic, with emphasis placed on monitoring respiratory function. Plasmapheresis and immunoglobulins have been trialled with good effect, for use early after symptoms occur (Van der Mech & Schmitz 1992). Immunoglobulin therapy is presently preferred, because of the risks of plasmapheresis which seem to be heightened in Guillain–Barré syndrome.

Nursing management

Respiratory function Detailed observation of respiratory status is required in these patients including vital capacity and tidal volume. Monitor cough and gag, encourage deep breathing and coughing. If doubt exists measure arterial blood gases, administering oxygen as required and with caution. Ventilation and/or tracheostomy may be required.

Neurological status Motor and sensory assessments, including cranial nerves especially facial (VII), vagus (X), for autonomic dysfunction, and glossopharyngeal (IX).

Monitor autonomic dysfunction Cardiac arrhythmias, hypo/hypertension, urinary retention, inappropriate ADH secretion.

Pain control Monitor characteristics of pain, positioning, analgesia, management of immobility. A pain chart is useful.

Immobility Pulmonary embolism, ileus.

Psychosocial aspects If the patient is unable to talk, establish a means of communication to ensure a level of independence, provide items to improve visual field such as mirrors and ensure a stimulating environment. Involve family and friends where possible, and ensure that the patient's dignity and privacy are respected. This area of care is perhaps the most important, once respiratory, autonomic and pain management are agreed. The patient with GBS may be in hospital for a protracted period of time, in some cases a year or more. It is therefore important, especially in the high dependency area, to ensure that the patient can take some degree of control in his care. This may require a great deal of planning and innovation on the part of the nurse and the multidisciplinary team.

PHARMACOLOGY

Many of the medicines used in the care of neurological patients are widely used for other conditions; these include sedatives and analgesics. In this section only the most commonly used neurological medicines such as anticonvulsants, osmotic diuretics and analgesia will be described.

Phenytoin

Uses Prevention and treatment of generalised seizures. It is sometimes used in conjunction with other therapy for the treatment of localised seizures. When administered intravenously it must be given slowly therefore limiting its use in status epilepticus, where diazepam is often the first-line treatment.

Dosage and administration Initial intravenous dose 10–15 mg/kg, delivered at no more than 50 mg/min. This would be followed up by 300–400 mg daily in divided doses either intravenously or orally. Patients receiving phenytoin intravenously should have cardiac monitoring throughout. It is therefore appropriate to move to the enteral route as soon as it is available. Phenytoin can be successfully given via the oro/nasogastric tube in its liquid form, although any enteral nutrition must be stopped usually 1 hour pre- and post-administration, to allow absorption. To maintain the patient's nutritional requirements it is better to administer once a day in the enteral nutrition rest period, if this is acceptable to maintain the patient's blood levels. Phenytoin is poorly and erratically absorbed from intramuscular sites; this route should therefore only be used with caution and as a last resort.

Contraindications Phenytoin should be used with caution in patients who have respiratory depression, myocardial infarction or who are pregnant. Bradyarrhythmias may be exacerbated during intravenous administration.

Side effects These are frequent and wide ranging, particularly during intravenous administration. Rapid i.v. administration causes hypotension and can cause arrhythmias. Patients metabolise phenytoin at different rates, therefore the dose is titrated against blood levels. Signs of toxicity include nystagmus, ataxia, diplopia, lethargy, drowsiness and in severe cases unconsciousness. Other side effects include nausea, vomiting, constipation, dysphagia, change in the patient's ability to taste, weight loss, blurred vision, dizziness, twitching, headache, shrinking of the gums, rashes, lymphadenopathy and haematological effects.

Carbamazepine

Uses Prophylactic management of localised and generalised seizures. It appears to be most effective in patients with complex localised seizures. It is also used for the control of neurogenic pain in a variety of conditions including trigeminal neuralgia, Guillain–Barré syndrome, multiple sclerosis, diabetic neuropathy and post-traumatic paraesthesia.

Dosage and administration Dosage is titrated according to individual requirements and response. Initial dosage is 400 mg daily in divided doses, increasing by 200 mg a day until optimum response is achieved. Treatment with carbamazepine should be introduced or reduced slowly, usually at weekly intervals. Any previous treatment should be maintained or reduced as the carbamazepine is slowly increased.

Carbamazepine is available as a tablet or in suspension; the latter will provide higher peak concentrations and is prescribed in more frequent smaller quantities. If administered via a nasogastric tube it can be mixed with an equal volume of dilutant, water or 0.9% sodium chloride, to prevent adherence to the PVC tubing.

Contraindications Carbamazepine should only be prescribed for patients with cardiac, hepatic, haematological or renal disease or in pregnancy after a risk benefit analysis.

Side effects These are many and varied but include decrease in platelet and leucocyte counts, adverse cardiovascular effects including aggravation of hypertension, hypotension, congestive cardiac failure, syncope, aggravation of coronary heart disease, arrhythmias and AV block, abnormal liver function tests, urinary frequency/retention, impotence, drowsiness, fatigue, ataxia, confusion, blurred vision, visual hallucinations, hyperacusis, speech disturbances, nausea, vomiting, constipation and rashes.

Mannitol

Uses To reduce raised intracranial pressure following trauma or during neurosurgery. There is evidence to show that there may be a rebound increase in intracranial pressure about 12 hours post-infusion and if the blood–brain barrier is not intact then mannitol could draw water back into the brain. For mannitol to work renal blood flow and glomerular filtration must be appropriately high to enable the drug to reach the tubules. It should not be used if serum osmolarity is > 320 mosm/l.

Dosage and administration 1.5–2 g/kg as a 20% solution, intravenously over 30–60 minutes.

Contraindications Renal failure, pulmonary oedema, dehydration and congestive heart disease. Mannitol should only be used during pregnancy where clearly indicated.

Side effects Electrolyte imbalance, dehydration, water intoxication (due to fast administration or poor urine output) and pulmonary oedema are the most severe effects. Other effects include blurred vision, nausea, vomiting, hypotension, tachycardia and thrombophlebitis. Extravasation can cause localised oedema and possible necrosis of the surrounding tissues.

Nimodipine

This is a calcium channel blocker similar to nifedipine. It has been unsuccessful in preventing vasospasm; however it does seems to have a significant effect in reducing ischaemic complications (33% to 22%) by opening up the collateral circulation and blocking calcium influx (Lindsay et al 1991).

Uses To reduce ischaemic neurological deficits following acute subarachnoid hemorrhage, it may also improve outcome following acute ischaemic strokes. In SAH, therapy should be commenced within 96 hours of the original bleed.

Dosage and administration Intravenously 1–2 mg/h continuously, usually starting at a lower dose and increasing according the patient's ability to maintain blood pressure. Orally 60 mg 4-hourly.

Contraindications Nimodopine should only be used in pregnancy when the benefits outweigh the potential risks.

Side effects Hypotension especially with intravenous use, flushing, headache and oedema.

Codeine phosphate

Uses Mild opiate analgesia, with minimal CNS depressant effects.

Dosage and administration Usually given intramuscularly or orally, 30–60 mg 4–6-hourly. Listed under Schedule 2 of the Misuse of Drugs Act 1968, in intramuscular in preparation.

Contraindications Respiratory depression.

Side effects Tolerance and physical dependence, CNS depression especially in the older patient.

There is much debate regarding the use of opiates in neurological patients. It is commonly agreed that opiates should be given if the patient's pain requires them. Codeine phosphate is only a mild opiate and may not be the best form of pain management.

CONCLUSION

The nervous system is fascinating and although complex, a basic understanding not only allows the nurse to provide well planned and proactive care, but also provides insight into potential problems and therefore the ability to react appropriately to those situations. This understanding assists in the care of many patients who may not be admitted with a primary neurological diagnosis, but who have previous pathology of the nervous system or may be at risk of CVA or seizure. More detailed information can be found in the articles and books listed as References and Further reading for those who would like to discover more.

REFERENCES

Bion J, Oh T E 1997 Sedation in intensive care In: Oh T E (ed.) Intensive care manual 4th edn. Butterworth Heinemann, London, p 673

Carola R, Harley J P, Noback C R 1990 Human anatomy and physiology. McGraw Hill, USA

Gennarelli T A, Spielman G M, Langfitt T W 1982 Influence of the type of intracranial lesion on outcome from severe head injury. Journal of Neurosurgery 56: 26–36

Hickey J V 1992 The clinical practice of neurological and neurosurgical nursing, 3rd edn. J B Lippincott, Philadelphia

Hudak C M, Gallo B M 1994 Critical care nursing: a holistic approach. J B Lippincott, Philadelphia

Lindsay K W, Bone I, Callander R 1991 Neurology and neurosurgery illustrated, 2nd edn. Churchill Livingstone, Edinburgh

McMahon-Parkes K, Cornock M A 1997 Guillain–Barré syndrome: biological basis, treatment and care. Intensive and Critical Care Nursing 13: 42–48

Purves D, Augustine G J, Fitzpatrick D et al 1997 Neuroscience

Sakas D E, Dias L S, Beale D 1995 Subarachnoid haemorrhage presenting as a head injury. British Medical Journal 310: 1186–1187

Sherman D W 1990 Managing an acute head injury. Nursing 20(4): 47–51

Teasdale G, Jennett B 1974 Assessment of coma and impaired consciousness: a practical scale. Lancet ii 81–84

Theodore J, Robin E 1975 Neurogenic pulmonary oedema Lancet. ii: 749–751

Thompson R F 1993 The brain: a neuroscience primer, 2nd edn. W H Freeman, New York

Van der Mech F G A, Schmitz P I M 1992 The Dutch Guillain–Barré study group. A randomised trial comparing intravenous immunoglobulin and plasma exchange in Guillain–Barré syndrome. New England Journal of Medicine 326: 1123–1129

Waldmann C S and Thyveetil D 1998 Management of head injury in a district general hospital. Care of the Critically Ill 14(2): 65–70

Worthley L I G 1994 Synopsis of intensive care medicine. Churchill Livingstone, Edinburgh

FURTHER READING

Gentleman D, Dearden M, Midgley S, MacLean D 1993 Guidelines for resuscitation and transfer of patients with serious head injury. British Medical Journal 307: 547–552

Johnson B P 1995 One family's experience with head injury: a phenomenological study. Journal of Neuroscience Nursing 27(2): 113–118

NHSE 1996 Admission to and discharge from intensive and high dependency care. Department of Health, London

Thomson R, Gray J, Madhok R, Mordue A, Mendelow A D 1994 Effect of guidelines on management of head injury on record keeping and decision making in accident and emergency departments. Quality in Health Care 3(2): 86–91

CHAPTER 8

Post-anaesthetic and post-operative care

Guy Young

Key learning objectives

The purpose of this chapter is to provide an insight into the needs of the patient following anaesthesia and surgery. The key objectives are that the reader will gain an understanding of:

- The importance of the pre-operative preparation of patients
- Anaesthetic techniques and their implications for post-operative care
- The use of supplemental oxygen in the post-operative period
- Airway management in the initial post-operative period
- The effective assessment and management of post-operative patients.

Prerequisite knowledge

A general knowledge of anatomy, physiology and the disease process is assumed. The reader might find the chapter more rewarding if they have a more detailed understanding of:

- The ABC of resuscitation (a basic life-support session would be particularly useful)
- Respiratory physiology, including blood gas analysis
- Cardiovascular physiology, including ECG interpretation.

INTRODUCTION

Patients who are in the initial stages of recovery from anaesthesia and surgery are naturally highly dependent. Whether unable to maintain their own airway or in pain, they require a significant level of nursing intervention. Nurses working in this field need to have a high level of knowledge and skill in order to provide a high standard of care. While technical expertise is essential, humanistic skill and professionalism are vital. During this period patients are extremely vulnerable and they rely very heavily on the nurse to act as their advocate.

The main focus of this chapter is the post-operative assessment and management of patients. Areas such as airway management, respiratory management and nausea and vomiting will be examined in some detail. There is a strong emphasis on patient assessment as this is seen to be key in providing appropriate and effective care. Assessment is approached from a systems perspective as this has made presentation easier. Towards the end of the chapter there are some brief pointers for the management of specific types of surgery. It is recognised that nurses working in these fields require a much deeper understanding of the specialty.

In order to make sense of much of the post-operative situation it is necessary to provide some insight into the pre-operative phase and anaesthesia. This then forms the basis of the first part of the chapter.

PRE-OPERATIVE ASSESSMENT

The need for high dependency post-operative care can be largely predicted. By seeing patients pre-operatively the nurse can help to ensure that the most appropriate post-operative care facilities are available.

Effective pre-operative assessment is vital in order to minimise the physiological changes and stresses that anaesthesia and surgery place on the patient (McKnight 1994). The anaesthetist will take a detailed history looking at issues such as past medical history, chronic illness, reaction to previous anaesthetics and current state of health. The American Society of Anesthesiologists (ASA) classification (Box 8.1) is the most common grading system currently used, and gives an overall assessment of anaesthetic risk. Patients who are in categories 3 and above may be predicted to need high dependency care, throughout the peri-operative and/or post-operative episodes. Effective communication between medical and nursing staff is therefore important to ensure that this facility is available. The development of collaborative care planning not only enhances communication, but also helps to predict and plan post-operative facilities (Swan 1994). There will inevitably be those cases where things do not go as planned and high dependency care is unexpectedly required. On the whole, however, the need can often be predicted.

It is widely accepted that the giving of pre-operative information can enhance post-operative recovery (Hayward 1975, Droogan & Dickson 1996;). For this reason patients who are anticipated to require high dependency care should be given relevant information pre-operatively. Although the focus here is on post-operative care it is suggested that the patient is prepared for the whole peri-operative process and that information is not limited to what will happen when they wake up. Examples of the type of information that could be given are shown in Box 8.2.

Particular emphasis should be placed on pain relief methods. It is crucial that patients understand that they need to inform staff if they are experiencing pain. This will enable staff to ensure that they receive the best possible pain relief.

Much of this information can be given by ward staff. Ideally they should themselves have some insight into the processes that take place within a high dependency area. This can be achieved by arranging short placements in high dependency areas for ward staff or by making it a part of any orientation programme.

Staff from the high dependency area could visit the patients pre-operatively. Although this can place considerable pressure on limited staff resources, every effort should be made to offer this facility. Patients themselves can visit the HDU. A recent study in intensive care found that patients would like this opportunity, although some felt that they would find the experience frightening (Watts & Brooks 1997). Therefore, the benefits of pre-operative visiting may be dependent on the individual and this should obviously be taken into account. Information can be given in other ways to those patients who would prefer not to visit the HDU.

■ **BOX 8.1** ASA physical status classification (adapted from: Dripps et al 1961)

ASA 1: Normal, healthy patient

ASA 2: Patient with mild systemic condition, e.g. well controlled diabetes, old age

ASA 3: Patient with systemic disease that limits activity but is not incapacitating, e.g. angina, chronic airway disease

ASA 4: Patient with an incapacitating disease that is a threat to life, e.g. advanced cardiac or pulmonary disease

ASA 5: Moribund patient not expected to survive 24 hours even with an operation

---

■ **BOX 8.2** Pre-operative information

Discussing the following issues with patients may help to reduce pre- and post-operative anxiety:

Pre-operative
- Fasting
- Removal of prostheses and cosmetics
- Pre-medication
- Repeated checking of identity and proposed operation
- The anaesthetic room, including personnel and procedures carried out there, e.g. insertion of lines, pre-oxygenation, monitoring

Peri-operative
- The possible need for additional shaving, e.g. to accommodate a diathermy plate
- Any particular position that they may be placed in or other intervention that would account for pain or discomfort post-operatively, e.g. a sore throat following intubation
- The possible need for medication to be administered via the rectal route while under anaesthetic (e.g. analgesia). With this example, the patient's consent should be sought.

Post-operative
- Attachments and monitoring, e.g. oxygen mask, endotracheal tube, intravenous lines, ECG electrodes, urinary catheters and drains
- Observations, particularly where they may be disruptive or unpleasant, e.g. neurological observations and pupillary reaction
- Pain relief methods
- What staff will be present and the degree of supervision the patient can expect
- Whether family and friends can visit.

These include booklets and videos prepared by the post-operative area. The process of giving information to patients, including details of pain relief methods, should start as early as possible, possibly at the pre-admission stage (Abbott & Glenn 1994). This is becoming increasingly common in the field of day surgery, where nurses are closely involved in the pre-operative assessment of patients (Murphy 1994).

ANAESTHESIA

Anaesthesia is the absence of normal sensation (Mosby's Dictionary 1994). It can occur as a result of traumatic or pathophysiological damage to nerve tissue or be induced in order to allow pain-free surgery. Broadly speaking, there are two types of surgical anaesthesia, general and regional (local). General anaesthesia depresses the central nervous system resulting in unconsciousness, loss of muscle tone and reflexes. Regional anaesthesia produces a loss of sensation in a specific area of the body without loss of consciousness.

General anaesthesia

General anaesthesia consists of four stages (Table 8.1). During induction of anaesthesia the patients pass through stages 1–3. Stage 4 is considered to be overdose and should be avoided. As the patient emerges from anaesthesia he passes through the stages in reverse order. It is during stage 2 (excitement) that undesir-

Table 8.1 Four stages of anaesthesia (adapted from Boulton & Blogg 1989)

Stage	Effect	Patient Response
1. Relaxation	• Amnesia • Analgesia	• Drowsiness • Dizziness • Exaggerated hearing • Decreased sensation of pain
2. Excitement	• Delirium	• Irregular breathing • Increased muscle tone, motor activity • Vomiting • Breath holding and struggling • Dilated pupils
3. Surgical anaesthesia	• Sensory loss	• Quiet regular breathing • Jaw relaxed • Loss of pain/auditory sensation • Decreased muscle tone • Eyelid reflex absent
4. Danger	• Medullary paralysis	• Paralysis of respiratory muscles • Fixed dilated pupils • Rapid thready pulse • Respiratory arrest

> Problems experienced by the patient during induction of anaesthesia can recur during emergence. Ask the anaesthetist about induction so that you can prepare for any likely problems.

> Anaesthetic agents have a wide variety of physiological effects. Try waking the patient up before actively treating symptoms such as hypertension and bradycardia.

able effects such as laryngospasm and vomiting may occur: this happens because voluntary control is temporarily lost. The patient becomes susceptible to uncontrolled and exaggerated response to almost any stimulus (Boulton & Blogg 1989). Although modern anaesthetics have shortened stage 2, induction and emergence remain two of the most critical periods of anaesthesia. It is important for the nurse caring for a patient during the immediate post-operative period to be aware of the patient's level of anaesthesia. By being able to assess that the patient is still at a level of surgical anaesthesia, because for example he requires airway maintenance, the nurse can be prepared for any problems such as vomiting as he passes through stage 2. It is important that the anaesthetist relays any problems experienced during induction to the nurse caring for the patient post-operatively as these may potentially occur on emergence.

General anaesthesia may be achieved using inhalational or intravenous agents (see Table 8.2 for examples). Inhalational agents can be gaseous or volatile (a vaporised liquid). These agents are easily absorbed and excreted through the lungs, resulting in rapid induction and emergence. Intravenous agents also produce rapid induction but unlike inhalational agents they need to be metabolised and excreted by the body, which can slow emergence. In practice a combination of inhalational and intravenous anaesthetic is normally used. Intravenous agents are used to produce rapid induction for the patient, which is more pleasant than breathing gas through a mask. Inhalational agents provide maintenance of anaesthesia and rapid emergence at the end of surgery. All anaesthetic agents can produce significant effects on cardiovascular, respiratory and neurological function. These will be covered later on in this chapter. When emergency surgery is required a technique known as rapid sequence or 'crash' induction is used (see Box 8.3 for more information).

Table 8.2 Examples of anaesthetic agents

Name	Type	Advantages	Adverse side effects
Propofol	• Intravenous	• Smooth induction • Rapid recovery, no hangover	• Bradycardia • Convulsions have been reported
Thiopentone sodium	• Intravenous	• Smooth, rapid induction	• Irritant to tissues • Effects may persist for 24 hours
Ketamine	• Intravenous/ intramuscular	• Analgesic properties • Patient maintains a patent airway	• Hallucinations • Relatively slow recovery
Nitrous oxide	• Inhalational • Gaseous	• Used for maintenance of anaesthesia • Inexpensive	• Cannot be used as sole agent, lack of potency
Halothane	• Inhalational • Volatile	• Rapid induction • Pleasant to inhale	• Bradycardia and other dysrhythmias • Liver damage
Isoflurane	• Inhalational • Volatile	• Rapid induction • Fewer cardiovascular effects than halothane	• Depressed respiration

■ **BOX 8.3** Rapid sequence induction

Rapid sequence (crash) induction is a technique used to anaesthetise patients who have a full stomach. Although seen primarily when dealing with emergency surgery it is a technique that is likely to be used when it becomes necessary to intubate a patient in an HDU. The technique follows four stages: pre-oxygenation, intravenous induction, relaxation with suxamethonium and intubation. Rapid sequence induction is almost always accompanied by cricoid pressure, a technique used to occlude the oesophagus to prevent gastric regurgitation. Oesophageal occlusion is achieved by applying direct backward pressure on the cricoid cartilage towards the cervical vertebrae (see Fig. 8.1). Although it appears relatively simple, cricoid pressure is not a technique that a novice should attempt, particularly in an emergency. It is suggested that HDU nurses practise the technique in controlled situations such as an anaesthetic room before assuming competence.

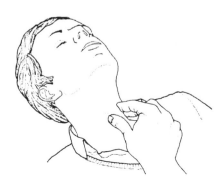

Fig. 8.1 Cricoid pressure. (Based on the ABC of Resuscitation reproduced by kind permission of BMJ Books.)

Muscle relaxant drugs such as suxamethonium and vecuronium are also used during anaesthesia and surgery. The main reasons for using these drugs are:

- To relax the vocal cords to allow endotracheal intubation
- To relax the muscles involved in respiration to allow effective artificial ventilation
- To relax striated muscle to facilitate surgery, e.g. laparotomy.

Insufficient reversal of muscle relaxants may lead to problems during the post-operative period. These are dealt with later in this chapter.

Regional anaesthesia

Regional anaesthesia aims to temporarily block nerve impulses from a particular area or region of the body. This can be very localised such as infiltrating a wound prior to suturing or widespread such as a spinal anaesthetic. The injection of local anaesthetic (e.g. lignocaine, bupivacaine) around nerve fibres results in blockage of nerve transmissions from a specific area of the body. The resulting anaesthesia can last for hours and provides the opportunity for pain-free surgery without the risks of general anaesthesia. This makes regional anaesthesia a good choice for patients with pre-existing medical problems such as chronic respiratory disease. It is not appropriate, however, for patients who are unable to co-operate or keep still, such as children or those with mental difficulties. Specific problems associated with regional anaesthesia are dealt with later in the relevant sections of this chapter.

The role of the anaesthetic assistant

It is not the intention of this chapter to examine the role of the nurse as anaesthetic assistant. This is an issue that arouses some debate (Preston 1996) and is a role that is more clearly developed in other countries such as the USA. However, it does appear that the skills required by an anaesthetic assistant or nurse anaesthetist are very similar to those held by a high dependency nurse.

OXYGEN THERAPY

The administration of oxygen will be frequently referred to during this chapter. Therefore, before discussing the assessment and management of the post-operative patient, it is worth considering oxygen therapy in more detail. The use of oxygen in the immediate post-operative phase is necessary to enhance the patient's recovery and to prevent potentially serious complications (Baxter et al 1993). The nurse caring for the post-operative patient needs to be aware of the reasons for administering oxygen, the methods of administration (see Box 8.4) and the potentially harmful effects. Traditionally oxygen has been treated as a drug to be given only when prescribed by a doctor. With the development of high dependency areas, pulse oximetry and easy access to blood gas analysis, however, nurses should be able to make informed judgements about when additional oxygen is necessary, at what percentage it should be given and when it can be reduced or discontinued.

By increasing the alveolar partial pressure of oxygen (PaO_2) the tension gradient of inhalational anaesthetic agents across the alveolar–capillary membrane is increased and, as a result, the elimination of anaesthetic is speeded up (Ashurst 1995). We will see later that hypoxia occurs for a variety of reasons following surgery and anaesthesia. The administration of supplemental oxygen in the immediate post-operative phase will help to reduce the risk of hypoxia occurring. The body's oxygen requirement will rise as a result of recent tissue damage.

■ **BOX 8.4** Oxygen delivery methods

Facemask

The most common form of O_2 delivery. Many types are available to allow the administration of different concentrations. Some are dependent on adaptors (e.g. Ventimasks) to provide a fixed percentage, others use the flow rate of O_2 to adjust the concentration delivered to the patient. **NB** The flows suggested are only an approximation and the actual percentage the patient receives is influenced by factors such as the fit of the mask and the patient's inspiratory flow rate. Using a reservoir attachment can achieve more stable and consistently higher concentrations. Some patients become claustrophobic when wearing a mask and others find the smell of the plastic unpleasant.

Nasal cannulae

These devices deliver low flows of O_2 but this is often sufficient to prevent hypoxia. Although they are less claustrophobic they can be uncomfortable and will dry out the mucous membranes of the nose. A more comfortable alternative is the nasal catheter which is held in place by a small cylinder of sponge in a single nostril. The side of the nose used should be changed regularly as this will reduce the drying effect.

T-piece

This device is used to deliver O_2 to self-ventilating patients who have endotracheal tubes or laryngeal mask airways in situ. By attaching the T-piece O_2 can be passed by the end of the tube/airway. Adding a short length of corrugated tubing creates a small reservoir of O_2 and helps to maintain a stable concentration. If use of the T-piece is required for any length of time continuous positive airway pressure (CPAP) should be considered as breathing against very little resistance can result in basal collapse.

Therefore, ensuring an adequate supply early on can have a positive effect on wound healing (Cooper 1990).

Following major surgery, oxygen may be required for 24 hours or more in order to optimise tissue oxygenation and minimise the risk of hypoxia (Catley et al 1985). It is important to note that the aim is to maintain normal levels of arterial blood gases and peripheral oxygen saturations, not unnecessarily high levels. Running an abnormally high arterial partial pressure of oxygen (PaO_2) is of no benefit to the patient, as once the oxygen capacity has been reached no further oxygen can be carried despite a rise in PaO_2.

It has long been thought that dry oxygen, given for long periods, dries out the mucous membranes of the upper airways. For this reason it is common practice to humidify the gas prior to the patient receiving it. This aims to reduce complications such as sputum retention and chest infection and improve patient comfort. Recent research has demonstrated however that there is no advantage, in terms of preventing chest infection and maintaining adequate oxygenation, in using cold water nebulising humidifiers rather than dry oxygen therapy (Kinoulty 1998). Indeed, patients receiving humidified oxygen were shown to have experienced more discomfort and disruption of sleep. Having said that, regular mouth toilet should be carried out on patients having long-term oxygen, i.e. more than about 4 hours. Adequate hydration is also essential in order to keep the mucous membranes moist.

Patients with chronic airways disease such as emphysema should have oxygen administered with care as their stimulus to breathe is a low PaO_2. They should be closely observed for signs of a rising $PaCO_2$ (see respiratory assessment) and, where there is concern, arterial blood gas analysis should be performed. As long as this group of patients is monitored and oxygen is used carefully, there is no reason why they should not have it. They are equally at risk of becoming hypoxic following surgery and so the idea that they should not have oxygen at all because of their chronic health is outdated and not in their best interests. The only patients who do not routinely require additional O_2 are those who have had their operation under local or regional anesthesia. However, many of these patients have had some sort of sedation and, as a result, may have depressed respiration. If this is the case, then they may also benefit from added O_2 until fully alert.

POST-OPERATIVE ASSESSMENT

The patient should arrive in the post-operative care unit (POCU) accompanied by the anaesthetist and another member of the theatre team, preferably the anaesthetic assistant or scrub assistant. A handover to the POCU nurse should be given which should include:

- Identification of the patient
- Relevant medical history, e.g. whether he suffers from respiratory disease or diabetes
- Details about the operation performed
- Type of anaesthesia used
- Any peri-operative problems
- Analgesia and any other drug therapy already given
- The presence of drains, intravenous cannulae, catheters or wound packs
- Any specific post-operative instructions, e.g. that the patient may require additional oxygen for an extended period.

This is also an opportunity for the POCU nurse to ensure that relevant documentation and prescription of analgesia, antiemesis, oxygen and intravenous fluid therapy has been completed.

During handover the nurse can make a preliminary assessment of the patient's general condition. When doing this it is useful to follow an ABC (Airway, Breathing, Circulation) model. The nurse should establish that the airway is patent and that the patient is breathing. Oxygen therapy and, if possible, pulse oximetry monitoring should be commenced. The patient's respiratory rate and pattern should be noted. Baseline observations of heart rate and arterial blood pressure should be made and recorded, and wounds and drains checked for excessive bleeding. The patient's level of consciousness and general demeanour should be noted.

Once this initial assessment has taken place, and the nurse considers it safe, the anaesthetist may leave the patient. A more detailed and methodical assessment of the patient should then be made. It is suggested that the ABC model is still followed but it is recognised that individuals may use variations such as 'top to toe' assessment. The important thing is that the nurse follows an assessment process that ensures that nothing is missed. The method outlined here will be based on a systems model although it is acknowledged that other models, adapted to the post-operative setting, may be equally effective.

> Using an ABC model of assessment will help the nurse to focus on the key priorities of care for a post-anaesthetic patient.

AIRWAY MANAGEMENT

Airway obstruction

Airway maintenance is of vital importance in the immediate post-operative phase. Unconsciousness, as a result of anaesthesia, means that the tongue can fall back and obstruct the airway. Even if anaesthesia has worn off, the peri-operative administration of opiates can have a similar effect.

Laryngospasm, as a result of upper airway irritation, causes airway obstruction even in a fully conscious patient. Regurgitation of stomach contents is possible during the immediate post-anaesthetic period and this is a real threat to airway maintenance. The patency of the airway is also at risk following any surgery in the region of the head and neck as a result of oedema or haematoma formation. Haemorrhage or foreign bodies – for example gauze packs used during dental surgery – can also obstruct the airway.

Assessment

An initial overview of the patient's condition can give vital clues as to the patency of the airway. There may be cyanosis present. There may be no movement of the chest or paradoxical (see-saw) breathing where the abdomen 'sucks in' as the chest expands and vice versa. The trachea may appear to suck inwards during inspiration (tracheal tug). Any of these signs can indicate severe or total obstruction. The breathing may be noisy as a result of soft palate obstruction indicated by snoring (stertor) or laryngospasm which results in a loud crowing noise on inspiration (stridor). It is important to remember that total obstruction is silent and so the absence of noisy breathing does not mean that the airway is clear. Confirmation of a patent airway can only really be achieved by ensuring that air is moving in and out of the nose and mouth by listening with your ear close to the patient's face, feeling with your hand over the nose and mouth or by looking, for example, at whether condensation is forming on the inside of the oxygen mask during expiration.

> Total airway obstruction is SILENT. A quiet patient is not necessarily a breathing patient: airway patency must be monitored continuously in an unconscious post-anaesthetic patient.

Airway adjuncts

The patient may arrive from the operating room with artificial airways in situ (Box 8.5). These should not be removed until the patient shows signs of being able to maintain his own airway. This would be indicated by, for example, an increase in conscious level, swallowing or gagging, or an attempt by the patient himself to remove the airway. Although it is safer to remove an endotracheal tube or laryngeal mask airway under controlled conditions, it is perfectly acceptable to let the patient remove a Guedel airway. This means that the nurse can be confident that he is ready to do without it. However, if there is evidence that the airway is causing the patient to gag it should be removed. This is because the situation can result in the patient vomiting – which in turn could lead to serious airway and respiratory complications.

■ **BOX 8.5** Artificial Airways

Guedel (oropharyngeal) airway (Fig. 8.2) – Curved plastic tubes with a flange at the oral end, they have a flattened shape so that they fit neatly between the tongue and hard palate. They come in a range of sizes and it is important to select the right one. Too large a size can cause vomiting and laryngospasm, too small will not maintain the airway. The patient's airway may still need to be manually opened even though a Guedel airway is inserted.

Nasopharyngeal airway (Fig. 8.3) – These are, made from malleable plastic with a bevel at one end and a flange at the other. Inserted where possible into the right nostril (because of the angle of the bevel end) using plenty of lubricant. A safety pin should be inserted through the flange to prevent the airway disappearing. This is better tolerated than the Guedel airway but risk of trauma is higher. Again, this may well require manual airway support as well.

Laryngeal mask airway (Fig. 8.4) – This device is essentially a mini-facemask that sits over the laryngeal inlet. An inflatable cuff creates an airtight seal allowing administration of anaesthetic gases and if necessary positive pressure ventilation. The major disadvantage is that, unlike a cuffed endotracheal tube, it does not protect the airway from aspiration of stomach contents. Left in situ following anaesthesia, however, it will prevent obstruction by the tongue. Although the manufacturers recommend that the cuff is deflated immediately prior to removal, this results in the displacement of secretions that have collected on the cuff and the nurse should be prepared for the patient to cough and should have suction equipment ready. There is a developing trend however to leave the cuff inflated during removal as this seems to remove pharyngeal secretions more effectively on the surface of the mask (Brimacombe et al 1996). This method should be used with care to avoid trauma to the teeth, mouth and the cuff itself. In practice the LMA is sometimes removed with the cuff partially deflated. This is less uncomfortable for the patient but retains most of the secretions.

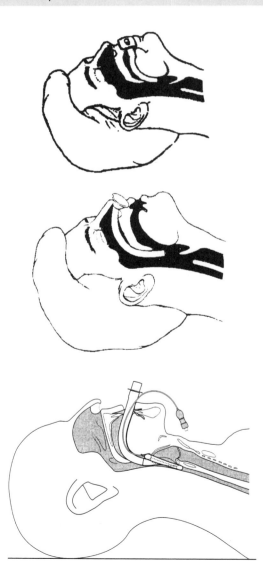

Fig. 8.2 Oropharyngeal airway in situ. (From Henry & Stapleton (1992) p 102 Reproduced by kind permission of the publishers W B Saunders.)

Fig. 8.3 Nasopharyngeal airway in situ. (From Henry & Stapleton (1992) p 104 Reproduced by kind permission of W B Saunders.)

Fig. 8.4 Laryngeal mask airway in situ. (From Eaton 1992, p 43. Reproduced by kind permission of the author.)

Intervention

When a patient is experiencing problems with his airway this should be dealt with immediately. In the unconscious patient, the airway should be manually supported until the patient is able to do so unaided. Placing the patient in the lateral (recovery) position (Fig 8.5) if his condition allows, is often sufficient to re-establish and maintain a patent airway. This may, however, make attachment of monitoring and assessment of vital signs and wounds more difficult.

Alternatively the nurse can move the tongue forward by using the head tilt/chin lift or jaw thrust methods (see Box 8.6). If the patient does not already have one, a Guedel airway can be inserted. However, if the patient is not completely unconscious this should be avoided because of the risk of stimulating a gag reflex and vomiting. The nurse should know that the successful insertion of a Guedel airway does not guarantee a patent airway, and that the patient may still require manual airway support. A nasopharyngeal airway can be used but the risk of epistaxis and the fact that they can be difficult to insert do not make them ideal in a situation where an airway needs to be established quickly. It is important to note that even if airway adjuncts are successful, patients who are unable to maintain their own airway should never be left unattended. Their condition can change rapidly and unpredictably.

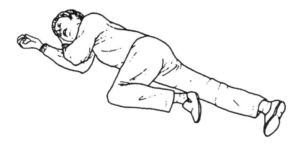

Fig. 8.5 Recovery position. (From *Resuscitation for the Citizen*, reproduced by kind permission of the Resuscitation Council.)

■ **BOX 8.6** Manual airway support (Resuscitation Council UK 1994)

Head tilt/chin lift (see Fig. 8.6)
1. Support the head on a small pillow.
2. Extend the head on the neck by pushing the forehead backwards and the occiput forwards.
3. Place two fingers under the tip of the mandible and lift the chin, displacing the tongue anteriorly.

(Cont'd)

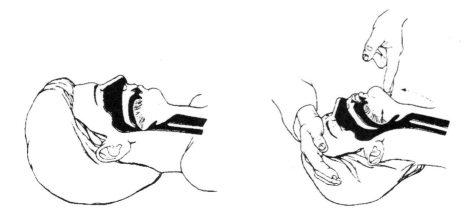

Fig. 8.6 Head tilt/chin lift. (From Henry & Stapleton 1992, p 51. Reproduced by kind permission of W B Saunders.)

(BOX 8.6 *Cont'd*)

Jaw thrust (see Fig. 8.7)
1. Hold the patient's mouth slightly open by pushing the chin down with the thumbs.
2. Place the fingers behind the angles of the mandible and apply steady upward and forward pressure to lift the jaw forward.

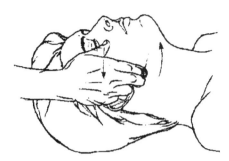

Fig. 8.7 Jaw thrust. (From Henry & Stapleton 1992, p 52. Reproduced by kind permission of W B Saunders.)

Laryngospasm

Laryngospasm is a protective reflex caused by irritation of the upper airway. It most commonly follows extubation or surgery in the area of the larynx or pharynx, for example tonsillectomy. It may also result from the presence of secretions or foreign bodies. It is characterised by a loud high-pitched crowing noise on inspiration.

When laryngospasm is present, it is vital to get help and to ensure that emergency equipment necessary for intubation and resuscitation is at hand. The patient's condition can deteriorate very rapidly as hypoxia develops. Treatment is initially aimed at maximising air entry and clearing the causative agent. If possible the patient should be sat up to make inspiration more effective and, if not already doing so, encouraged to cough to try and clear any secretions or foreign bodies. Oropharyngeal suction with a large bore (Yankauer) catheter should be performed if the patient is unable to clear the irritant himself. A high concentration of oxygen should be given via facemask to reduce the risk of hypoxia. If it is certain that the airway is clear then a bag and mask oxygen delivery system can be used to apply positive pressure in an attempt to relieve the laryngospasm (Murray-Calderon & Connolly 1997). In the semiconscious or unconscious patient, manual support of the airway should also be performed. If these methods are unsuccessful then the patient will require intubation and the condition allowed to settle before extubation is retried. It is important to remember that laryngospasm with moderate to severe airway obstruction can be present in a conscious patient and, as a result, he is likely to be extremely frightened. Not only might the patient experience difficulty breathing but he may also find the noise that he is making distressing. The nurse must be aware of this and provide appropriate support. The patient may be very sensitive to his surroundings and be aware of the potential severity of his condition, and it is important for the staff to remain calm and efficient as this can help to make the patient feel safe. A patient with laryngospasm who starts to panic and hyperventilate can be extremely difficult to manage. This patient is more likely to deteriorate faster than one who is able to maintain a slow, regular breathing pattern.

Summary

Airway maintenance must be the prime objective for the nurse during the immediate post-operative period. If a patient is experiencing airway problems that are not easily dealt with, such as the presence of a foreign body or acute swelling of the neck, help should always be summoned. A potentially manageable situation can rapidly develop into a very serious one if an airway is not established quickly and effectively. This can be prevented by having a more experienced nurse and/or anaesthetist/surgeon involved at an early stage.

RESPIRATORY FUNCTION

Once a clear airway has been established, the patient's respiratory function needs to be assessed. Respiratory management is covered in detail in Chapter 5 and this section will focus on the immediate post-operative period and management specific to anaesthesia and surgery.

Anaesthesia depresses respiration and, as the deep stages of anaesthesia are reached, breathing will actually cease. Some surgery, for example abdominal, requires muscle paralysis which, because of its effects on the respiratory muscles, causes respiratory arrest. Opiates given during surgery may depress respiration. The anaesthetist aims to have reversed these effects, with the exception of analgesia, by the time the patient leaves the operating room. There is, however, potential for severe respiratory depression to be present in the immediate post-operative period, if all of these things are not fully achieved.

Respiratory assessment

In order to make a comprehensive assessment of respiratory function the nurse needs to view the patient holistically. The patient's general demeanour should be noted. Restlessness, confusion or a decreased level of consciousness can have many causes in the post-operative patient. However, hypoxia and hypercapnia should be considered until proven otherwise. Pallor or cyanosis can indicate hypoxia. In patients with dark skin, the nailbeds and mucous membranes of the mouth should be looked at in order to make an accurate assessment. This is one of the reasons for removing nail varnish before surgery. Because carbon dioxide causes vasodilatation, a patient with a flushed appearance and very warm peripheries may be hypercapnic.

The respiratory rate and pattern should be assessed. A slow rate may be caused by opiate overdose or deep anaesthesia, and this may be accompanied by shallow breathing with resultant diminished tidal volumes. Shallow respirations may also be associated with tachypnoea (a rapid respiratory rate) and this most commonly results from pain, particularly following abdominal or thoracic surgery. A shallow respiratory pattern may also be the result of the continuing effects of muscle relaxants. If the nurse suspects this she can gain further information by asking the patient, if conscious, to open his eyes wide, stick out his tongue or grasp the nurse's hand tightly. An inability to do these things or an obvious lack of power could indicate that there are some continuing effects from the paralysing agents. Confirmation can be made by the use of a nerve stimulator. This battery-powered device delivers small electric stimuli via two skin electrodes placed over a peripheral nerve. The resulting motor responses to stimuli give an idea as to the extent of neuromuscular blockade. This technique should only be used by people who have been trained to use the device safely.

Movement of the chest wall should be assessed. Both sides of the chest should move upwards and outwards during inspiration. Uneven movement indicates that one lung is inflating less effectively that the other. This can be due to lobar collapse as a result of sputum retention, pneumothorax or haemothorax. The position of the trachea should be noted, as a deviation from the midline can indicate a tension pneumothorax, which will develop into a potentially life-threatening situation if not treated promptly. Palpation of the chest wall can help to assess the symmetry of movement. One can also feel coarse crepitations which indicate sputum in the larger airways. Surgical emphysema, a condition usually associated with pneumothorax (where air leaks from the pleural cavity into the subcutaneous tissues), may also be felt as a crackling sensation under the skin. Severe surgical emphysema around the neck can, in itself, cause airway obstruction.

Auscultation of the lung fields provides valuable information. In addition to confirming decreased air entry and the presence of loose secretions, fine crackles may indicate pulmonary oedema as a result of, for example, left ventricular failure or fluid overload. Wheezes or loud musical sounds indicate bronchospasm. This is most commonly associated with pre-existing respiratory disease such as asthma and chronic obstructive airway disease but may also result from anaphylaxis due to drug or blood product administration.

Pulse oximetry is a useful adjunct to assessing lung function and a reduced peripheral oxygen saturation (SPO_2) can indicate decreased gas exchange at alveolar level. An accurate measurement is however dependent on a good signal at the site of the probe. An unreliable reading may result from a patient with poor peripheral circulation – for example, someone who is cold or shocked. Changing the monitoring site and using a dedicated probe on the nose or earlobe may produce a better signal. Ambient light sources can also interfere with the signal and a reduction in the amount of light interference by, for example, placing the hand under the bedclothes can help to achieve a more accurate reading. It is essential to view the plethysmographic wave on the pulse oximeter produced by the patient's pulse in order to ensure that an accurate reading is being achieved. It is important not to accept the numerical display as being accurate unless there is a clearly defined and supportive plethysmographic waveform. Although pulse oximetry gives useful information about oxygenation, it does not necessarily give any information about how well the lungs are being ventilated. There have been cases where patients with a normal SpO_2 have been found to have dangerously high blood levels of carbon dioxide as a result of hypoventilation (Davidson & Hosie 1993). Where hypoxia or hypercapnia is suspected it is essential to confirm this by taking an arterial blood sample for blood gas analysis (see Ch. 5).

In order to complete the picture of the patient's respiratory status a chest X-ray can be performed. This can confirm the cause of diminished respiratory function, in particular pneumothorax, lobar collapse due to sputum retention and pulmonary oedema. It will also give valuable information regarding the position of endotracheal tubes, pleural drains and central venous lines.

Ensure that you have a clearly defined waveform on the pulse oximeter before you are confident that you have a correct numerical reading. Also remember that pulse oximetry measures O_2 saturation not CO_2 levels: a satisfactory SpO_2 does not necessarily mean that the patient is breathing effectively.

Respiratory management

While the majority of patients in the immediate post-operative period will not have respiratory problems, it is said that hypoxia is the most common and dangerous cause of damage to patients during this period (Hatfield & Tronson 1996). While the nurse has a vital role to play in detecting respiratory insufficiency as outlined above, her main role must be to prevent it occurring in the first place. Where decreased respiratory function is present, it is important to establish the cause and treat it appropriately (see Box 8.7). However, as every patient has the potential to develop breathing problems the nurse can reduce the risks substantially by intervening early.

■ **BOX 8.7** Causes of decreased respiratory function and initial interventions

Anaesthesia
Maintain airway, give O_2, monitor SpO_2, provide stimulus to wake (shake patient gently and call name). Consider giving flumazenil if benzodiazepines have been used in surgery or as pre-medication.

Opiate effects
Maintain airway, give O_2, monitor SpO_2, encourage patient to take deep breaths. Consider naloxone but expect patient to wake in pain; alternatively use doxapram to increase respiratory rate and depth.

Residual paralysis
Maintain airway, give O_2, monitor SpO_2, provide reassurance if patient awake. Give neostigmine to reverse paralysing agents.

Basal collapse
Give O_2, monitor SpO_2, encourage deep breathing and coughing exercises, sit patient up, change position regularly, consider CPAP, involve physiotherapist.

Pneumothorax
Give O_2, monitor SpO_2, prepare for chest drain insertion. If tension pneumothorax develops with acute deterioration in patient condition consider needle thoracocentesis.

Pain
Give O_2, monitor SpO_2, give adequate analgesia or consider alternative analgesia if present method not effective. Change patient's position, show patient how to support wound to aid deep breathing.

Heart failure
Give O_2, monitor SpO_2, sit patient up, consider diuretics, vasodilators and inotropic support.

Once the patient is awake a series of regular exercises, sometimes known as the 'stir-up' regimen, can be used to minimise the risk of respiratory problems. This is where the patient is encouraged to take deep breaths and cough at regular intervals. In practice, it is easy to incorporate this into the regular assessments that the nurse makes of the patient. Although recovered from anaesthesia, the patient may still be sleepy: co-ordinating stir-up exercises with other assessments helps to minimise interruptions to necessary rest. The nurse can help the patient to deep breathe effectively by placing her hands on the chest wall and encouraging the patient to try and push the hands away by taking the deepest breath possible. When maximum inspiration is achieved, asking the patient to hold his breath, close his mouth and take a small 'sniff' will help to prevent areas of lung collapsing as well as reinflating those areas that might have collapsed already. In addition to this, the patient should be encouraged to cough which will again help to prevent atelectasis and reinflate collapsed areas of the lungs. When abdominal or thoracic surgery has been performed the patient should be instructed to hold his wound, having first covered it with a folded towel or small pillow, as this can make it less painful and helps to reduce the patient's fear of 'bursting his stitches'. Both of these exercises are easier to perform with the patient in the sitting position unless this is contraindicated, for example, following surgery on the spinal column. Unless otherwise specified or indicated, the patient should be helped to sit up as soon as he is awake enough to do so. Sitting up will also improve expansion of the lung bases. It should be noted that following certain types of surgery, such as ophthalmic or neurological, coughing should not be encouraged as the resultant

Encouraging early deep breathing and coughing helps to reduce post-operative respiratory complications.

Table 8.3 Cardiovascular effects

Effect	Possible cause
Dysrhythmias	• Anaesthetic agents and drugs • Hypoxia • Hypokalaemia
Hypotension	• Anaesthetic agents and drugs • Hypovolaemia/haemorrhage • Epidural/spinal anaesthesia
Hypertension	• Fluid overload • Peripheral vasoconstriction • Pain/anxiety • Pre-existing hypertension
Haemorrhage	• Incomplete surgical haemostasis • Ruptured suture line/slipped tie
Heart failure	• Fluid overload

rise in local pressure can be detrimental to the patient's condition. This is important because the high intrathoracic pressures generated during coughing can be transmitted to, for example, the blood vessels in the brain. Following neurosurgery, where maintaining a low intracranial pressure is critical, this is clearly undesirable.

These exercises will be difficult, if not impossible, for patients to perform if they are in a lot of pain. This is particularly true following abdominal and thoracic surgery. The importance of adequate pain relief in preventing post-operative respiratory problems cannot be stressed strongly enough (Aitkenhead 1996).

CARDIOVASCULAR SYSTEM

Anaesthesia and surgery can have major effects on the cardiovascular system (Table 8.3).

Assessment

When first accepting a patient the nurse should carry out a general assessment of the patient's cardiovascular status. Pallor, clammy skin, weak peripheral pulses and cool extremities can all be signs of a poor cardiac output and/or hypovolaemia. Wounds should be checked for any obvious bleeding or haematoma formation and volumes of blood in any drainage systems should be noted. The patient's temperature should be taken, preferably using a tympanic thermometer, to ensure that the patient is not hypothermic. There is a vast range of techniques available for monitoring cardiovascular parameters, such as ECG monitoring and automated non-invasive blood pressure measurement, and choice depends upon patient need and the availability of equipment. It is important, however, that nurses do not become over-dependent upon technology and forget, for example, how to use the manual palpation of pulses, manual auscultation of blood pressures and water CVP manometers as measurement tools. It will after all be these techniques that will have to be employed in the event of equipment failure or non-availability. It is also important to use these techniques to check the accuracy of automated equipment, as such equipment can often be inaccurate, especially if not regularly serviced or checked. Nevertheless, the bare minimum is regular monitoring of heart rate and blood pressure as these give fundamental information about cardiovascular status. Changes in these parameters can be a good indicator of impending problems. The frequency of these measurements is really dependent on the condition of the patient but the important thing is to measure and record them regularly so that any trends can be seen. 'One-off' measurements can be highly subjective and give little useful information.

Advanced cardiovascular monitoring is covered in more detail in Chapter 6. However, the following may be useful in the immediate post-operative period, when the patient can be particularly unstable and may require warming and/or rapid replacement of fluid volume:

- ECG
- Invasive arterial blood pressure
- Central venous pressure
- Urine volume measurement
- Peripheral temperature.

Drugs

Virtually all anaesthetic agents and drugs used during surgery have the potential to cause cardiovascular changes. A look at all the possibilities is beyond the scope of this chapter. Nonetheless, the anaesthetic record should always be checked to see what drugs and types of anaesthetic have been used, as this can often help in determining the treatment of post-operative problems. It is also important to check which drugs have been given during the operation, for example antiemetics, in order to ensure that they are not given again in the immediate post-operative period, as this could represent overdosage.

Dysrhythmias

The majority of dysrhythmias seen immediately post-operatively tend to be sinus tachycardia or bradycardia. These are normally related to drug therapy, hypovolaemia, pain and anxiety. The main aim of management should be to treat the causative factor, not the rhythm. It is also worth looking at the pre-operative ECG, if available, as this can save a lot of anxiety for the staff as the patient may have a pre-existing abnormal ECG. Many patients with hypertension are treated with beta-blockers and bradycardia is normal for them. Again, the important thing is whether or not the patient's condition is compromised. A patient with a heart rate of 120 who is otherwise stable should be observed and the tachycardia not treated unless there is a deterioration in condition. A patient with a heart rate of 50 who is hypotensive and complains of feeling light-headed may need to have the rate speeded up with drugs such as atropine or glycopyrrolate. However, in such an instance the opinion of a medical colleague should be sought.

Atrial fibrillation is frequently seen and its treatment depends on the patient's pre-operative state and whether or not it is causing problems. The serum potassium should be checked and digoxin given if necessary. Ventricular extrasystoles (ectopics) are usually due to hypokalaemia and this should be corrected. Antiarrhythmic drug therapy is only usually used if the extrasystoles are frequent and may potentially compromise the patient's condition. Very often, the more common dysrhythmias are benign and do not need treatment (Aitkenhead 1996).

Less common arrhythmias associated with pre-existing heart disease or peri-operative myocardial infarction are covered in Chapter 6 and so will not be dealt with here.

Hypo- and hypertension

Hypotension is often directly related to anaesthesia and, as such, usually ceases to be a problem as the anaesthesia wears off. The overall condition of the patient needs to be assessed before treatment of hypotension is initiated. A sleeping

■ **BOX 8.8** Malignant hyperpyrexia

Malignant hyperpyrexia is a hereditary disorder of calcium metabolism. Following administration of a triggering agent, usually inhalational anaesthetic agents or depolarising muscle relaxants, there is an excess release of calcium ions in the muscle tissues. This results in massive and continuous skeletal muscle contraction with associated buildup of heat. The temperature can rise rapidly by as much as 6°C/hour. Left untreated, the patient will die. The only effective treatment is sodium dantrolene which inhibits calcium ion release. The nurse working in the post-operative care unit must be aware of where the stock of this drug is kept. Other measures include stopping the administration of the triggering agent and active cooling of the patient. This is immediately life threatening and expert medical help should be summoned without delay.

patient who is stable, except for a systolic blood pressure of 80 mmHg, should be allowed to wake before a decision to treat the blood pressure is made.

Patients having spinal anaesthesia are often hypotensive as the blocking of the sympathetic nerves, due to this technique, can cause peripheral vasodilatation. The reason that these patients should not sit up until they regain feeling in their legs is that they cannot vasoconstrict and would consequently pass out, or at least feel very unwell, as the blood drained from their heads. As chronic respiratory or heart disease is often the reason for using spinal anaesthesia, it is not wise to treat the hypotension with large volumes of fluid. More commonly ephedrine, a vasoconstrictor, is used to raise the blood pressure.

Patients who are cold following surgery can become hypotensive as they warm and peripherally vasodilate. This is managed by giving colloid solutions, preferably while monitoring central venous pressure. Where hypotension is as a result of cardiac insufficiency, it may be necessary to use inotropic agents (see Ch 6). A rare but serious cause of hypotension is malignant hyperpyrexia (see Box 8.8). Although most commonly seen during anaesthesia, it is important for the post-operative care nurse to be aware of it and its treatment.

> Patients who have had spinal anaesthesia should be sat up gradually to avoid dizziness and syncope. They should not stand up until full sensation has returned to their legs.

The two most common causes of hypertension in the immediate post-operative period are pre-existing peripheral vascular disease and pain. Unfortunately, it is quite common for oral antihypertensive drugs to be omitted on the morning of operation as the patient is nil by mouth. Although evidence suggests that it is safe for the patient to take a small volume of fluid prior to surgery (Haines 1995) this is not widely practised and, as a result, normal medication is often not given. The result is that the normally well-controlled patient can become hypertensive during or after surgery. When patients are taking regular antihypertensive drugs, the ward nurse should contact the anaesthetist if there is any doubt as to whether the drugs should be given. Unless their blood pressure is at a dangerous level the best treatment is to recommence their normal drug therapy as soon as they can tolerate fluids. Pain control will be covered later in this chapter but suffice to say that the provision of adequate analgesia can greatly reduce the blood pressure.

> Unless specifically requested, regular medications should not be omitted on the grounds that the patient is 'nil by mouth'.

Following certain types of surgery, for example cardiac and vascular, it is important to keep the blood pressure below a certain level to protect the integrity of vascular suture lines. In order to achieve this it can be necessary to use intravenous vasodilators, such as glyceryl trinitrate or sodium nitroprusside.

Haemorrhage

Nearly all surgery involves some degree of blood loss and the degree of post-operative bleeding is dependent on the type of surgery. For example, there can be significant blood loss expected following knee replacement whereas one would not expect this following thyroidectomy.

When assessing post-operative bleeding the overall cardiovascular status should be taken into account rather than simply looking at the volume of ooze or drainage. Techniques such as girth measurement and drawing around the ooze on dressings do not give a very reliable indication of the degree of bleeding. Take, for example, a patient who is cardiovascularly stable and peripherally warm following orthopaedic surgery, but continues to drain 200 ml/hour into vacuum drains. This patient would cause no real concern as long as he is given blood to replace the losses. However, there should be great concern about a patient following laparotomy who is persistently tachycardic, hypotensive, cold and oliguric despite continued colloid filling.

The management of haemorrhage should aim at preventing complications by maintaining an adequate circulating volume and haemoglobin content. Observed losses, for example into drains, should be replaced with colloid, preferably blood. Where bleeding is less obvious, filling should be guided by vital signs and, where possible, central venous pressure measurements. Haemoglobin levels should be measured, particularly when large volumes of plasma have been infused. If felt appropriate, a clotting screen should be performed and, where indicated, clotting agents such as fresh frozen plasma given. Following surgery where heparin is used, such as cardiac and vascular, the administration of protamine sulphate aims to stop any continuing heparinisation.

Obvious oozing from a wound should be treated by applying a pressure dressing which should then be monitored closely. When bleeding from a wound is heavy or sudden, direct manual pressure should be applied and maintained while a surgeon is summoned. If this does not stem the flow, it is likely that exploration of the wound in theatre will be required. A return to theatre may be necessary where bleeding is suspected but not visible, for example, intra-abdominally. In certain cases, wounds may need to be opened quickly as haematoma formation may put the patient at risk – for example following thyroidectomy – where a patent airway could be threatened. For this reason, wounds for this type of surgery are often closed with clips or staples which are easier to remove than sutures. The nurse caring for these patients should have clip/staple removers easily to hand. Occasionally, sudden catastrophic haemorrhage may occur – following vascular surgery for example. As well as the measures outlined above, rapid fluid administration will be necessary including non-crossmatched blood (O negative) if indicated. It may also be necessary to initiate cardiopulmonary resuscitation if the patient either becomes pulseless or ceases to have an effective cardiac output.

If large volumes of stored blood need to be given because of a major haemorrhage, patients can become hypothermic and it is best to give the blood through a warming system where possible. Clotting problems may also develop, as stored blood is deplete of clotting factors, and it is common to give fresh frozen plasma after every few units of blood to try and reduce this problem.

Hypothermia

Hypothermia is said to exist when the body temperature drops to 35°C or less (Surkitt-Parr 1992). There are many reasons why hypothermia develops in the surgical patient, including the effects of anaesthesia, insufficient covering, the ambient temperature of operating theatres (21–24°C), the length of surgery and pre-operative fasting (McNeil 1998). Although measures are often taken in theatre to reduce the risk of hypothermia, such as the use of warming mattresses and blankets, it is common for patients to be hypothermic post-operatively. It is important to monitor the patient's temperature frequently during the initial period. Mild hypothermia (35°C) can be managed by using woollen blankets and ensuring that the patient is not unnecessarily exposed; for example, ensure that arms and shoulders are covered with bedclothes. At temperatures below 35°C active warming should be performed. This can be done using forced warm-air technology. This involves the use of a warm air blower and an inflatable quilt. The quilt is placed next to the patient and warm air escapes from the underside. This has been shown to be the most effective way of warming post-operative patients (Giuffre et al 1991) and is becoming increasingly popular. However, because the technique is so effective, care should be taken not to overheat the patient and so avoid the problems of sudden rewarming, as mentioned earlier.

NEUROLOGICAL STATUS

Assessment

During anaesthesia there is obviously a marked change in neurological status. At the lower stages of anaesthesia the patient is deeply unconscious and loses many of the normal reflexes. When anaesthesia is stopped, the patient emerges from unconsciousness passing through the stages of anaesthesia in reverse. This is important as it gives the nurse dealing with a waking patient an idea of what stage of recovery has been reached. It also gives some insight into the reasons for the patient's behaviour. Generally, the lines of distinction between the stages are blurred and the patient simply wakes up without difficulty. Reactions are sometimes very marked, however, and it is important to remember that a restless, confused or aggressive patient may simply be passing through the delirium stage.

Formal assessment of a patient's neurological function is only really necessary if he does not wake as expected or remains confused or distressed. Neurological assessment is dealt with in detail in Chapter 7 and so will not be discussed here. From the point of view of immediate post-anaesthetic assessment, the patient's name should be called and, if necessary, he can be gently shaken by the shoulders. If this fails to elicit a response then he should be left to sleep and another attempt made to rouse him a few minutes later. Painful stimuli – for example rubbing the sternum, twisting ear lobes or even slapping the face – should *never* be used to wake the patient up! Indeed nurses should, in general, avoid these altogether. They are extremely painful and potentially harmful and, if not done for good reason, are tantamount to assault. The application of controlled painful stimuli, such as applying pressure to nailbeds or testing palmar reflexes, should be used only as part of a full neurological assessment when there is genuine concern about the patient's level of consciousness. In addition, these techniques should only be carried out by staff who are proficient and skilled in this area. The point at which one should become concerned about the patient not waking up is dependent on many factors. These include the type and length of anaesthetic, whether or not pre-medication was given, what analgesia was given in theatre, and the patient's age, general health and pre-operative neurological state.

It is important to make the distinction between the sleeping and the unconscious patient. Where reflexes are present, the airway is being self-maintained and there is some response to stimuli, it is likely that the patient is in a deep sleep, possibly due to opiate analgesia. It could also be due to pre-medication still having an effect or merely because the patient is physically exhausted. It tends to be forgotten that patients may have very little rest in the days leading up to surgery, often as a result of anxiety, sleeping in an unfamiliar environment and constant interruptions. If they have undergone emergency surgery they may well have endured days of discomfort or pain. It should not be surprising then, that when it is all over and their pain is well controlled, they can sleep deeply for a considerable time. The sleeping patient may stir from time to time and respond to stimuli, although he may not be able to keep his eyes open or talk coherently. However, the unconscious patient will not respond and may well require assistance to maintain a patent airway. An unconscious patient for example will tolerate a Guedel airway, while a sleeping patient will tend not to. It is the patient who remains unconscious for a long time who should cause concern.

Serious neurological problems following anaesthesia are rare (Boulton & Blogg, 1989) but some people do have over-sensitive reactions and can remain unconscious for hours; this is sometimes referred to as delayed emergence (Hatfield & Tronson 1996). Treatment of this condition is mainly supportive, including artificial ventilation if necessary. More commonly, the combination of pre-medication, anaesthetic and opiate analgesia is the cause of prolonged unconsciousness. If it is felt necessary, the administration of naloxone will usually wake the patient. Naloxone acts by blocking the effects of opiates which means that, unless used very carefully, the patient can wake rapidly in a large degree of pain. Its judicious use can however establish that there is no serious neurological problem. It is important to appreciate that naloxone has a very short half-life, and repeated doses may be required to maintain satisfactory levels of neurological and respiratory function. The use of benzodiazepines (e.g. diazepam) as pre-medication can also delay a return to consciousness, particularly if they are given very near the time of surgery. If this is suspected, flumazenil (Annexate) may be used as an antidote.

As in every situation, the level of consciousness should not be viewed in isolation and the patient's general condition should be carefully assessed before treatment is initiated. For example, in a patient who is profoundly hypotensive, getting the blood pressure up is more likely to improve the conscious level than administering naloxone. This also avoids the undesirable reversal of analgesia.

Neurological assessment during the immediate post-operative period is not confined to the central nervous system. A large range of regional and local blocks may be used instead of general anaesthesia or as post-operative pain relief. These should be assessed not only to make sure that they are working but also to protect the patient from injury. Following spinal anaesthesia, for example, the patient should not be allowed to stand until full sensation has returned to his legs otherwise he is likely to fall over. Because of reduced sensation and mobility, these patients are also at risk of pressure-related injuries, in the same way as a paraplegic might be. It is essential for the nurse to ensure that areas at risk, for example heels and the sacral area, are diligently assessed. Where necessary, pressure-relieving devices, such as low airloss beds, should be considered. However, as the effects of the block are transient, regular monitoring and changes of position should be effective. Where local blocks have been used the affected area should be protected until sensation returns in order to avoid injury. The nurse should be particularly aware of this as it is all too easy to trap an anaesthetised hand between a bed and trolley without any reaction from the patient.

> Painful stimuli should be used only as part of a formal neurological assessment: never use them simply to wake a patient up.

FLUID MANAGEMENT

The management of fluid balance will be covered in detail in Chapter 10. There are certain things that should be borne in mind when looking after the post-surgical patient. It is important to establish the amount and type of fluid that has been given and lost in theatre as this can have a bearing on the patient's overall condition. Colloid will only normally be given if there has been significant blood loss in theatre. Generally crystalloid such as Hartmann's solution is given as necessary to maintain the patient's blood pressure, replace insensible losses and to rehydrate them following a period of fasting.

Post-operative fluid regimens are dependent on factors such as weight, age, measured blood loss and the anticipated time before oral fluids will be taken. It is now fairly standard practice following major surgery to give fluid based on measurement of central venous pressure and urine output, where appropriate, rather than simply giving a certain volume over a period of time. This approach is often safer, more effective and better geared to the individual.

Following major surgery it is common for the patient to have an indwelling urinary catheter. This allows better assessment of fluid requirements and cardiovascular status. The urine output may be low following surgery. This is often due to the fact that no fluids have been taken by the patient for up to 16 hours as it is still common practice, although largely unnecessary, to allow nothing by mouth from midnight on the day before the operation. If the urine is very concentrated or volume is small it is usually no real cause for concern as long as the patient is not cardiovascularly compromised. It is likely that it will improve as the patient starts to take oral fluids or is rehydrated intravenously. It may be necessary to increase the rate of intravenous fluids or give a fluid challenge if the urine output is very low. As a rule of thumb, a urine output of 0.5–1.0 ml/kg/h is aimed for.

When there is no urine output at all it is best to check for mechanical problems before pouring fluid into the patient. The position of the catheter should be checked to make sure it is correctly sited. A bladder washout with saline can be performed in case a blood clot or debris is blocking the catheter lumen. If fluid can be injected but not aspirated it indicates that there is some form of obstruction. This may be caused by the retaining balloon and removing a few ml of water from it may improve the situation. If the problem persists then the catheter may well need changing.

If the urine output remains poor despite the patient being adequately filled, with a reasonable blood pressure and a patent catheter, a dopamine infusion at a rate which will improve renal perfusion (2–5 mcg/kg/min) should be commenced. Diuretics such as frusemide should only be used if there is evidence of fluid overload or retention or signs of heart failure. Using diuretics simply to improve the figures on the chart without resolving the cause results in a dehydrated patient who will stop passing urine later on.

PAIN CONTROL

Good pain control is vital following surgery. Uncontrolled pain not only is distressing for the patient but delays recovery and increases the risk of post-operative complications (Hauer et al 1995). Pain assessment and management will be dealt with in detail in Chapter 11. This section will focus on the relief of immediate post-operative pain.

Analgesic drugs are usually given during surgery to keep the patient pain free during the procedure and, in an ideal situation, this should continue into the immediate and later post-operative periods. In practice, analgesia given in theatre, apart from epidural and spinal, will have lost some of its effectiveness by the time the patient wakes up. The anaesthetist has to balance the positive side of good post-operative analgesia against the negative aspects of the patient not waking up or breathing effectively. It is therefore common for nurses to have to deal with patients waking up in some degree of pain, varying from mild to very severe. Dealing with pain often becomes the priority as the distress it causes makes any accurate assessment of the patient's condition impossible. Fortunately, there are a number of types of pain control available which are very effective in the immediate post-operative period:

- Non-steroidal anti-inflammatory drugs (NSAIDs)
- Opiates
- Regional and local blocks.

NSAIDs

This group of drugs – it includes paracetamol, coproxamol and diclofenac – is useful for mild to moderate pain. Although they are not the first choice in treating acute severe pain, they are extremely effective in treating deep aching pain as seen following orthopaedic or gynaecological surgery, for example. Given either during surgery or at the same time as opiates, they can provide an excellent, long lasting combination of analgesia. There are many preparations available and they can be given by a variety of routes. One of the most commonly used is diclofenac (Voltarol). Voltarol may be given rectally as well as orally which is useful if the patient is nauseated or vomiting.

Opiates

Opiates are by far the most common type of analgesia used for acute post-operative pain. Although there are many preparations, the two most commonly used are morphine and diamorphine. The usual routes of administration are intramuscular, intravenous and epidural. Intramuscular (i.m.) injection remains popular. It gives good pain relief for moderate to severe pain within 15–30 minutes of administration. The duration of analgesia is dependent on the preparation but i.m. morphine, for example, can last for up to 3–4 hours. The drawback to the intramuscular route is that there are peaks and troughs of effectiveness. Ideally, the drug should be given regularly whether the patient has pain or not. What tends to happen, however, is that the doses are given when the patient requests them, meaning that the patient has to experience pain in order to get analgesia, which is far from ideal.

Constant analgesia can be achieved by running a continuous infusion. The infusion can be run subcutaneously but the intravenous route is felt to be slightly more effective for acute post-operative pain. The problem with using opiates by continuous intravenous infusion is that the effect is cumulative and the risk of overdose is high unless the patient's conscious level is carefully monitored. As this would effectively mean waking the patient every 30–60 minutes, it rather defeats the object of providing good analgesia. A technique rapidly growing in popularity in the area of post-operative analgesia is patient controlled analgesia (PCA). This involves intravenous opiate being delivered via a device which allows the patient to administer regular analgesia as he requires it. There are many different devices on the market but effectively they all do the same thing, which is to allow the patient to deliver a fixed dose of analgesia at set intervals. These parameters either are fixed as in some of the disposable systems or may be determined by nursing and medical staff. The great advantage of PCA over continuous infusion is that it puts the patient in control. It also makes overdose virtually impossible as the patient has to be conscious in order to deliver a dose. It is important to note that in order for this method to be fully effective, the patient will require full, and quite possibly repeated, explanation of how it works. It is also essential that the nurse undertakes regular assessment of the patient and the effectiveness of the analgesia. The fact that analgesia is patient controlled does not mean that the nurse is not involved in its management.

Giving statutory intravenous doses of opiate has a place in the immediate post-operative period in order to rapidly control pain. The doses should be small and given regularly until the pain is relieved. It is important to achieve good analgesia by this method before commencing continuous infusion or PCA otherwise they will simply not be effective. In the case of continuous infusion, this will allow the rate to be set at a reasonable level. The temptation otherwise will be for the nurse to increase the rate to the maximum prescribed dose, and as a result the patient gets far more of the drug than he actually needs. If a patient in pain is simply connected to a PCA system he will end up demanding doses more frequently than he is able to get them Not only will the pain not be controlled but he will grow frustrated and disillusioned with the system.

Epidural administration of opiates, usually by continuous infusion, is particularly effective for surgery of the lower limbs, pelvis and abdomen. Pain from thoracic surgery can also be well controlled by an epidural sited at cervical level. Less commonly, epidural analgesia is managed with a PCA system, although this tends to be most often used with obstetric patients.

Opiates depress the central nervous system. Of particular importance is depression of the respiratory centre. Any patient receiving opiates, particularly by continuous infusion, should have his conscious level and respiratory function closely and regularly monitored. This should involve regular checks on conscious level and respiratory rate at the very minimum. Where possible, the peripheral oxygen saturation should be continuously monitored. It is standard practice for a patient having an opiate infusion to be prescribed naloxone. This is often instructed to be given if the respiratory rate falls below a certain level, but this is often an arbitrary figure and it is wise to perform a thorough assessment of the patient and to try and rouse him before giving naloxone. Obviously, if the patient is unrousable with a slow respiratory rate, then the opiate effects should be reversed. Whenever the nurse is attending to post-operative patients, particularly those having opiate analgesia, it is good practice to encourage them to take a few deep breaths and to cough. This will greatly reduce the risk of atelectasis (collapse of alveoli) and chest infection.

Regional and local blocks

Epidural administration of opiates has already been mentioned; however, local anaesthetic can also be given by this route. This blocks pain impulses in the peripheral nervous system and so has the advantage of not creating drowsiness or respiratory depression. It does, however, produce paraesthesia and so decreases patient mobility and, as mentioned earlier, can cause hypotension. In practice, epidural infusions tend to be made up of local anaesthetic and opiate mixed together. This allows smaller doses of each to be used, reaping the benefits of both, but minimising the unwanted side effects.

Local or regional blocks are achieved by infiltrating the area around a nerve with local anaesthetic. These can be very localised such as a ring block or can cover a wider area such as spinal anaesthetic. These blocks are very effective and completely numb the area. This means that the actual surgery can be performed using them, so avoiding the risks of general anaesthesia. Even if the patient does have an anaesthetic they provide good analgesia post-operatively. The effects last anything up to 4–6 hours but it is wise to commence some other form of analgesia once sensation starts to return, so that the pain does not get out of control. In certain situations a catheter can be left in situ through which local anaesthetic may be given by continuous infusion. This is particularly effective following thoracic surgery where the tip of the catheter is situated near the nerves supplying a specific area of the chest wall (paravertebral block). A growing practice is for surgeons to instil the tissues with local anaesthetic before the wound is closed. This can mean that the patient is completely pain free for a couple of hours post-operatively which is a great benefit, particularly in terms of the necessary deep breathing and coughing in the initial recovery phase.

Pain control is one of the most important aspects of post-operative care and the nurse has a primary role in ensuring that it is achieved. A patient in pain is difficult to manage and this can make other aspects of his condition harder to assess. By effectively controlling pain, recovery can be quicker and complications reduced.

WOUND CARE

Wound management is a huge subject, and detailed examination is beyond the scope of this book. There is a massive range of proposed strategies (Moore 1997, Courtenay 1998, Lait & Smith 1998;) and of products available on the market. Every hospital is likely to have an infection control team who are instrumental in developing local wound-care protocols. In addition to this, surgeons will have their own preferences as to how wounds should be managed. With this in mind, this chapter will not go into specifics but will concentrate on the basic principles of management of fresh surgical wounds and the more common post-operative complications.

Wounds should be checked regularly as part of the overall post-operative assessment. More often than not this is a cursory glance at the dressing to make sure that there is no obvious bleeding, swelling or reddening of the skin. Immediately following surgery there are unlikely to be any signs of infection, but reddening may occur because of an allergic reaction to the dressing itself and/or the skin preparation. Although most dressings are now hypoallergenic, elastoplast is still used where it is necessary to apply pressure to the wound and many people are allergic to this. If an allergic reaction is suspected the dressing should be removed and an alternative used. Care should be taken when removing the dressing as skin can be pulled away at the same time, particularly in the elderly or where blistering has occurred.

The main complication associated with fresh wounds is haemorrhage. This may be obvious, or may result in haematoma formation. Where there is overt bleeding from the wound, direct pressure should be applied and a surgical opinion sought. Initially, the pressure should be applied over the existing dressing but this may have to be removed for either better assessment or renewal. The aim should be to keep any contact with the wound aseptic. If the bleeding is heavy, however, the priority is to stop it and so a clean technique is acceptable. At the very least, universal precautions (such as wearing gloves) should be followed to protect staff. Often a period of direct pressure, followed by some form of pressure dressing is sufficient to stop the bleeding. If this is not the case then re-exploration of the wound in theatre may be necessary. It should be remembered that a little blood goes a long way, and that what may appear to be a significant bleed may only amount to a few millilitres. Surgical dressings are designed to absorb blood, thereby taking it away from the wound; a bloodstained dressing pad is best left alone as it is doing what it is supposed to do. Only if blood is seeping through should one consider changing it. Even then, it may be better to apply a pad over the top of the existing dressing. Each time a fresh wound is exposed it increases the risk of infection.

Haematoma formation can be very obvious and, again, direct pressure should be used to prevent the haematoma getting larger and a surgical opinion sought. Where drainage devices are present, their patency should be confirmed and vacuum systems should be checked to ensure that a vacuum is present. Removing a proportion of the wound closure system can sometimes allow the haematoma to drain but more often than not the wound will require surgical re-exploration. Early detection and treatment of haematoma formation is particularly important following surgery around the head and neck – for example carotid endartarectomy or thyroidectomy – as the patient's airway can be compromised. If this occurs, the nurse may often have no option but to remove some or all of the wound closure in order to prevent a life threatening situation.

POST-OPERATIVE NAUSEA AND VOMITING (PONV)

Nausea and vomiting are two of the most common complications following anaesthesia and surgery (Naylor & Inall 1994). The physiology of PONV is multifaceted and complex and beyond the brief of this chapter. A number of factors are thought to affect its incidence, such as age, gender, obesity, anxiety and previous history of PONV (Tate & Cook 1996a). The type of surgery also has an effect – for example, laparoscopic procedures have been found to have a high incidence of PONV (Pataky et al 1988). Drugs used during anaesthesia and opiate analgesia are thought to be major contributory factors in PONV (Palazzo & Evans 1993).

Although often seen as a relatively minor complication PONV is distressing for patients and potentially dangerous as it increases, for example, intracranial and intraocular pressure. This is particularly so if the surgery has been performed in these areas. Prevention of PONV is desirable and anaesthetists will often give prophylaxis before or during surgery.

Treatment of PONV with antiemetic drugs is common (see Box 8.9) and often very effective. There are however measures that the nurse can take to reduce PONV. These include keeping movement to a minimum, ensuring adequate pain relief and reducing anxiety. Maintaining oxygenation, hydration and blood pressure will also help prevent PONV. Less orthodox treatments such as acupressure, herbal remedies and aromatherapy have been shown to be effective (Tate & Cook 1996b) but do not appear to be widely practised in the acute hospital and immediate post-operative setting.

Patients experiencing PONV should have their airways closely monitored as they are at risk of obstruction and aspiration. Patients who have vomited should be given the opportunity to rinse their mouths or brush their teeth. Efforts should be made to make them comfortable and any vomit should be removed. The smell of vomit does nothing to help a nauseated patient. If patients are diaphoretic (sweaty) they can be washed and bedclothes changed, although very often patients will prefer to be left alone and not moved around too much.

> Post-operative nausea and vomiting (PONV) is unpleasant and distressing for the patient. It is not a 'minor' complication or something that can be left to get better on its own: make treating it a priority.

FACTORS SPECIFIC TO TYPE OF SURGERY

Whatever type of surgery has been performed, the basic principles of management as outlined in this chapter will apply. However, there will be certain areas that will require special consideration depending on the type of surgery. The following information is provided for guidance only and is not meant to be exhaustive.

General surgery

Abdominal wounds are common following general surgery making good pain relief vital in order to prevent respiratory problems secondary to hypoventilation. Epidural analgesia is particularly effective. Significant fluid imbalance can occur following major gut surgery, and central venous pressure and urine output should be closely monitored during the immediate post-operative period. If surgery is likely to prevent eating and drinking for some time then parenteral feeding should be considered sooner rather than later.

■ **BOX 8.9** Antiemetic agents

Phenothiazines
Most common is prochlorperazine. Can cause Parkinsonian type symptoms at high doses. Also known to cause sedation and hypotension particularly if given intravenously.

Dopamine antagonists
Such as metoclopramide. Metoclopramide can also cause extrapyramidal effects but can be given intravenously without hypotension and so is useful for rapid treatment.

Butyrophenones
Such as droperidol and haloperidol. These have an antiemetic effect but are major tranquillisers and so will produce drowsiness. Tend to be used for prophylaxis rather than treatment.

Antihistamines
Cyclizine is sometimes used for PONV but its duration is short and it can cause sedation.

5-HT$_3$ antagonists
These drugs have already been widely used in the prevention of chemotherapy-induced nausea and vomiting. Their use in the treatment of PONV is becoming more common although they are not always the first choice because of their high cost. The most commonly used are ondansetron and granisetron.

Thoracic surgery

Good pain relief is again particularly important in order to facilitate chest expansion. Sitting patients up and encouraging deep breathing as soon as they are conscious is also useful in maximising ventilation. An early visit from the physiotherapist can be very beneficial. The patients will have underwater seal drains (see Ch. 5) and may well require early chest X-ray to check for lung re-expansion.

Vascular surgery

Haemorrhage, sometimes major, is the most important complication associated with vascular surgery. Wounds and drains should be closely monitored and the blood pressure maintained within any prescribed limits. Formation of thrombus at the site of operation can cause ischaemia. Circulation to the limbs should therefore be closely monitored following surgery on the vessels in the lower part of the body, and pulses distal to the site of the surgery, for example pedal, should be checked regularly. The use of a Doppler machine may be necessary if pulses are weak. Regular neurological observation should be carried out following carotid endarterectomy. The urine output should be closely monitored following abdominal aortic aneurysm repair, especially where the aorta has been clamped above the renal arteries during surgery.

Orthopaedic surgery

Blood loss tends to be great during and after orthopaedic surgery, particularly joint replacement. Wound and drains should both be closely monitored. Checking the haemoglobin level post-operatively will indicate whether or not blood transfusion is required. Correct positioning of these patients is vital, particularly following spinal and hip surgery. Expert advice should be sought if there is any doubt. It is worth noting that many emergency orthopaedic operations are on the elderly and so particular care may need to be taken when moving them. Following orthopaedic surgery, many patients will also have plaster casts and it is important to check regularly for good circulation to the distal limb. As this type of surgery often imposes a degree of immobility, close attention to pressure areas and the use of pressure relieving devices is therefore vital.

Gynaecological surgery

It is important to check for any bleeding from the vagina as well as from wounds and drains. It is best to avoid tipping these patients head down as this can result in blood pooling in the vagina and hence go unrecognised. Emergency gynaecological surgery is often as a result of miscarriage or ectopic pregnancy and signifies, therefore, the loss of a baby. Patients and partners will be very distressed and require tactful and sensitive support.

Genitourinary (GU) surgery

Careful management of fluid balance is obviously required following renal surgery. Surgery on the prostate gland may result in major bleeding and this needs careful monitoring. Continuous bladder irrigation is required to prevent clots forming in the bladder and urinary retention. Cold irrigant can significantly lower body temperature and this should be measured regularly. Irrigant can also be absorbed, resulting in fluid overload and hyponatraemia (TURP syndrome). This is potentially life threatening and requires rapid treatment.

Plastic surgery

There are many types of procedures undertaken within the field of plastic surgery; however, the key post-operative issue is wound management. Where flaps have been grafted it is important to monitor their temperature and circulation. Keeping the patient warm, well hydrated and well oxygenated will give the flap the best chance of success. When surgery is on the head or neck, the airway should be closely monitored.

Ear, nose and throat (ENT) surgery

The major consideration following ENT surgery is maintenance of the airway. Nursing patients on their side and with the head slightly down, until the patient is conscious, helps prevent inhalation of blood. Bleeding can also be masked if it is going into the patient's stomach – excessive swallowing is a sign of bleeding and should be investigated further. This tends to be seen most often following tonsillectomy or septorhinoplasty. Following surgery of the inner ear nausea and vomiting are common and distressing problems. Antiemetics should be given as appropriate.

Cardiac and neurological surgery are not discussed here as their management is very specific and detailed. The principles involved are covered in Chapters 6 and 7.

CONCLUSION

This chapter has aimed at providing an insight into the needs of the patient during the initial post-operative period. It can be seen that patients are highly dependent throughout the whole peri-operative process. Nurses caring for patients during this time need to possess a broad range of human, clinical and technical skills in order to provide the highest quality care. The ability to act as the patient's advocate is essential, as this is a time when the patient is particularly vulnerable. The nurse must be aware of and proactive in ensuring the patient's safety, comfort and welfare.

The modern operative process involves a considerable use of high technology. It is essential that the post-operative nurse be technically knowledgeable and skilled. However, it should be remembered that technology is there to enhance the delivery of nursing care, not replace it. The skilled high dependency nurse will selectively utilise technology to make the fullest assessment possible, and provide the most appropriate patient interventions. But only by using the fundamental assessment and practice skills such as looking and listening, as well as the nurse's own experience and intuition, will she be able to provide the highest standard of care.

> Technology enhances the delivery of nursing care: it does not replace it.

REFERENCES

Abbott D, Glenn E 1994 Patient education in a pre-admission clinic. Surgical Nurse 7(2): 5–8

Aitkenhead A R 1996 Postoperative care. In: Aitkenhead A R, Smith G (eds) Textbook of Anaesthesia, 3rd edn. Churchill Livingstone, London

Ashurst S 1995 Oxygen therapy. British Journal of Nursing 4: 508–515

Baxter K et al 1993 Are they getting enough? Meeting the oxygen needs of post operative patients. Professional Nurse 8: 310–312

Boulton T B, Blogg C E 1989 Ostlere and Bryce-Smith's anaesthetics for medical students. Churchill Livingstone, Edinburgh, ch 13

Brimacombe J R, Brain A I J, Berry A M 1996 Instruction manual on the use of the laryngeal mask airway in anaesthesia, 3rd edn. Intravent Research Limited, ch 16

Catley D M et al 1985 Pronounced episodic oxygen desaturation in the post operative period: its association with ventilatory pattern and analgesic regimen. Anesthesiology 63: 20–28

Cooper D M 1990 Optimising wound healing: a practice within nursing's domain. Nursing Clinics of North America 25: 165–180

Courtenay M 1998 Choosing wound dressings. Nursing Times 94(9): 46–48

Davidson J A, Hosie H E 1993 Limitations of pulse oximetry: respiratory insufficiency – a failure of detection. British Medical Journal 307: 372–373

Dripps R D et at 1961 Role of anesthesia in surgical mortality. Journal of the American Medical Association 178: 261

Droogan J, Dickson R 1996 Pre-operative patient instruction: is it effective? Nursing Standard 10(35): 32–33

Eaton C J 1992 Essentials of immediate medical care. Churchill Livingstone, Edinburgh

Giuffre M, Finnie J, Lynam D, Smith D 1991 Rewarming postoperative patients: lights, blankets, or forced warm air. Journal of Post Anaesthesia Nursing 6(6): 387–393

Haines M H 1995 AANA journal course: update for nurse anesthetists – Pulmonary aspiration revisited: changing attitudes toward preoperative fasting. AANA Journal 63: 389–396

Hatfield A, Tronson M 1996 The complete recovery rroom book, 2nd edn. Oxford University Press, Oxford

Hauer M et al 1995 Intravenous patient controlled analgesia in critically ill postoperative/trauma patients: research based practice recommendations. Dimensions of Critical Care Nursing 14: 144–153

Hayward J 1975 Information – a prescription against pain. Royal College of Nursing, London

Henry M C, Stapleton E R 1992 EMT prehospital care. W B Saunders, Philadelphia

Kinoulty S 1998 A study to compare the effects of humidified oxygen to dry oxygen in postoperative cardiothoracic patients. Unpublished BSc dissertation

Lait M E, Smith L N 1998 Wound management: a literature review. Journal of Clinical Nursing 7(1): 11–17

McKnight C 1994 Pre-operative assessment of the surgical patient. Care of the Critically Ill 10(1): 35–38

McNeil B A 1998 Addressing the problems of inadvertent hypothermia in surgical patients. Part 2: Self learning package. British Journal of Theatre Nursing 8(5): 25–31

Moore Z 1997 Continuing education: wound care. World of Irish Nursing Series of articles Feb 1997–Oct 1997

Mosby's Medical, Nursing and Allied Health Dictionary 1994 4th edn. Mosby, St Louis

Murphy S J 1994 Preoperative assessment for day surgery. Surgical Nurse 7(3): 6–9

Murray-Calderon P, Connolly M A 1997 Laryngospasm and noncardiogenic pulmonary edema. Journal of Peri-Anesthesia Nursing 12: 89–94

Naylor R J, Inall F C 1994 The physiology and pharmacology of postoperative nausea and vomiting. Anaesthesia 49 (suppl): 2–5

Palazzo M, Evans R 1993 Logistic regression analysis of fixed patient factors for postoperative sickness: a model for risk assessment. British Journal of Anaesthesia 70: 135–140

Pataky A O, Kitz D S, Andrews R W, Lecky J H 1988 Nausea and vomiting following ambulatory surgery: are all procedures created equal? Anaesthesia and Analgesia 67: S1–S266

Preston R 1996 Anaesthesia – room for advancing nursing practice? British Journal of Theatre Nursing 6(6): 5–7

Resuscitation Council UK 1994 Advanced Life Support Manual. Resuscitation Council UK, London

Surkitt-Parr M 1992 Hypothermia in surgical patients. British Journal of Nursing 1(11): 539–545

Swan B A 1994 A collaborative ambulatory preoperative evaluation model. AORN Journal 59: 430–437

Tate S, Cook H 1996a Postoperative nausea and vomiting. 1: Physiology and aetiology. British Journal of Nursing 5: 963–973

Tate S, Cook H 1996b Postoperative nausea and vomiting. 2: Management and treatment. British Journal of Nursing 5: 1032–1039

Watts S, Brooks A 1997 Patients' perceptions of the preoperative information they need about events they may experience in the intensive care unit. Journal of Advanced Nursing 26: 85–92

FURTHER READING

Boulton T B, Blogg C E 1989 Ostlere & Bryce-Smith's anaesthetics for medical students. 10th edn. Churchill Livingstone, Edinburgh.

Drain C B 1994 The post anesthesia care unit: a critical care approach to post anesthesia nursing, 3rd edn. W B Saunders, Philadelphia.

Litwack K 1995 Post anesthesia care nursing, 2nd edn. Mosby, St Louis

Medical emergencies

Jo Norman
Andrew Cook

Key learning objectives

- To gain confidence of the general principles of care when faced with a sudden deterioration in the condition of a patient.
- To gain an understanding of clinical situations in which patient well-being may become compromised.
- To gain an understanding of how to systematically assess the systems of life, in the correct order, in a manner that maximises the patient's potential for recovery.
- To gain an understanding of the value of a cyclical approach to patient assessment, care and reassessmentce.
- To gain an understanding of how to prioritise patient problems, and how to deal with them in the first instance.
- To understand how reflective practice is beneficial to the management of emergency situations.

INTRODUCTION

Patients with medical emergencies present the nurse with a wide range of problems and challenges which test knowledge, abilities and skills. In the early stages of dealing with such a patient, the nurse must respond quickly and effectively to prevent further harm. The knowledge, abilities and skills that are required centre primarily around assessment.

Perceptions of what constitutes an emergency vary widely, dependent upon knowledge, work environment and patient/client profiles. Broad definitions of the term medical emergency do, however, exist and serve as a foundation upon which to develop a discussion.

Emergency may be defined as: 'A serious situation that arises suddenly and threatens the life or welfare of a person ... as a medical crisis' (Glanz 1986). Alternatively:

> Emergency means different things to different people. Traditionally, health care professionals have defined a true emergency as any trauma or sudden illness that requires immediate intervention to prevent imminent severe damage or death.

> (Ford 1986)

Overall there seems to be agreement that an emergency involves, to a greater or lesser extent, themes of 'seriousness', 'life threatening' and 'sudden'. It is essential for the nurse to establish the exact nature of the presenting emergency in order to initiate the appropriate intervention. The reasons for this are:

1. To prevent further deterioration
2. To work towards improving the patient's status.

In order for the above objectives to be met, effective systems of assessment should be brought into action quickly and efficiently. It is vital that these systems are clearly understood by the nurse dealing with, and often leading the management of, such situations.

This chapter aims to demonstrate the development and application of an assessment system that will assist the nurse when dealing with a medical emergency.

SYSTEMS OF PATIENT ASSESSMENT

Systems of assessment already exist within both nursing and medical practice. These have been established and tested extensively in a variety of situations and have proven themselves to be effective. While these methods of rapid assessment are most commonly practised within the accident and emergency setting, the principles they use may easily be applied to any clinical setting, such as medical assessment wards, minor injuries units, high dependency areas, observation wards and acute admission wards. What is important is that the clinical setting makes the system work for them, rather than allowing the system to dictate their practice. Such assessment tools should be used as sets of guidelines, therefore, upon which to further develop best clinical practice. The simplest model in use is that of reversed triage. This has been defined as:

> 'the formal process of assessment of emergency patients on arrival by a trained nurse, to ensure that they receive appropriate attention with the requisite degree of urgency (George et al 1992).

> Or: ... [although] each A&E unit may implement different triage systems, the process usually seems to concentrate on early patient assessment, priority rating, .first aid and control of infection (Jones 1993).

Triage has its origins on World War I battlefields in France where casualties were 'sorted' according to the gravity of their injuries, with treatment concentrated upon those most likely to survive. In the modern hospital triage reverses this process so that treatment is primarily given to those with the gravest illnesses. Therefore it is, technically, reversed triage.

Triage has recently been formalised into a national policy. The Manchester triage system (Mackway-Jones 1997) allows the nurse to use one of 52 patient triage protocols. These are set out in flowchart format in order to facilitate ease of use, and ensure that the appropriate triage decision is made quickly, effectively and in a methodical manner. Depending upon their presenting problem and condition, each patient is assigned to one of five categories, where 1 is most urgent and 5 is least urgent.

While triage can be seen as a simple model of rapid patient assessment, its fundamental principles can be applied, through other models, to any clinical setting. These are pertinent for all high dependency areas.

The treatment of patients who have sustained significant traumatic injuries are currently assessed and treated according to a rapid systematic process known as advanced trauma life support (ATLS) (Alexander & Proctor 1993). ATLS directs the medical team to assess and treat the systems of life in strict order:

A Airway (with C-spine control)
B Breathing
C Circulation
D Disability
E Exposure (with temperature control).

It is of no benefit to have a neatly dressed wound if the patient is not breathing. Advanced trauma life support directs the medical team to treat the systems of life in strict order of priority.

Thus, a patient with a major external haemorrhage would only have this problem dealt with once the airway had been secured and respiratory function had been assured. Clearly it is of no benefit to have a neatly dressed wound if the patient is not breathing.

In this way oversights can be avoided through routinised assessment, so that the team does not simply focus upon the most dramatic, 'eye-catching' injury or event, which may in itself not be life threatening.

Within nursing knowledge, the most widely utilised systems of assessment are the numerous nursing models. These aim to highlight the patient's problems: physical, psychological and social, so that a comprehensive and holistic package of care can be developed. This variety of models includes the original Roper, Logan and Tierney Activities of Daily Living to the patient-dependent systems such as Roy's, Orem and Peplau (Aggleton & Chalmers 1986). However, all nursing models aim to make a thorough assessment using a systematic process. This helps to prevent the nurse from focussing simply upon the primary reason for admission. Following a systematic nursing model, the nurse can be prevented from ignoring those issues which may give the patient greater concern, or cause greater harm. For example: a patient admitted post-operatively – where the nurse may feel that his post-operative care is the greatest priority – may, in fact, feel that his embarrassment about using a bedpan is his greatest worry. All patient issues are of importance, and the role of a nursing model is to highlight them all, and allow the nurse to structure her care to meet all of the patient's needs.

These concepts can easily be applied to both the high dependency and other settings. There is clearly a need to develop a systematic approach to the assessment of the presenting medical emergency in the high dependency area. This system must be user-friendly within the environment and not simply a transferral of one system from one setting to another. The peculiarities and specific needs of each care environment should be considered when adapting any model of assessment that has previously been used in a different setting. By incorporating elements from a range of assessment systems, a comprehensive tool can be developed in order to assist with the assessment of the medical emergency in the high dependency area.

In simple terms, there are three stages to the treatment of the medical emergency:

- Understanding
- Identifying and prioritising problems
- Action and evaluation.

Understanding

This refers to the process of realising that an emergency exists from the initial signs the nurse encounters: signs that indicate that the patient has suddenly become worse and is deteriorating rapidly. The nurse may not know the exact nature of the problem, only that a major problem exists and that a rapid, systematic response should be initiated. A post-operative patient for example, may suddenly exhibit marked pain, changes in skin colour and a deterioration in conscious level, looking increasingly unwell.

Identifying and prioritising problems

This second stage endeavours to isolate the exact nature of the problem in a manner which ensures that the most vulnerable systems of life are protected before progressing to the next. As each system is assessed the cause of the emergency should, hopefully, become apparent.

Action and evaluation

This final stage refers simply to the interventions which are put in place primarily to resolve the problem and stabilise the patient. The nurse hopes this will conclude in a resolution of the cause and stabilisation of the patient's condition.

Although this is a sequential, systematic approach to patient care, as with all other examples of assessment, the implementation of the stages is a fluid process. In practice, action to resolve a problem highlighted in the early stages of identification should be implemented while examination of further systems of life takes place. For example, a patient with no cardiovascular output will require immediate cardiopulmonary resuscitation (CPR) at the same time as assessments are made of the various systems of life. Further to this is the notion of continual reassessment which should take place for the duration of the emergency. This can be regarded as the process of evaluation, and recognition of this important step closes the circle of care, or initiates another. Evaluation should continue in the post-emergency phase so that a further emergency may be recognised with speed.

The patient with left ventricular failure (LVF) clearly requires the administration of diuretics and nitrates to resolve the pulmonary oedema as soon as this has been identified; nonetheless, the assessment of the cardiovascular and neurological systems should carry on simultaneously. The respiratory system should also be reassessed following this treatment to ensure that a beneficial outcome has been achieved.

Furthermore, as the nurse working in the high dependency area gains knowledge and experience, the process of reflective practice can develop. This involves utilising prior knowledge, experience and reflection in the assessment and subsequent treatment of the next emergency patient presented. Reflective practice should be actively nurtured by the multidisciplinary team as a whole and is more complex than simply working from experience (Atkins & Murphy 1993, Johns 1995, Greenwood 1993). The benefits of reflective practice are numerous, and include:

- An understanding of why we do something, rather than simply how
- The development from practitioner into expert
- The ability to gain empathic insight into the experience of others
- An acceptance that mistakes should be regarded as a positive learning opportunity, rather than a negative cause for discipline
- Room for the consideration of alternative ways of caring, in a non-judgemental environment.

Drawing on everything that has been identified, a spiral model which shows both the fluid nature of the treatment process as well as the notion of reassessment may be utilised to demonstrate these principles (Fig. 9.1). The model shows the pillars of the three stages, while the upward spiral demonstrates the passage of care and assessment over time. As the patient is assessed and problems are identified, the action of giving restorative treatment leads the team back to another stage of understanding, and so to prioritisation of new problems and so on until the patient is restored to a more stable status.

Stages 1 and 2 (Understanding and Identifying and prioritising the patient's problem) will now be explored further.

STAGE 1 – UNDERSTANDING THAT AN EMERGENCY EXISTS

The purpose of this mini-assessment is to allow the nurse to gain basic but tangible evidence of the existence of an emergency, even if it may not identify exactly what

Understanding   Taking action

Fig 9.1 Spiral model

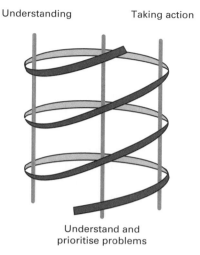

Understand and
prioritise problems

has caused it. It may be seen as a 'snapshot' assessment that takes only moments to perform. Nonetheless, it is imperative in order to trigger any alarm bells! From this assessment, the second stage should be initiated as specifics of the emergency are identified. The second stage is often applied almost instantaneously. For example, the patient found in a collapsed state may well require instant initiation of CPR once the absence of a pulse is noted. However, should the patient simply have fainted from the heat of a stuffy summer ward, a blood pressure reading and a glass of cool water may be all that is necessary.

Stage 1 can be broken down into three elements, all of which provide the nurse with tangible evidence that allows for an informed decision to declare an emergency situation. These are 'know', 'see' and 'find' (see Box 9.1).

Consider, for example, the 6-hour post-operative surgical patient who suddenly develops agitation, sweating, pallor, confusion, hypotension and tachycardia and who may also have developed internal haemorrhage. These presenting symptoms

■ **BOX 9.1** 'Snapshot' assessment

Know	What the nurse is told	• Present and past medical history • Social history • Previous medical interventions, e.g. surgery • Parameters of patient's known 'normals'
See	Quick visual assessment	• Pallor • Sweating • Mental state • Posture • Facial expression • General constitution
Find	Quick physical assessment	• Airway patency • Respiratory rate • Blood pressure • Pulse • Obvious haemorrhage • Temperature • Vomiting • Monitor changes

will alert the nurse to consider many causes, but what is important is that he identifies that an emergency of some kind exists, and then initiates the appropriate emergency action. This is followed by a more thorough assessment in stage 2.

STAGE 2 – IDENTIFYING AND PRIORITISING THE PATIENT'S PROBLEMS

There are five key areas in this stage. These are ordered in strict priority and should be addressed in this order irrespective of the clinical setting. It is widely accepted that the order of assessment presented here is that which maximises the patient's potential for survival. For example, it must be accepted that to 'bag and mask' ventilate a cyanosed patient is of little use if the physical airway is totally obstructed.

While these key areas of assessment are ordered in strict priority, it is necessary to note that in practice the process is undertaken with such speed that they are often examined almost simultaneously. Furthermore, as problems are identified within each area it is vital that the appropriate treatment is initiated immediately, or as soon as is reasonably practicable. It is clear therefore, that the patient with a medical emergency should be cared for by a number of appropriately qualified healthcare professionals, and maximising the patient's potential can often only be achieved by directing great resources to that patient. This point should be considered carefully when planning and managing any high dependency area, to ensure that appropriate support mechanisms are available as and when required.

For each key area three points are explored:

- The outcome goal
- Factors to consider
- Tools of assessment.

AIRWAY

Goal To achieve a patent and secure airway that allows adequate ventilation to the lungs.

Obstruction

The most common airway problem is that of obstruction, either total or partial. Before considering complex causes, the nurse should examine the position of the patient's head, and thus airway, and ensure that the patient is positioned in such a way as to maximise the patency of the tract. Initially, the nurse should attempt to resolve the problem by simple 'chin-lift' or 'jaw-thrust' movements (see pp. 193–194) and then reassess airway patency. Should this be unsuccessful, the mouth should be examined for foreign bodies such as food bolus, false teeth or vomit. Should a foreign body be identified, resolution can be attempted by performing a gentle 'finger-sweep' of the buccal cavity, as long as this does not put the nurse's fingers at risk. If the foreign body does not come away with ease, it may be possible to achieve a result by use of Magill forceps. Foreign bodies lodged low in the upper airway may well require removal under general anaesthetic. This will leave the team with no option but to form an emergency surgical airway as a life-saving measure, for example, a crycothyroidotomy or a mini-tracheostomy.

In the event that the patient is mechanically ventilated, the nurse should initially consider the most simple causes of obstruction such as ventilator failure and mucus plug obstruction. These may be resolved through suction and interim manual ventilation. Nonetheless, there is no excuse for not using as many preventative measures as possible in order to prevent the situation occurring in the first place; for example:

1. Regular airway perfusion assessment – chest auscultation, expansion of all lung fields
2. Prophylactic suctioning and physiotherapy, if indicated by previous, copious sticky secretions
3. Setting ventilator airway pressure alarms to within reasonable parameters and regular assessment of ventilator delivery/efficacy.

Tools of assessment

The tone and sound of the patient's respiratory efforts may well change in the emergency situation. The *development of respiratory stridor* is a clear indication of obstruction at some point of the respiratory tree, and should be investigated until a clear cause has been identified. Causes may include bronchospasm, laryngeal spasm and foreign body.

Examination of the buccal cavity for foreign bodies and swelling should be performed rapidly with the aid of a tongue depressor and light source. A definitive airway should quickly be established if there is any sign or suspicion that the airway problem is the result of oedema at any point along the upper airway. In the event of the patient having airway adjuncts in situ, these should be examined for mucus plug formation and checked to ensure correct assembly and size.

BREATHING

Goal To achieve adequate lung/respiratory function, providing oxygenation within life-sustaining levels.

Bronchial constriction

There are numerous causes of respiratory compromise associated with the lower regions of the respiratory tree. All have the potential to become life threatening but the incidence may vary greatly. Clear understanding of each problem is necessary to ensure that a prompt and appropriate response is initiated.

> All instances of respiratory compromise can be life threatening. Understand each possible problem clearly.

Bronchial constriction may result from an underlying past medical history of asthma, emphysema, chronic obstructive, airways disease (COAD), allergy, asbestosis, bronchitis or psittacosis (parrot's disease). Acutely, bronchoconstriction may result from respiratory trauma caused by heat (fire), chemical inhalation, particulate foreign body (dust, powders, etc.) or anaphylaxis.

Pneumothorax

The development of a pneumothorax will result in a partial or complete collapse of either or both lungs. The causes of pneumothorax are numerous, but can be divided into traumatic or spontaneous. Traumatic pneumothorax may be caused by:

- Blunt chest trauma (road traffic accident, fall or assault)
- Penetrating chest injury (thoracic surgery, stabbing or bullet injuries).

However, the cause rarely influences treatment, and it is more common for treatment to be determined by the type of pneumothorax presenting (see Box 9.2).

Extra caution should always be used with the ventilated patient as spontaneous collapse of a lung can create a tension pneumothorax due to positive pressure ventilation being forced into a reduced vital capacity.

■ BOX 9.2 Types of pneumothorax

Simple pneumothorax
Refers to the collapse of a lung, where the lung is rendered inactive and there is no tidal flow of gases through it.
Haemothorax
Similar to a simple pneumothorax, but a collection of blood forms in the resulting cavity of the thoracic cage.
Tension pneumothorax
This occurs when a 'one-way valve' air leak develops from either the lung or chest wall into the pleural cavity as a result of transferring a negative pressure environment into one of positive pressure, with no means of escape. Pressure within the chest increases causing the chest contents to be displaced to the opposite side of the chest. This constitutes an absolute emergency, as cardiac function will rapidly become compromised due to the exerting external pressure. This is known as tamponade. Along with respiratory distress the trachea shifts from the midline position and can thus be easily identified. Immediate treatment is required and this may be delivered by the insertion of a large-bore cannula into the chest wall at the second intercostal space, the mid-clavicular point of the tensioned side of the chest. This helps to render the pneumothorax simple as a result of providing an exit point for the accumulating positive pressure. This should remove the patient from immediate danger. A chest drain should then be inserted in order that resolution of the pneumothorax may commence. This may be facilitated by the use of thoracic suction to aid the removal of the accumulated gas and/or causative fluid.

Presentation of a surgical emphysema (where respiratory gases collect in the subcutaneous layer, creating a 'bubble-wrap' crackling upon touch pressure; with swelling to the upper chest and possibly the face, and possible patient discomfort) may result from injury, either traumatic or surgical, and may predispose the patient to the development of a pneumothorax. The patient presenting with surgical emphysema may have no initial respiratory problem, but should be monitored closely for the possible development of such an event.

All pneumothoraces can be classed as either 'open' or 'closed'. This simply refers to whether there is a traumatic hole through the chest wall, in which case the pneumothorax is classed as open. If the chest wall is intact then the pneumothorax is said to be closed. A tension pneumothorax can be open, where the 'hole' concerned creates the flap valve allowing air to flow inwards only. This is often described as a 'sucking' wound.

Pulmonary oedema

Pulmonary oedema can result from cardiac failure where the back pressure of blood through the pulmonary circuit of the cardiovascular system is such that fluid leaks into the bronchial spaces. The causes of such cardiac failure include myocardial infarction, left ventricular failure (LVF), congestive cardiac failure (CCF), *cor pulmonale* and cardiomyopathy.

Pulmonary oedema may also result from trauma to the bronchial membranes as a result of smoke inhalation, heat, chemical inhalation, vomit aspiration, water aspiration or anaphylaxis. In the case of near drowning, pulmonary oedema will result when the water inhaled has a high electrolyte concentration. These concentrates, if hypertonic to the blood, cause the osmotic flow of fluids from the vascular space into the bronchiole.

Neurological failure

Neurological failure, both traumatic and neuro-medical in origin, typically results in bradypnoea as a result of compression to the respiratory centre by rising inter-cranial pressure (ICP). This can be severe enough to result in hypoxia, thus compromising the brain. If unattended, this will inevitably progress to respiratory arrest. The patient with bradypnoea will, therefore, require immediate artificial ventilatory support.

Tools of assessment

The initial methods of assessing the respiratory function primarily involve observation of whether the patient's respiratory effort is aided by the accessory muscles, primarily the external intercostals, but may also involve the sternomastoids, scalene and pectoralis muscles. The position of the patient should also be considered, taking note of whether the patient is grasping the sides of the bed in order to give added upward support to the chest, whether he has a desire to sit forward, and whether he displays 'air hunger' (gasping). The ability of the patient to speak in complete sentences, rather than in broken sets of one or two words, is a subjective – although a reasonable – indication of the degree of respiratory distress. The patient's complexion may also indicate severe respiratory distress. Typically, the distressed patient will present with pale, clammy skin, often described as 'ashen' or 'waxy'.

The importance of respiratory rate recording cannot be stressed too strongly. The average adult takes between 12 and 20 respirations per minute. Respiratory rates outside these limits can indicate respiratory problems and, therefore, its recording must be included as one of the vital sign observations.

> The importance of respiratory recording cannot be stressed enough.

Mechanically, the assessment of respiratory function can be aided by use of the pulse oximeter, arterial blood gas analysis and peak expiratory flow rate (PEFR) measurement.

Constant pulse oximetery allows for continuous monitoring of the patient's arterial oxygen saturation. In addition, it may also be used as an indicator of adequate or inadequate peripheral perfusion (plethysmographic waveforms). It must be remembered that the pulse oximeter should be used only as a guide, and that in certain circumstances the oxygen saturation recording may not be a true reflection of gaseous activity. Carbon monoxide poisoning is such an example. Here, false readings are likely be given as carboxyhaemoglobin appears the same to the pulse oximeter as oxyhaemoglobin. More commonly, artificially low saturation monitor levels will be noted in the patient who is peripherally shut down for whatever reason. As blood supply to the nailbed is poor a true reflection of saturation levels will be difficult to achieve. It is also important to bear in mind that simple measures such as removing nail varnish, trimming of long nails and removal of dirt may all improve the accuracy of the monitor readings.

Accurate analysis of gases within the blood, and thus accurate assessment of respiratory gas exchange, can only be identified through arterial blood sampling. In order to obtain a precise picture of the patient's gaseous exchange activity over time, repeated ABGs must be taken approximately every 30 minutes initially, until the acute 'emergency' stage has passed. Repeated ABGs indicate the success or failure of the treatment given to the patient during the crisis. If repeated ABG samples are required, it is more reasonable for the patient to have an arterial line inserted for this purpose, rather than to have to endure repeated random needle stabs. This can be a cause of significant discomfort to the patient as well as causing significant trauma to blood vessel walls.

Peak expiratory flow rate (PEFR) can clearly only be measured on the patient capable of co-operating with the procedure. However, in such cases the PEFR will indicate the lung capacity and respiratory strength of the patient and is a valuable method of identifying a gradual decline or improvement in respiratory status.

CIRCULATION

Goal To adequately perfuse the brain and vital organs ensuring adequate transfer of gases, nutrients and waste products.

Shock

Emergencies concerned with the circulatory system result in shock, which can be defined as an abnormal condition of inadequate blood flow, resulting in diminished organ perfusion. While this may at first be a life-saving physiological response to overwhelming physiological insult, it will quickly deteriorate into a life-threatening condition.

The physiology of shock is a complex collection of changes, both biochemical and physical. Together these allow the body to compensate for dramatic alterations in homeostasis. From a nursing perspective however, the patient presenting with shock constitutes an absolute emergency.

There are five categories of shock: hypovolaemic, cardiogenic, neurogenic, septic and anaphylactic. All types present with dramatic changes in some or all of the patient's vital signs. The presenting combination of changes will assist the nurse in identifying the type. Therefore, it is important that all vital signs are thoroughly and frequently assessed.

> Shock allows the body to compensate for dramatic alterations in homeostasis. But for the nurse a patient in shock is always an absolute emergency.

Hypovolaemic shock

Hypovolaemic shock is caused by an acute loss of circulating blood volume, either because of direct blood loss, or by a loss of body fluids which results in an indirect reduction in circulating volume. The latter may result from burns or body water content depletion caused by diarrhoea and vomiting from gastrointestinal infection.

The direct loss of circulating blood volume, either externally or internally, may be as a result of direct trauma through accident or assault, or as a post-operative complication. Existing pathology may also result in sudden blood loss, such as a dissecting aortic aneurysm or carcinoma advancing into a major vessel. Hypovolaemia as a result of haemorrhage may be subdivided into four classes, dependent upon the percentage of total volume loss (see Table 9.1).

The indirect loss of circulating volume will result when fluid from the blood volume is lost selectively as opposed to a loss of blood 'per se'. In the trauma situation, this is most likely to be the result of serous fluid loss from burns.

Fluid management in patients with burns If over 20% of the total body surface area has incurred burns of either partial or full thickness, the patient is at great risk of developing hypovolaemic shock. This could equate to partial thickness burns to one whole leg only. Caution should be used when administering replacement fluids for a burns patient. This must be carefully calculated using the following formula: 2–4 ml Hartmann's lactate per kg body weight per percentage of body surface burn over 24 hours from time of initial burn injury. For example: a 70 kg man with a 20% partial thickness burn will require: $(4 \times 70 \times 20 = 5600$ ml/24 hours $= 233$ ml/h.

The method of assessment for calculating the percentage of body area burnt is commonly known as the 'rule of nines' (see Fig. 9.2).

Table 9.1 Estimated fluid and blood losses based upon patient's initial presentation

	Class I	Class II	Class III	Class IV
Blood loss (ml)	Up to 750	750–1500	1500–2000	> 2000
Blood loss (% BV)	Up to 15%	15–30%	30–40%	> 40%
Pulse rate	<100	>100	>120	>140
Blood pressure	Normal	Normal	Decreased	Decreased
Pulse pressure (mmHg)	Normal or increased	Decreased	Decreased	Decreased
Respiratory rate (per minute)	14–20	20–30	30–40	> 35
Urine output (ml/h)	> 30	20–30	5–15	Negligible
CNS/mental state	Slightly anxious	Mildly anxious	Anxious or confused	Confused and lethargic
Fluid replacement (3 : 1 rule)	Crystalloid	Crystalloid	Crystalloid and blood	Crystalloid and blood
Severity	Mild	⟵————————⟶		'Emergency'

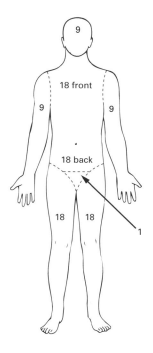

Fig. 9.2 The 'rule of nines' assessment of body area burnt. (After Alexander & Proctor 1993.)

Consideration should be given to the patient with gross fluid loss from the GI tract. Persistent diarrhoea and/or vomiting can rapidly result in dehydration and severe electrolyte imbalance, which will leave the patient with hypovolaemic shock. Clearly, adequate replacement of fluids to prevent such shock should be considered as a preventative intervention.

The treatment of hypovolaemic shock will involve the replacement of fluids rapidly, although this should be controlled and carefully measured. The choice of fluid is pivotal to the success of the treatment. Colloids are now widely felt to be of little use, and may even be detrimental, as they only expand the fluid volume in the

■ BOX 9.3 Hypovolaemic shock

SIGNS AND SYMPTOMS

System	Likely effect
Blood pressure	Gradual decrease
Temperature	Unchanged/slow decrease owing to vasoconstriction
Pulse	Rapid increase
Respirations	Gradual increase

IMMEDIATE INTERVENTIONS

Intervention	Rationale
• Massive fluid replacement: whole blood for blood loss, crystalloids for non-blood, fluid loss	• To replace lost vascular volume • To increase cardiac preload, improving stroke volume and blood pressure
• Via two 14FG venous cannulae, sited in each anticubital fossa, or by i.v. 'cut-down' of the long saphenous veins	• To prevent cellular dehydration • To ensure adequate perfusion of cerebral tissue and gaseous exchange in the pulmonary circuit
• Identify the source of fluid loss	• In order that a plan for the definitive resolution of the source of fluid loss can be initiated
• Stemming the flow of the fluid either by compression in the case of haemorrhage, or by covering broken skin surface with polythene food wrap (cling film) in the case of the burns patient	• To prevent continued volume loss, this being the primary solution to the emergency
• Fluid loss due to internal haemorrhage can only be stemmed surgically, thus transfer to theatre must not be delayed	• To prevent further deterioration, sepsis and/or death

vascular space. Colloids take considerable time to pass into the cellular space. As an initial physiological response prior to treatment, the body will have forced fluid out of the cellular space into the vascular space in an attempt to compensate for the drop in circulating volume. The cells are thus left dehydrated and their full function will be impaired until that fluid is replaced. Colloid fluids, while addressing the vascular deficit, do little initially for the cellular losses. For this reason, the fluids of choice are either crystalloid Hartmann's lactate solution or whole blood, as these address both the vascular and cellular loss. If hypovolaemia is a result of direct blood loss, there should be no delay in the administration of whole blood, even if this means that only type specific or even universal O negative blood is given.

See Box 9.3 for the signs and symptoms of shock and immediate interventions.

Cardiogenic shock

Cardiogenic shock occurs when the heart, for whatever reason, ceases to function as an effective pump. There are three main causes of cardiogenic shock:

- Physiological
- Iatrogenic
- Traumatic.

Physiological and iatrogenic The physiological disease processes of myocardial infarction and chronic lung disease may leave the heart so damaged that it ceases

---

■ **BOX 9.4** Cardiogenic shock (iatrogenic)

SIGNS AND SYMPTOMS

System	Likely effect
Blood pressure	Rapid decrease
Temperature	Unchanged or decreased due to vaso constriction and hypothermia
Pulse	Rapid increase
Respirations	Rapid increase culminating in audible 'bubbly' chest sounds and foaming pink expectoration

IMMEDIATE INTERVENTIONS

Intervention	Rationale
• Administration of immediate high dose intravenous diuretics	• To deplete vascular volume, reducing cardiac preload allowing the heart to function more effectively (See note below)
• Chest physiotherapy and/or suctioning, if indicated	• To maximise the patient's respiratory status and to ensure comfort
• Intravenous administration of opiates	• To improve cardiac function and stroke volume • To make the patient more comfortable and less distressed
• Intensive psychological support	• To prevent anxiety and panic, both of which can exacerbate the strain already placed upon the heart

Note Current research has questioned this traditional method of treatment. There is some evidence to suggest that intravenous loop diuretics are effective only because they have a mild consequential vasodilatory effect, and not because of their diuretic effect. Vasodilation causes a drop in cardiac preload. Preload is related to the volume of blood coming from the circuits leading to the heart. It increases when the ventricle concerned is unable to pump the blood through the heart at a sufficiently rapid rate. The blood builds up in the vessels, and capillary beds behind the affected ventricle cause an increase in capillary pressure and, eventually, oedema. If the right side of the heart fails, this pressure builds in the peripheral capillary beds, causing peripheral oedema. If the left ventricle fails then the pressure is exerted on the pulmonary capillary beds, causing pulmonary oedema. Vasodilatation creates further capacity for the blood. This reduces the pressure upon the affected ventricle to move the blood through the heart and in turn reduces the pressure on the capillary beds. Overall, preload is said to have been reduced, as a result of removing some of the 'potential' work of the heart. It is this effect which allows the heart to stabilise and resolve the symptoms. Thus it has been suggested that a similar, if not better, result will be obtained by high dose administration of sublingual glyceril trinitrate (GTN) spray. This creates widespread vasodilatation which reduces the preload and thus resolves the symptoms.

■ BOX 9.5 Cardiogenic shock (traumatic)

SIGNS AND SYMPTOMS

System	Likely effect
Blood pressure	Rapid decrease. This is commonly unresponsive to fluid replacement therapy
Temperature	Unchanged
Pulse	Rapid increase and a thready nature
Respirations	Gradual increase

IMMEDIATE INTERVENTIONS

Intervention	Rationale
Rapid pericardiocentesis to drain the blood collection. This cannula should be left in situ and capped in order to facilitate regular drainage if required	To relieve pressure exerted upon the heart by the fluid, so allowing the heart to pump effectively

to function effectively. In an emergency situation this may deteriorate into left ventricular failure, leaving the patient not only in cardiogenic shock but also with lung consolidation as a result of pulmonary oedema.

Iatrogenic causes of cardiogenic shock centre mainly around the over-zealous use of intravenous fluid infusion. This again may induce left ventricular failure. Fluid monitoring is of particular importance in the patient with a known cardiac pathology, who will clearly be unable to tolerate a substantial increase in vascular volume. The signs and symptoms of iatrogenic cardiogenic shock and immediate interventions are given in Box 9.4.

Traumatic A traumatic cause of cardiogenic shock is a cardiac tamponade (other causes include drug overdose, electric shock and anaphylaxis). This results from either direct penetrating thoracic trauma (accidental or surgical) or, secondary to pneumothorax, major diaphragmatic rupture and/or surgery. Blood, or occasionally some other fluid, collects around the body of the heart within the mediastinum, resulting in an increase of pressure applied to the heart muscle. The heart is compressed to the point where effective contraction ceases to be possible. Special care and thorough examination of the patient are vital as a cardiac tamponade can convincingly mimic a tension pneumothorax. The differential diagnosis can be quickly made by auscultation of the chest where a cardiac tamponade is more likely to give normal breath sounds, with muffled heart sounds and an in-line trachea, whereas a tension pneumothorax is more likely to give clear, normal heart sounds but a deviated trachea.

See Box 9.5 for the signs and symptoms of traumatic cardiogenic shock and immediate shock and immediate interventions.

Neurogenic shock

The most likely patient to develop neurogenic shock in a high dependency environment will be the patient with a simple, closed head injury who is initially stable but requires monitoring. In this scenario, an insidious increase in intracranial pressure (ICP) may result from slow bleeding into the closed box of the skull. Raised ICP may also result from cerebral oedema because of a variety of intracranial pathologies:

• Hypoxia
• Cerebrovascular accident

■ BOX 9.6 Neurogenic shock

SIGNS AND SYMPTOMS	
System	Likely effect
Blood pressure	Gradual hypertension with a widening pulse pressure
Temperature	Drastic swings between hypo and hyperthermia
Pulse	An increasing bradycardia
Respirations	Fluctuating respiratory function

- Space-occupying lesion
- Traumatic head injury
- Drug/alcohol intoxication
- Meningitis/encephalitis
- Hypo-/hyperglycaemia
- Inter-/intracerebral haemorrhages.

Whatever the cause, a rise in intracranial volume results in an increase of direct pressure upon the mass of the brain. In this situation the brain's activity is rapidly compromised resulting in a classic clinical picture. The signs and symptoms of neurogenic shock are listed in Box 9.6.

These standard observations need to be accompanied by a full neurological assessment, including an assessment of sensory and motor function, the principles of which are detailed in Box 9.7.

Spinal and general anaesthetic can also cause neurogenic shock. This is because of a sudden suppression of sympathetic nervous activity. This allows for unchecked parasympathetic activity resulting in overwhelming vasodilatation for which even a healthy/normal vascular volume is inadequate. This leads to a 'relative hypovolaemia' and all the classic signs therein. Interventions and rationale are described below.

In the case of anaesthesia-induced shock, traditional methods of addressing hypovolaemia may prove ineffective. The only definitive treatment is to resolve the cause of the neurological disturbance. It may be possible to reverse the effect of the anaesthesia by administration of pharmocological reversal agents, but this is not always possible and is dependent upon the anaesthesic used. It is commonly a short-term problem which will self-resolve as the anaesthesia is eliminated from the body, either by reversal drug therapy or by natural metabolism. However, supportive care will be required during the interim, with particular reference to the respiratory and cardiovascular systems. If the respiratory system is suppressed sufficiently, the patient will require ventilatory support and so transfer to a more intensive environment may need to be considered, if not resolvable within the HDU itself.

In cases of raised ICP the use of cerebral diuretics have only a limited place, usually to 'buy time'. Establishing the underlying cause of the rise in ICP – for example: surgical aspiration of haematoma or removal of a tumour – and resolving it accordingly, is the only effective way to treat this form of shock. This type of patient will inevitably require urgent liaison with a neurosurgeon, and may be transferred to a specialist neurosurgical intensive care facility.

Septic shock

Septic shock results from the body's inability to manage and cope with an overwhelming infection. The source of the infection can be from any route, but early identification of the microbiological cause will be important in terms of the administration of appropriate drug therapy. Certain patients will be at greater risk of

■ **BOX 9.7** Principles of assessment

Parameter	Good practice
Eye opening	The patient should be observed quietly for a short period to look for spontaneous eye opening. His name should then be called loudly to see if a response can be elicited, followed by strong, but non-marking, painful stimuli.
Verbal response	The patient may only vocalise once a stimulus is applied. This should again be that of a loud calling of his name, followed by pain (e.g. nailbed compression (see Think point))
Motor response	A clear simple command should be given to the patient such as 'Touch your nose'. If there is no response here, approved painful stimuli (see Think point) should be applied and the response observed.
Temperature	This sign is not usually monitored well by nurses. The temperature must be recorded with every set of observations. Fluctuations may occur early in cerebral pathology as the hypothalamus is particularly sensitive to intracranial disturbance, and are of significant importance.
Pulse	While external monitors are a simple way of monitoring pulse rate, the rhythm should also be periodically assessed, either by direct palpation or by a minute of closely watching the cardiac monitor rhythm.
Respiratory rate	This should be counted for at least 30 seconds and multiplied, but preferably taken over a full minute as respiratory changes may include an irregular pattern.
Blood pressure	Changes in blood pressure are a late sign as it is affected by a number of physiological influences, e.g. baroreceptors in the aortic arch and carotid sinus. It is always considered of high value by assessing nurses, despite this lateness. If a blood pressure change is the first noted alteration, then it is probably true that the other parameters have not been tested correctly and changes have been missed.
Pupil reaction	The room should be darkened. A powerful light source, not an ophthalmoscope, should be brought into the eye from the outside margin. The response of the pupil should be observed on both sides, as in normal health pupils always work in unison, known as 'consensual reflex'. The other eye should then be in tested the same way, again observing the effect on both pupils.
Power of response	If the patient is co-operative then all four limbs should be tested for both extension and flexion strength. This can be achieved by asking the patient to push *and* pull each limb against pressure exerted by the nurse in a 'tug-of-war' manner. If unco-operative, the strength of involuntary or combative limb movements can be observed as a less objective measure.

Approved painful stimuli are those methods which cannot be regarded as an assault upon the patient. 'Nipple tweaking', periorbital pressure and pre-sternal rubs should be avoided as there is potential for leaving the patient bruised or his dignity compromised. Preferred methods are those which are neither an affront to the person nor injurious. These include nailbed pressure and reflex testing. The stimuli should begin at a low level and increase gradually until a response is established, or considered absent.

During the acute stage of shock vital signs should be assessed every 15 minutes or when any treatments are given – whichever is sooner.

infection than others, for example, those who have undergone invasive surgery, especially in cases of abdominal surgery where the peritoneal cavity is exposed to bowel contents.

■ BOX 9.8 Septic shock

Signs and Symptoms

	Skin	Heart rate	Respirations	BP	Urine output	General applications
Stage 1 **Hyperdynamic**	Warm, flushed, moist	↑↑ Bounding	↑	Normal	Normal, up or down	• Restless • Chills and, fever
Stage 2 **Normodynamic**	Cool	↑↑ Weaker	↑↑	Slight ↓	↓	• Thirst • Pulmonary and peripheral oedema • Drowsy
Stage 3 **Hypodynamic**	Cold and clammy	↑↑ Thready	Failure	↓↓↓	Absent	• Unconscious • Severely unwell

IMMEDIATE INTERVENTIONS

Intervention	Rationale
• High flow oxygen administration	• To prevent or to address hypoxaemia and so adequate cerebral tissue oxygenation
• Rapid intravenous fluid therapy	• To resolve or to prevent sudden hypotension • To address dehydration caused by fevers
• Rapid initiation of antibiotic therapy	• Initially to abate the continued proliferation of the bacterial agent • To begin the destruction of the organisms

■ BOX 9.9 Anaphylactic shock

SIGNS AND SYMPTOMS

System	Likely effect
Blood pressure	Rapid hypotension
Temperature	Mild pyrexia
Pulse	Tachycardia
Respirations	Rapid increase

IMMEDIATE INTERVENTIONS

Intervention	Rationale
• Withdrawal of the cause of the reaction, if known	• To prevent further allergic response by the body
• Rapid drug therapy including intravenous antihistamine, intramuscular adrenaline and intravenous steroid (only if required)	• To begin to reverse the life threatening affects of the immunological allergic response of the body
• Maintenance of the airway is paramount, and the securing of a definitive surgical airway should be considered early if there is any suspicion of airway obstruction	• To allow the passing of respiratory gases along the respiratory tree. The passing of an ET tube early in treatment is simpler than having to perform an emergency crycothyroidotomy later

Theoretically, there are three possible stages within the septic shock cycle. A patient may present with one or all of the following symptoms described in Box 9.8.

Early diagnosis of septic shock and rapid intervention are vital if the process is to be broken.

Anaphylactic shock

Anaphylactic shock is the result of overwhelming systemic allergic reaction to a known or unknown antigen. This usually causes catastrophic and rapid respiratory distress and cardiovascular collapse. It may also be associated with oedema of the mucous membranes, most worryingly to those membranes of the respiratory tract. Furthermore, it may also cause widespread dermatological changes.

See Box 9.9 for the signs and symptoms of anaphylactic shock and immediate interventions.

Tools of assessment

Much attention has already been given to the variation in presentation of vital signs dependent upon the type of shock. However, it is of paramount importance that vital signs are assessed frequently during the acute stage of any shock episode, ideally at intervals of 15 minutes or when any treatments are given, whichever is sooner.

The patient's appearance will be useful in assessing shock. With the exception of the hyperdynamic stage of septic shock, the patient's skin will appear sweaty, cold and grey. This is due to the rapid peripheral vasoconstriction which occurs during shock as a physiological means of conserving the body's resources. This vasoconstriction will also result in a reduction in capillary refill times (CRT). CRT is assessed by pinching the nailbed of an elevated finger. The nail will blanch under pressure but should flush pink again within 2 seconds of the release of pressure. Increased CRT is indicative of poor perfusion and thus suggestive of shock.

The mental, cognitive status of the patient may be an early indication of shock. Patients may become restless, confused, anxious and disorientated in the early stages, leading to drowsiness and coma later. Thus the confused or mildly disoriented patient should never be dismissed without some assessment. Where there is a possibility of neurogenic shock, suggested by the patient's history, a full nursing and medical neurological assessment must be performed.

Many high dependency patients will already have indwelling urinary catheters in situ, and the opportunity this presents to monitor renal function should be taken. In most cases of shock, urinary output decreases. Wherever possible, it is helpful if patients are catheterised early in treatment so that renal function can be monitored more accurately or efficiently. A minimum urinary output of 0.5 ml/kg/h should be expected for an adult. Renal failure will dramatically complicate the patient's care (and increase the risk of mortality) and must be prevented wherever possible. Any predisposing renal symptoms must be treated as soon as they occur.

Patients with shock that cannot easily be resolved will require central venous cannulation. This not only allows for the administration of fluids and drugs, but also the monitoring of central venous pressure. The CVP reflects the balance between venous return to the heart, venous tone and heart function. CVP can be measured from a number of anatomical sites:

- Mid-axillary line
- Mid-axillary line at fourth intercostal space (phlebostatic axis)
- Sternal notch
- Xiphoid sternum.

It is not the site chosen that is of importance, but rather that the same site is used for all subsequent measurements once the first has been taken. It is also important to know the agreed measurement parameters of 'normal' according to the scale that is chosen. The position of the patient at the time of measurement should also be noted as this can influence the results. This allows for accurate continuity of care and, more importantly, accurate understanding of changes in measurement findings or trends. Other parameters can be assessed for changes which may influence the patient's care. These include routine blood screening and arterial blood gas measurement.

DEFICITS IN NEUROLOGICAL STATUS

Goal: To establish accurate assessment of neurological status, identifying a cause where possible and to initiate care to stabilise the patient's condition.

There are a number of reason for change in a patient's neurological status. Some examples are given in Box 9.10.

Despite the cause of the conscious level change, the process of assessing these patients will generally be the same. Changes in neurological status may be the result of a rise in intracranial pressure (ICP). The first objective is always to notice that such a rise is occurring, secondly to maximise the patient's potential for recovery and finally to ascertain the cause and to treat this urgently. However neurological changes can result from a variety of other causes, so while the ICP is of great importance it is not the only parameter to be considered.

■ BOX NO 9.10 Change in neurological status

Cause	Reason
Hypoxia	Reduces overall cerebral activity as cells unable to metabolise effectively and so function
Cerebrovascular accident	Ischaemia to vital cerebral tissue, reducing cerebral function
Space-occupying lesion	Causes an increase in ICP. Invasion of vital cerebral tissue by tumour, reducing activity of that portion of the brain
Traumatic head injury	Causes either haemorrhage and so raised ICP, or disruption of tissue structure breaking vital pathways
Drug/alcohol intoxication	Interferes with chemical activity of cerebral tissue so reducing normal functioning
Meningitis/encephalitis	Because of tissue and meningeal inflammation secondary to microbial infection resulting in raised ICP
Hypo/hyperglycaemia	Reduce tissue metabolism and so function in hypoglycaemia, and because of resulting acidosis in hyperglycaemia
Inter/intracerebral haemorrhages	Cause a rise in ICP exerting intolerable pressure on the tissues

One of the most common causes of neurological change will be simple hypoxia, especially that which is a consequence of a non-cerebral illness or injury. Such problems should be easily identified through the basic airway, breathing and circulation assessment.

For the patient with a traumatic head injury, the risk of changes in neurological status should never be underestimated. The signs of such changes may be sudden, as in the case of subdural bleed, or may develop slowly over several hours, as with extradural bleeds. However, it is clearly safer to assume rapid deterioration when signs are first noted. The exact location of the bleed is of limited consequence in the emergency situation, the immediate treatment being the same. Such patients will require close, continual observation and reassessment, with urgent CT scanning as a priority. Neurosurgical team involvement is essential at this stage as urgent Burr holes may need to be performed, as with extradural bleeds. This procedure will hopefully allow the rapid evacuation of collected fluids, and therefore resolve the rising ICP. It must be remembered that the cavalier performing of Burr holes without a previous CT scan should not be considered.

There are a number of non-traumatic causes of neurological deterioration. The exact cause of the changes is again of limited consequence in the emergency situation, with the nursing interventions remaining broadly similar. A finite diagnosis is obviously necessary eventually, and this could be:

- Space-occupying lesion
- Cerebrovascular accident
- Subarachnoid/dural haemorrhage (spontaneous)
- Meningitis/encephalitis
- Hypo-/hyperglycaemia
- Alcohol/drug misuse (including the over prescription of opiates).

Only a limited number of interventions in such patients can resolve the neurological deficit immediately. These include the reversal of hypoglycaemia with rapid infusion of glucose (by administration of either 50 ml 50% glucose intravenously over 3–5 minutes, or preferably 500 ml 20% glucose intravenously over 15 minutes), and the administration of naloxone (400 mcg intravenously if possible or intramuscularly, as a bolus dose for the reversal of opiates). This may be repeated several times if required or a continuous infusion commenced. It is also important to note that naloxone has a relatively short half-life for patients with excessive blood levels of opiates. Other than the above, such patients will require close observation and supportive treatment. CT scanning in these circumstances may well be considered. It may be necessary to discuss the management of complicated overdose patients, for example, with the local Poisons Information Centre, and their advice should be followed closely and may need to be sought on several occasions for each patient. Some overdose patients may require referral to or discussion with a regional centre of specialised care. For example, paracetamol overdose which results in altered blood liver function test results, should be discussed with the Regional Liver Unit and their advice followed. Equally, the patient exhibiting renal failure secondary to an aspirin overdose should be discussed with the nearest renal medical team. It is important to remember that both renal and hepatic failure may, ultimately, result in deterioration of the patient's conscious level leading to coma, if not successfully treated.

Psychological changes may result in an apparent neurological deficit, and must always be considered. The elderly may experience disorientation and confusion as a result of anaesthetic, prescribed drugs and environmental changes (removal from the familiar home environment for a hospital admission). They may also have a pre-existing dementia which cannot be resolved. Any patient may have an underlying psychiatric disorder, such as schizophrenia, which can be exacerbated at any time and create an apparent neurological change.

All patients with an altered neurological status will require similar and immediate nursing care. This will include thorough assessment, administration of high flow oxygen and maintenance of a patent airway. Asking the patient to lie flat will ease assessment, and it is also the safest position should the patient's condition continue to deteriorate dramatically. This is also useful if procedures such as CPR and intubation become necessary.

For patients with a rise in ICP, the administration of cerebral diuretics should be considered. Such administration should never be seen as a definitive treatment in its own right, only as a temporary or interim measure. Cerebral diuretics such as mannitol and loop diuretics such as frusemide may also be considered as a temporary stabilisation method until the opinion of a neurosurgeon is sought. Ultimately, the use of diuretics should only be as a precursor to neurosurgical procedures. If diuretics are to be used, urinary catheterisation and renal function monitoring are obligatory in order to accurately monitor intake, output and effects of treatment.

Tools of assessment

It is clearly sensible to first eliminate or treat those causes which can be rapidly reversed, such as hypoglycaemia and simple opiate overdose. All patients with a sudden change in neurological status should therefore have a blood glucose analysis, oxygen saturation level recording and consideration given to recent administration of opiates, muscle relaxants, sedatives or anaesthetics. If any problem is identified from these observations, immediate treatment to reverse this should be given; for example, the administration of intravenous glucose, high flow oxygen and/or intravenous naloxone.

Following on from this, assessment will be based upon the standard hospital neurological observations chart. Nine parameters are tested, all of which require accurate assessment at each observation episode (as referred to earlier). Typically, nurses are better at performing the more technical observations such as blood pressure and pupil size, neglecting the simpler, but often more telling, signs such as temperature (Wilson et al 1988; Sullivan 1990; Ellis & Cavanagh 1992). It is important to remember that the best level of response, even if only momentary, should be recorded.

Other assessment procedures will include CT scanning and lumbar puncture where an infective cause is suspected. However, this should be performed with caution where an intracranial bleed is suspected. General blood screening will also be performed to seek biochemical changes that can be resolved – for example, evidence of acidosis on arterial blood gas analysis.

ENVIRONMENT (EXPOSURE)

Goal: To maintain a core temperature within life-sustaining parameters.

Hypothermia

Patients in the HDU are susceptible to the effects of the ambient environment, and consideration should be given particularly to the patient who has recently undergone surgery, or is in any form of shock, who arrives with an existing hypothermia. Many surgical procedures, especially in cardiac surgery, involve purposeful lowering of core temperature with ice and/or cardiopulmonary bypass in theatre, while other patients may gradually lower their core temperature as a result of inadequate bedding, room heating, or limb/body exposure during long or difficult surgery. Hypothermia has an overall detrimental effect on the patient's stability and recovery, and can mask symptoms of haemorrhage and hypovolaemia in particular. This is a result of vasoconstriction from the associated hypothermia.

Tools of assessment

The monitoring of core temperature is obligatory when a peripheral temperature of less than 35.5°C is recorded. The use of rectal, oesophageal or tympanic (with caution until more definitive research has been published) thermometers should be considered.

The subjective temperature ascertained by touch is a useful guide to the onset of hypothermia but must always be followed up by objective temperature assessment.

Peripheral perfusion will decrease in hypothermia, an indicator to this being by assessing capillary refill time. This is tested by raising the hand above the level of the heart, depressing a fingernail firmly for 2 seconds and then releasing. The return from the blanching effect of depression to a perfused, pink nailbed should take less than 2 seconds. A capillary refill of more than 2 seconds is indicative of reduced peripheral perfusion.

Patients with a noted hypothermia should be rewarmed slowly at a rate of no more than 1°C per hour. This should be achieved by the use of blankets and warmed i.v. fluids, with consideration to warmed peritoneal lavage or dialysis being given in extreme cases. The use of reflective 'space blankets' must be avoided where possible, as they may cause rapid peripheral warming with subsequent peripheral vasodilatation and hypotension. Some units may have access to a controlled patient warming system. These should only be used by skilled operators. Cardiopulmonary bypass can also be used as a method of rewarming patients with profound hypothermia.

TRANSFERRING THE PATIENT

Goal: To ensure the safe transfer of the patient from print of transfer to receiving point.

Each individual unit should give consideration to its own limits of care capability. The development of local guidelines should be seen as a joint responsibility by all professional disciplines. This will ensure early recognition of the patient who requires transfer to a hospital or unit which can provide optimal care.

Transfer, as a term, is as applicable to the movement of a patient from HDU to CT scanning as it is to the movement from one healthcare institute to another. The patient should be prepared safely for transfer and staff should consider all possible complications that could arise en route. They should ensure that safeguards are put in place to minimise risk. It must be presumed that it is better to over-treat than to under-treat, to save compromising patient care or to perform any relevant procedures in the event of a further emergency developing in transit, e.g., portable defibrillator, suctioning, etc. Such safeguards must be deemed appropriate as transfer must not be unnecessarily delayed. Remember the overall aim is to *do no further harm*.

Always remember that it can prove practically very difficult to perform certain medico-nursing procedures en route. If there is a possibility that a patient may require, for example, urinary catheterisation at some point, it would be prudent to consider performing that procedure prior to transfer, even if it is not entirely indicated at that time. Such medico-nursing procedures include:

- Establishment of a definitive airway
- Adequate i.v. access (peripheral and central)

- Arterial line access
- Immobilisation (spinal: either total or C-spine only)
- Pharmacological paralysation
- NG tube insertion
- Limb splinting or immobilisation
- Administration of analgesia +/− sedation/antiemetics.

Factors to consider

Personnel

Perhaps the most important consideration is the availability and skill level of the people undertaking the transfer. A balance has to be reached that is compatible with both the safety of the patient undergoing transfer and the effects of depleting staffing levels within the HDU for the period of the transfer.

Equipment

Equipment plays a key role in the management of the transfer. While it is clearly foolish to depart 'with everything bar the kitchen sink', it is probably more fool-hardy to leave with such minimal equipment that you would be unable to deal with even the most basic of situations. Every patient will have very different needs, influenced by his illness, distance of travel and mode of transport. It is therefore vital to spend some time prior to departure anticipating the possible situations that could arise for an individual patient. Equipment taken should reflect the plans formed to address those situations. Equipment is of no use if it does not function when required. Spending a few moments checking that it is in working order, including stored battery life, prior to leaving may well save not only face, but also the patient's life. In addition, if the patient has any drug infusions in progress, it will be necessary to consider the 'lifetime' of the infusions and whether backup supplies are required.

Distance

The level of preparation is almost always comparable to the distance the patient must travel. A move from HDU to CT scanning down a short, single corridor, will clearly require less preparation than a move by helicopter over 300 miles. Principles of patient safety and staff preparation must, however, be applied to all movements involving the critically ill. The 'quick dash down the corridor' must always be avoided, for everybody's sake.

Mode of transfer

In selecting a mode of transport, it is vital to remember the principle of 'do no further harm'. The mode of choice is dependent upon the availability of the desired vehicle and the personnel required to staff it. Distance is a major influencing factor. The movement to CT scan of some 50 metres can best be undertaken on a trolley bed, while a transfer from London to Manchester may best be undertaken by air. This is further influenced by extraneous factors such as time of day and prevailing weather conditions. The overall consideration should be in favour of the most rapid method of transfer. If an ambulance could deliver your patient in 2 hours, whereas a helicopter could deliver him in 20 minutes but is not available for 3 hours, clearly the ambulance would be the mode of choice.

Communication

Communication, verbal and written, between both the transferring and receiving areas must be clear, accurate and concise. The safety of the patient will without doubt depend on good, two-way discussion. Communications should cover:

- Demographic patient details
- Patient's problem/condition
- Patient's previous medical and nursing history (including notes and care plans)
- Treatment already given, including medication and fluids
- Vital signs
- Investigation results (including those pending and method of accessing results later)
- Names of both medical and nursing staff in charge of the transfer, at both the transfer and receiving points
- Next of kin details.

The family

While you may have provided excellent care to the patient, the relatives may be less than well served. Their emotional involvement must not be underplayed, and full explanations regarding the transfer should be given in a clear, unhurried fashion. This means the avoidance of medical jargon unless you are sure that the relatives have a background that will allow them to understand. The discussions should include:

- Reason for transfer
- Current condition with honest prognosis
- Details of receiving unit
- Assistance with arrangements to travel
- Offering of religious support
- Assistance with contacting relatives and friends.

It is probably prudent to assign one nurse to act as liaison with the relatives, so that the experience can be as personal as possible. The nurse should have proven communication skills, and be equipped with all the pertinent details of the case, so that she may answer the relatives' questions honestly.

REFERENCES

Aggleton P, Chalmers H 1986 Nursing models and the nursing process. Macmillan Press, London

Alexander R, Proctor H (eds) 1993 Advanced trauma life support: course for physicians. First Impression, USA

Atkins S, Murphy K 1993 Reflection: a review of the literature. Journal of Advanced Nursing 18: 1188–1192

Ellis A, Cavanagh S 1992 Aspects of neurosurgical assessment using the Glasgow Coma Scale. Intensive and Critical Care Nursing 8: 94–99

Ford 1986 Emergency care handbook. Springhouse Corporation, Pennsylvania

George et al 1992 Evaluation of nurse triage in a British accident and emergency department. British Medical Journal 304: 876–878

Glanz W (ed) 1986 Mosby's medical and nursing dictionary. Mosby, St Louis

Greenwood J 1993 Reflective practice: a critique of the work of Argyris and Schön. Journal of Advanced Nursing 18: 1183–1187

Johns C 1995 The value of reflective practice to nursing. Journal of Clinical Nursing 4: 23–30

Jones C 1993 Triage decisions: how are they made? Emergency Nurse 1(1): 13–14

Mackway-Jones K (ed.) 1997 Emergency triage. BMJ Publishing, London

Sullivan J 1990 Neurologic assessment. Nursing Clinics of North America 25(4): 795–809

Wilson S et al 1988 Determining interrater reliability of nurses' assessments of pupillary size and reaction. Journal of Neuroscience Nursing 20(3): 189–192

Fluid and electrolytes

CHAPTER 10

Heather Carroll

Key learning objectives

In relation to maintaining fluid and electrolyte balance, this chapter aims to identify:

- The underpinning physiological principles.
- Specific causes of fluid and electrolyte excess and deficit.
- Specific patient assessment data required in fluid and electrolyte excess and deficit.
- Specific nursing interventions required in fluid and electrolyte excess and deficit.

INTRODUCTION

In high dependency care a patient's fluid and electrolyte status can change rapidly and the need to be vigilant and alert to these changes is of paramount importance. Methodical collection of patient assessment information is vital for quick and efficient intervention at any stage of patient care. Fluid and electrolyte imbalance can occur insidiously, without obvious presenting problems. To be alert to these requires the use of invasive and non-invasive measurement techniques, acute patient observation skills, interpretation of biochemical indicators, and prioritisation of patient care needs. In health, fluids and electrolytes are finely tuned and constantly maintained by various physiological processes. In ill health there are many sources of fluid and electrolyte loss and gain, which can result in an overall imbalance. The nurse plays a vital role in monitoring and assessing these. The aim of this chapter is to provide relevant information and underpinning principles that may inform assessment and intervention in maintaining fluid and electrolyte balance. For the purpose of organisation, fluid and electrolytes will be considered separately.

FLUID AND ELECTROLYTE BALANCE

Evidence that a balance is maintained between the intake and output of body fluids in a healthy person is shown by the fact that body weight remains constant from day to day. If this balance is altered, the consequences will depend on the degree of imbalance incurred.

A reduction of 5% in body fluids will cause thirst, a reduction of 8% will result in illness, and a 10% reduction will result in death.

Sources of fluid intake and loss are shown in Box 10.1.

BODY FLUID COMPARTMENTS

Total body water constitutes approximately 60% of body weight in males and 52% in females, the latter being slightly less due to the higher fat content. Total body water is

■ **BOX 10.1** Sources of fluid intake and fluid loss

Fluid intake is derived from three main sources:
- Ingested fluids = 1500 ml/24 h
- Water in food = 500 ml/24 h
- Metabolic water resulting from oxidation of food amounts to approximately 400 ml/24 h

Total fluid intake = 2400 ml/24 h

Water is lost from the body in three main ways:
- Urine output = 1500 ml/24 h
- Evaporation (via lungs and skin) = 800 ml/24 h
- Alimentary tract = 100 ml/24 h

Total fluid output = 2400 ml/24 h

Fig. 10.1 Tank model fluid compartments. (Based on Smith (1980), with kind permission.)

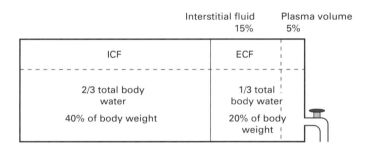

less in obesity and in the elderly. These are important factors for consideration when estimating overall fluid balance in individuals. Body fluids are distributed between two compartments: the intracellular fluid (ICF) and extracellular fluid (ECF) compartments. Smith (1980) utilises the tank model (Fig. 10.1) to depict the respective compartments, pointing out that in reality the ECF surrounds the ICF like a shell:

1. The intracellular fluid (ICF) is contained within the cells and accounts for two-thirds of total body water (40% body weight).
2. The extracellular fluid (ECF) surrounds the cells and accounts for one-third of total body water (20% total body weight). The ECF is distributed between:
   - The interstitial space, that is fluid outside the vessels, bathing the cells. This compartment accounts for three-quarters of total ECF volume.
   - The plasma compartment which constitutes 'plasma volume', that is the 'vascular space' (fluid within the vessels). This compartment accounts for one-quarter of total ECF volume. Adult blood volume is approximately 5 litres, 75 ml/kg.

Expansion or contraction of either of these compartments will result in presenting clinical features detailed in Table 10.6. Any infused intravenous fluids will directly enter the ECF compartment, primarily the vascular space, and will then be distributed into the respective fluid compartments, according to their composition. When considering fluid balance in the highly dependent patient it is important to be aware of the potential development of a 'third space', that is movement of fluid into body cavities, e.g. in paralytic ileus (fluid pools into the bowel). Metheny (1996) provides a useful microscopic visualisation of body fluid distribution (Fig. 10.2).

The various fluid compartments are separated by semi-permeable membranes; continuous exchange of water and solutes occurs within the body, transported by diffusion and osmosis to maintain constant balance.

> With age, the body increases its fat content and loses a significant amount of muscle mass. Because muscle holds 40% of total body water, the water content of the older person reduces to around 45–50% – mostly due to the loss of muscle mass. Any stressor or disease will therefore more easily lead to dehydration in the older person.

> Other examples of 'third space' include peritonitis, burns, crush injuries, and in increased capillary permeability states. The development of a third space can represent a hidden site of circulating volume, causing signs of ECF loss without any obvious external loss.

Composition of body fluid compartments

The composition of the fluid compartments varies in relation to their respective electrolyte content. An electrolyte is defined as a substance that develops an

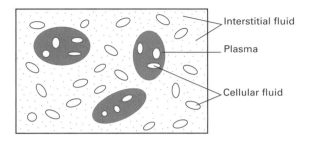

Interstitial fluid

Plasma

Cellular fluid

Fig. 10.2 Microscopic visualisation. (Based on Metheny 1996, with kind permission.)

Table 10.1 The ionic concentration of body fluids in a typical 70 kg man			
Solute	**Plasma**	**ECF**	**ICF**
Sodium (mmol/l)	142	145	12
Potassium (mmol/l)	4	4.1	150
Chloride (mmol/l)	103	113	4
Bicarbonate (mmol/l)	25	127	12
Proteins (g/l)	60	0	25
Osmolality (mOsmol/kg)	280	280	280

Table 10.2 Summary of major electrolyte functions (Metheny 1996)	
Electrolyte and plasma level	**Functions of electrolytes**
Sodium (135–145 mmol/l)	• Major cation in ECF, maintains osmotic pressure and volume in this compartment • Essential for nerve impulses and muscle contractions • Influences acid–base balance, chloride and potassium levels
Potassium (3.5–5.0 mmol/l)	• Major cation in the ICF compartment, maintains osmotic pressure and volume in this compartment • Essential for transmission and conduction of nerve impulses, for the contraction of skeletal, cardiac and smooth muscles • Necessary for movement of glucose into cells
Calcium (4.5–5.5 mmol/l)	• Promotes normal nerve and muscle activity • Increases contraction of the myocardium • Maintains normal cellular permeability and promotes blood clotting • Bone development and healing
Chloride (96–106 mmol/l)	• A major anion in the ECF helps maintain ECF osmotic pressure and water balance • Influences neutrality between cations and anions • Digestion – essential for production of hydrochloric acid
Phosphate (0.8–1.4 mmol/l)	• A vital component in the structure of bone tissue and teeth • Essential in the metabolism of all cells • As a buffer – maintains acid–base balance
Magnesium (1.5–2.5 mmol/l)	• A major ICF cation closely related to potassium • Vital for ICF enzyme reactions involving ATP • Implicated in neural control, neuromuscular transmission and cardiovascular tone

electrical charge when dissolved in water – ions are collectively referred to as electrolytes. Electrolytes that develop a positive charge are cations, e.g. sodium (Na^+), potassium (K^+) calcium (Ca^+) and magnesium (Mg^{2+}). Electrolytes with a negative charge are anions, e.g. chloride (Cl^-) and bicarbonate (HCO_3^-).

The composition of body fluid varies between compartments (Table 10.1).

In all body fluid anions and cations are always present in equal amounts, as positive and negative charges must be equal – an electromechanical fact (Metheny 1996).

MECHANISMS INVOLVED IN THE REGULATION OF FLUID AND ELECTROLYTE BALANCE

Movement and maintenance of fluid compartments

Movement of water and solutes between fluid compartments is continuous. In health the actual concentration of solutes and amount of water in each compartment remains relatively unchanged. In order that movement can take place cell membranes have to be crossed, and these membranes are described as partially or semi-permeable. Water and small electrolyte molecules pass easily, larger colloid substances and protein are held back. Body fluids are maintained at a constant level by several homeostatic mechanisms, namely osmosis, diffusion and active transport. Maintaining a constant internal environment involves fluid and electrolytes being able to continuously move between fluid compartments, across cell membranes. Movement of water is governed by two principal forces: (1) osmotic pressure – pressure that must be applied to a solution on one side of a membrane to prevent osmotic flow of water across the membrane from a compartment of pure water (Vander, et al 1994); pressure is exerted by electrolytes and blood proteins. (2) Hydrostatic pressure of blood – the pressure exerted by fluid against the wall of its container. When osmotic pressure changes in one fluid compartment water moves across the semi-permeable membrane from an area of lesser osmotic pressure to that of greater osmotic pressure until equilibrium is achieved. The volume of blood flowing through the vessels creates hydrostatic pressure which is the driving force causing filtration of fluid through the semi-permeable membranes of the capillaries.

Small molecular solutes diffuse passively through cell membranes either across a selectively permeable membrane or down a concentration gradient within cells. Their continuous random movement results in transfer in both directions; the net movement tends to be to the compartment having the lower solute concentration. The end result of diffusion is the equilibrium of substances on both sides of the membrane (Fig. 10.3).

Fig. 10.3 Movement of water between body fluid compartments by osmosis in dehydration.

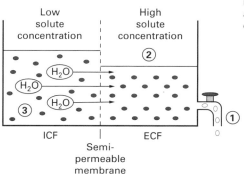

Dehydration commonly occurs as a result of a multitude of clinical scenarios (see Box 10.2)

1. Excessive loss of water from ECF compartment
2. Osmotic pressure increases in the ECF compartment
3. Water leaves ICF compartment by osmosis, moving into ECF, thereby maintaining osmolarity and ECF volume (total body fluid volume is reduced)

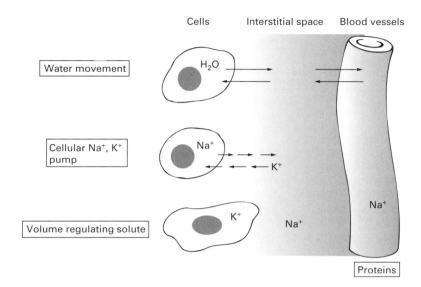

Cells   Interstitial space   Blood vessels

Fig. 10.4 Basic principles controlling solute and fluid exchange between compartments

Water movement

Cellular Na$^+$, K$^+$ pump

Volume regulating solute

Active transport

Sodium is the most important electrolyte for the maintenance of osmotic pressure and volume in the ECF compartment. Any change in sodium concentration will lead to fluid volume changes (water follows sodium). Potassium is the main intracellular cation and maintains the ICF osmotic pressure. Electrolytes do not move between the cell walls and capillaries as easily as water. Na$^+$ and K$^+$ ion concentrations in ECF and ICF are nearly opposite (Table 10.1). This reflects the activity of the chemical substance known as adenosine triphosphate (ATP) on dependent Na$^+$/–K$^+$ pumps. ATP is released from the cell wall which gives the electrolyte the energy required to pass through semi-permeable membranes. The membrane is selectively permeable, so that what is transported in or out of the cell at any time depends on the body's current metabolic condition. The respective N$^+$ and K$^+$ concentrations are maintained inside and outside the cells through active transport. Na$^+$ is pumped out of the cell (keeping intracellular Na$^+$ low) and K$^+$ is pumped into the cell (maintaining high intracellular K$^+$ levels). Renal mechanisms reinforce this distribution, regulating Na$^+$ excretion. If dietary intake of Na+ is low the urine contains virtually no Na$^+$; if it is high the urine is heavily laden with Na$^+$. As Na$^+$ is reabsorbed from the filtrate K$^+$ is secreted. In spite of an enormous variation in dietary intake, K$^+$ levels are kept constant. This constancy is achieved by the renal tubular absorption of potassium and the secretion of variable amounts of potassium. Movement of potassium across cell membranes regulates plasma potassium levels. When potassium is lost from the body – for example in urine – potassium moves out of the cells into the ECF to maintain potassium equilibrium between ICF and ECF.

In the ECF compartment there is exchange of water and electrolytes between the interstitial fluid compartment and the intravascular compartment (Fig. 10.4). The principal difference in composition between these compartments (highlighted in Table 10.1) is the presence of proteins in the plasma. Proteins cannot pass the capillary membrane, therefore function as osmotically active substances holding fluid in blood vessels. The osmotic pressure exerted by plasma proteins is referred to as oncotic pressure at approximately 20–30 mmHg. With Na$^+$, the plasma proteins control intravascular volume.

Table 10.3 Plasma osmolality and ADH response

Plasma osmolality	ADH response	Physiological effect
Normal	Present	Maintenance of normal balance
• Lowered – in fluid excess Plasma osmotic pressure reduced	• Reduced stimulation of osmoreceptors – inhibited release of ADH	• Increased kidney tubule excretion of water, large volumes of dilute urine produced
• Increased – in fluid loss/excessive intake of electrolytes Plasma osmotic pressure increased	• Stimulation of osmoreceptors – increased release of ADH	• Increases kidney tubule reabsorption of water, fluid retained in circulation, small volumes of concentrated urine produced

Osmolality

Water balance disorders are manifested by alterations in plasma osmolality. Osmolality refers to the number of dissolved particles per kilogram of solvent. Normal plasma osmolality is 280–290 mOsmol/kg of water and this provides an environment which is favourable for cellular activity. The major determinant of plasma osmolality is sodium. The osmolality of the ICF compartment must balance that of the ECF compartment in order to maintain a correct and orderly distribution of fluid between the cell and its environment (Colbert 1993).

> There is a diminution in thirst perception with age, so that even in the face of volume depletion or hyperosmolality, which serve as stimuli for the intake of fluid, these stimuli are less effective.

- Osmolality is regulated so precisely that + or – 3 mOsmol/kg water will activate the body's osmolality regulating mechanisms.
- Changes in plasma osmolality are detected by osmoreceptors located in the hypothalamus. These receptors regulate the release of anti-diuretic hormone (ADH) from the posterior pituitary as well as having an effect on thirst.
- The two primary regulators of ADH are osmotic (plasma osmolality) and haemodynamic (blood volume and pressure).
- ADH is removed from the plasma by the liver and kidneys.

Electrolytes are the major factor in maintaining the osmolality of body fluids, upon which the integrity of the body fluid compartments – and ultimately the ability of individual cells to function – depends (Colbert 1993, p 58).

- **Cardiovascular system.** Plasma needs to reach the kidneys in sufficient volume and at adequate pressure for regulation of water and electrolytes to take place. This results in the production of urine in appropriate volume and concentration relative to the body's needs. This will be affected in cardiac/volume insufficiency and renal impairment.
- **Renal system.** The kidneys play a primary role in maintaining fluid and electrolyte balance. The cardiovascular system provides the plasma volume to enable regulation of water and electrolyte content of body fluids. The distal tubules of the nephron selectively excrete unwanted solutes by active transport (sodium is retained and potassium is excreted), maintaining normal osmolality and blood volume. The kidney also has an important role in acid–base regulation: the distal tubules have the ability to form ammonia and exchange hydrogen ion (in the form of ammonia) for bicarbonate to maintain the carbonic acid–bicarbonate ratio (Weinstein 1993).
- **Respiratory system.** The lungs maintain the composition of the blood oxygen and carbon dioxide levels, and therefore play an important role in regulating acid–base balance in extracellular fluid. The lungs also influence loss of fluid through ventilation (Chandler 1991).

Table 10.4 Hormones involved in the maintenance of fluid and electrolyte balance

Hormone	Trigger for response	Actions
Aldosterone secreted by the adrenal glands	• Stimulated by ↑ K^+ levels & ↓ Na^+ levels • Major trigger for release is renin–angiotensin mechanism	• Promotes reabsorption of sodium by the distal tubules in the kidney, and from the colon. • Promotes hydrogen ion secretion, and responds to changes in potassium levels
ADH secreted by the pituitary gland	• ↓ Plasma osmolality inhibits ADH release • ↑ Plasma osmolality stimulates ADH production	• Increases kidney tubule excretion of water • Increases kidney tubule reabsorption of water.
Renin → angiotensin Released by juxta-glomerular cells in kidney nephrons	• ↓ BP/circulating volume • Change in solute concentration	• Vasoconstriction • ↑ Peripheral resistence • Na^+ & H_2O retention
Parathyroid hormone Produced by parathyroid gland	↓ Calcium levels ↑ Calcium levels	• Parathyroid hormone secreted and depressed • Maintains level of ionised calcium in plasma

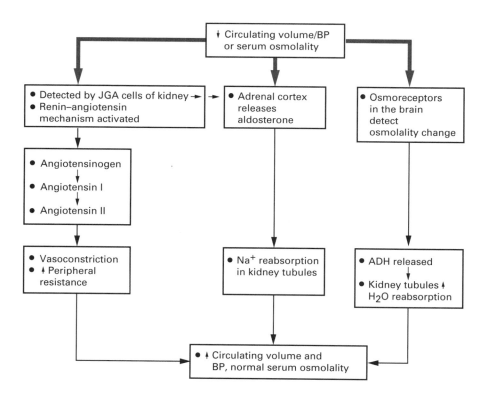

Fig. 10.5 Flow diagram outlining interrelated role of ADH, aldosterone and renin–angiotensin.

ADH, aldosterone and the renin-angiotensin system

These play major and interrelated roles in the maintenance of fluid and electrolyte balance (Table 10.4, Fig. 10.5)

In the normal ageing individual the release of ADH appears to be increased in response to a variety of stimuli which can result in the retention of fluid.

Atrial natiruretic hormone

Sodium can also be altered by other hormones called natiruretic hormones. The actions of these hormones are not clearly understood except for the atrial natiruretic hormone. This is released from the walls of the atria. It appears only to respond to severe changes in fluid volume, not to small changes in sodium intake. It does not therefore appear to play an important part in regulating sodium from day to day. It causes the reduction of renin release which in turn reduces the amount of aldosterone secreted. It is also known to reduce the level of ADH release by the posterior pituitary. The level of physiological concentration that influences the release of atrial natiruretic hormone is not known.

Acid–base balance

Metabolism results in the production of waste products, necessitating the maintenance of acid–base balance within body fluids. The respiratory system is responsible for this as are the blood and the kidneys. Blood is normally alkaline at a pH range of 7.38–7.42. This range is essential for the function of processes such as enzyme function, muscle contraction and blood clotting. The maximum deviation from this range that is compatible with life is 6.8 (extreme acidosis) – 7.8 (extreme alkalosis). The hydrogen ion concentration of blood is measured as pH. These parameters reflect the level of alkalinity or acidity.

Ingested food produces hydrogen ions during metabolism and carbon dioxide is continually entering the blood as an end product of carbohydrate and fat metabolism (Davidson 1987, p 13).

Three interrelated and well integrated mechanisms work within the body to preserve the appropriate pH of blood and maintain acid–base balance: chemical buffer systems in ECF and within cells, removal of carbon dioxide by the lungs and renal regulation of hydrogen ion concentration.

Physiological buffers

A buffer is a substance which accepts hydrogen ions from an acidic solution and donates hydrogen ions to an alkaline solution, thus minimising a change in pH. In essence blood buffers (present in all body fluid) provide the means for hydrogen ions to be transported from their site of production to their site of elimination with a minimum alteration of blood pH. These consist chiefly of bicarbonate, phosphate and protein, particularly haemoglobin i.e. (see Table 10.5).

The bicarbonate buffering system is of primary importance and is well described in texts such as Metheny (1996) and Smith (1980). It precisely regulates the concentration of carbon dioxide by the lungs and the kidneys by the following reaction sequence:

$$CO_2 + H_2O = H_2CO_3 = H^+ + HCO_3^-$$

A change in ECF hydrogen will stimulate peripheral chemoreceptors resulting in an increased respiratory rate and depth. In the lungs oxygen will associate with haemoglobin, resulting in the release of hydrogen which then combines with bicarbonate to form carbonic acid.

Table 10.5 The main physiological buffers

Buffer	Body compartment		
Bicarbonate	Blood	ICF	ECF
Plasma protein	Blood	ICF	ECF
Haemoglobin	Blood	–	–
Phosphate	Blood	ICF	ECF

Carbonic acid dehydrates to form carbonic anhydrase, releasing carbon dioxide which diffuses out of the erythrocytes and into the alveoli. In this way, carbon dioxide elimination removes hydrogen ions from the blood.

A change in hydrogen ion concentration in the blood will also cause the kidneys to excrete an acidic or alkaline urine which helps restore the normal pH balance. Respiratory compensation restores normal pH within minutes, whereas renal restoration is a slow process which may take hours or days to achieve. The largest source of buffer capacity in the body is found in the tissues and plasma proteins; haemoglobin is of particular importance.

In the vascular compartment carbon dioxide dissolves in water producing carbonic acid that dissociates to release hydrogen ions which is buffered by haemoglobin. The amount of bicarbonate produced in this way depends on the partial pressure of carbon dioxide (PCO_2) in the blood. Once the bicarbonate is produced it leaves the red blood cells by passive diffusion across the cell membrane into the plasma. As bicarbonate is an anion, its movement out of the cell is compensated by the inward movement of chloride. This movement is called the chloride shift. In this way the buffering capacity of haemoglobin greatly assists in the maintenance of a normal plasma pH. These acid bases provide a source of one of the most predominant buffers in the ICF – phosphate. Two forms of phosphate are involved:

- NaH_2PO_4 which is a weak acid
- Na_2HPO_4 which is weakly alkaline.

Buffering occurs when the alkaline phosphate combines with hydrogen to form the acid phosphate. This process takes place in the kidneys and is probably more important during chronic disturbances such as renal failure.

If the mechanisms and buffer systems fail, the resultant changes in blood pH will become life threatening.

FLUID VOLUME LOSS AND GAIN

Fluid volume loss

Most clinical situations potentially threaten an individual's fluid and electrolyte balance: water imbalance rarely occurs alone, and is usually accompanied by sodium imbalance. Loss of fluid volume may be sudden and acute, requiring immediate resuscitation, or gradual and insidious as a consequence of disease, infirmity or surgical intervention. This can result in fluid loss due to reduced input, increased output, or both. Dehydration (depletion of body water) results from fluid deprivation or loss of water. Individuals who are otherwise healthy may become dehydrated if deprived of water. Clinically significant volume loss results from loss of water, sodium and other electrolytes. Fluid volume loss is usually described in terms of serum sodium concentration: that is, hyperosmolar, isosmolar or hypo-osmolar volume depletion (Box 10.2).

In response to reduced fluid volume, homeostatic mechanisms will attempt to compensate for fluid loss. Antidiuretic hormone will reduce water loss from the body by retaining fluid and consequently reducing urine volume. The kidneys will also attempt to expand volume through activating the renin–angiotensin–aldosterone mechanism, resulting in sodium and water retention.

How fluid volume loss will manifest itself will depend on the severity of loss and how quickly it has occurred. Irrespective of the cause of fluid loss, cardiac output will be impaired because of diminished preload. Presenting patient problems will reflect the effects of reduced cardiac output, disruption of normal cellular metabolism and the resulting activation of homeostatic mechanisms to compensate.

> Many clinical situations threaten fluid and electrolyte balance. The results of such a loss can be sudden and acute, or gradual. In either case, assessment is the key to effective intervention.

■ **BOX 10.2** Fluid loss and possible causes

Type of fluid deficit	Possible causes
Hyperosmolar due to body water losses The ECF compartment is depleted, initially increasing the osmolality (creating an osmotic gradient) – fluid becomes hypertonic. In response fluid moves out of the ICF compartment into the ECF compartment, thereby maintaining intravascular volume.	• Food and water deprivation • Increased body or environmental temperature • Diabetes mellitus with hyperglycaemia • Hyperalimination • Diuresis in diabetes insipidus
Isosmolar (due to loss of fluids and electrolytes) Water and electrolytes are lost in equal proportions. ECF remains isosmolar, but volume decreases in all fluid compartments if not replaced.	• Loss of body fluids containing salt e.g. gastrointestinal loss from vomiting, diarrhoea, nasogastric loss • Haemorrhage, burns, peritonitis
Hypo-osmolar (solute loss in excess of water excretion) Reduced serum sodium and osmolality cause the ECF to become hypotonic. This results in an osmotic shift of fluid from the ECF compartment into the ICF compartment.	• Excessive use of diuretics, causing solutes to be lost in excess of water, and hypertonic urine • Gastrointestinal secretion loss

Fluid volume excess

Excess fluid volume (overhydration) is usually iatrogenic, but may be exacerbated by certain diseases, and in the presence of impaired heart, renal or liver function (Box 10.3).

Oedema is defined as the accumulation of abnormal quantities of fluid in the interstitial tissues (see below). However, the presence of oedema does not always indicate true fluid overload. A loss of albumin from the vascular compartment can cause peripheral oedema, yet the patient may be hypovolaemic (Urden et al 1992). The origins of oedema formation are extensive and valuable texts include Marieb (1994) and Vander et al (1992). In cases of fluid volume excess oedema can manifest itself generally, peripherally, or as pulmonary oedema.

NURSING ASSESSMENT IN FLUID AND ELECTROLYTE BALANCE

Fluid balance may be viewed as a dynamic entity, where assessment and intervention overlap, and where there are no clearly distinguishable boundaries as to where one starts and the other ends. It is the findings of assessment that inform nursing intervention and therefore through efficient analysis of assessment findings interventions can be anticipated and promptly instigated.

Identification of sources of fluid and electrolyte loss and gain in the highly dependent patient are imperative for continuous safe and effective monitoring (Box 10.4 on p. 248). Loss or gain of relatively small amounts of fluid and electrolytes can tip a very delicate balance in an unstable patient.

■ BOX 10.3 Fluid gain and possible causes

Type of fluid excess	Possible causes
Hypertonic Can result from increased solutes in the ECF compartment, leading to water being drawn out of the cells.	• Excessive administration of sodium bicarbonate (a greater proportion of sodium and protein) and of glucose (in hyperglycaemia)
Isotonic Resulting from increased fluid and electrolyte gains. Expansion of both ICF and ECF compartments occur.	• Excessive infusion of isotonic solutions • Congestive heart failure, acute renal failure, nephrotic syndrome, liver cirrhosis
Hypotonic (water intoxication) Excess water in the ECF compartment has a dilutional effect, reducing the osmotic gradient (sodium content is normal but excess water is present leading to hyponatraemia). Water moves from the ECF causing overhydration and swelling of cells.	• Excessive fluid intake, orally or infusion of 5% dextrose • Renal impairment, retention of irrigation fluid (urological surgery) • Physiological stress, e.g. as a result of trauma or surgery (ADH production is affected and increases rapidly, overriding normal regulation). This can result in reduced urine output and osmolality, leading to water retention and hyponatraemia

COLLECTION OF ASSESSMENT DATA

Records of fluid intake and output All fluid losses and gains need to be recorded on a fluid balance chart to provide a comprehensive record of fluid balance over a period of time. The time of day, volume and nature and sources of loss and gain need to be clearly identified.

Patient weight Significant fluctuations in body weight can occur over a matter of days and an important assessment of fluid status is patient weight. Daily measurement, at the same time, and on the same scales, provides essential comparative information over a period of time. The appropriateness of this assessment measure would be relative in individual cases. The use of bedscales will facilitate this in the highly dependent patient.

Cardiovascular assessment

Blood pressure and pulse

Assessment of blood pressure and pulse provides vital information on the patient's fluid balance status.

Pulse rate In general fluid loss the pulse rate will increase – with a loss of less than 10% blood volume (500 ml in an adult) there is often no clinical indication of hypovolaemia. With increasing loss of blood volume the first sign is tachycardia, followed by peripheral vasoconstriction resulting in pale cold extremities and a thready pulse. In general, fluid volume excess would normally be accompanied by tachycardia.

■ **BOX 10.4** Potential sources of fluid loss and gain

Sources of increased fluid loss

Urinary

Polyuria

- In certain conditions e.g. excess solutes from uncontrolled diabetes mellitus
- Excessive infusion of glucose or sodium bicarbonate
- Diabetes insipidus and ARF
- Overuse of diuretics

Respiratory

- Normal loss increases in a dry environment as a result of increased respiratory rate (tachypnoea)
- Lack of humidified oxygen

Skin

- With increased body temperature
- As a result of burns

GI Tract

- Diarrhoea and vomiting
- NG tube drainage
- Intestinal wound drains
- Ostomies, fistulae
- Haematoma and abscess formation
- Increased capillary permeability
- Paralytic ileus
- Peritonitis

Sources of increased fluid gain

Retention of fluid

- Renal, cardiac and liver failure

Oral fluids

- Excessive intake

Fluid replacement

- i.v. infusion, parenteral nutrition
- Gastrointestinal feeding
- Drugs in large fluid volumes

Blood pressure Ultimately this will decrease in continued fluid volume loss; however, initially it will be maintained by peripheral vasoconstriction. Blood volume loss in excess of 20% causes hypotension with systolic blood pressure less than 90 mmHg and diastolic often unrecordable (Davidson 1987). Estimations most notably change in cases of volume depletion. An increased pulse rate is usually the first sign, with a decreased blood pressure relative to loss. In fluid volume excess blood pressure is usually raised related to underlying cause of excess and often proportional to volume of excess.

Central venous pressure

- CVP estimates pressure in the right atrium with a range of 0–4 cm water. CVP recording enables monitoring of the effectiveness of fluid replacement therapy,

Table 10.6 Systemic signs and symptoms in fluid loss and gain

System	Signs in fluid loss	Signs in fluid gain	Monitoring and nursing observation
Cardiovascular	• Increased heart rate • Irregular thready pulse • Reduced blood pressure and CVP	• Increased heart rate, BP, CVP • Neck vein distension may be evident	• Pulse • Blood pressure • CVP
Respiratory	• Increased respiratory rate • Hyperventilation	• Increased rate • Dyspnoea and pulmonary oedema may be evident	• Nature and frequency of respirations • Signs of waterlogging of pulmonary circulation • Oxygenation status – skin colour • Saturation, i.e. pulse oximetry/blood gases
Urinary system	• Urine output decreased, or increased in diabetes insipidus	Output may be increased or decreased, depending on the underlying cause and renal function.	• Volume of urine output/24 h period
General orientation behaviour	• Apprehension • Restlessness	• Confusion • Irritability	• General orientation status
Skin	• Texture is dry and lax, under-perfusion of tissues and reduced vascularity leading to skin colour change, dry mucous membranes and evidence of thirst. • Excessive perspiration accompanies increased body temperature	• Dependent, generalised, and/or pitting oedema. • The skin may be warm, moist and swollen, with the appearance of being tight and shiny	• General appearance/ hydrational status • Colour • Temperature • Condition of mucous membranes

and recurrent fluid losses and gains. In uncomplicated fluid loss this is a reliable indicator of blood volume.

- General trends in CVP measurement need to be assessed.
- CVP monitoring aids assessment of the degree of volume depletion. Effective refilling of the circulation should be reflected by a normal reading.
- A low CVP may indicate decreased blood volume or drug induced vasodilatation, causing pooling of blood in the peripheral veins.
- A high CVP may indicate increased blood volume or heart failure, or vasoconstriction (causing the vascular bed to become smaller) (Metheny 1992).
- The frequency of CVP recordings will be titrated in relation to fluid administration and blood pressure. Overloading of the circulation needs to be observed when kidney function is compromised, and in pre-existing cardiac and respiratory conditions. CVP in conjunction with other parameters reflects the ongoing fluid status of the patient.

Systemic symptoms and signs in fluid loss and gain are given in Table 10.6.

Skin

Gently pinching the skin can reveal information about the interstitial fluid volume and skin elasticity. Normally, after pinching, skin will immediately return to its usual position. With fluid volume deficit, skin can remain 'raised' for several seconds. With age however, skin elasticity is lost, and this assessment alone will not truly reflect a fluid deficit.

Examination of the oral cavity should reveal a moist mouth and tongue. In cases of fluid loss the mucous membranes and tongue will appear dry; this may also be caused by mouth breathing as a result of hyperventilation.

Oedema

Oedema is defined as the accumulation of abnormal quantities of fluid in the interstitial spaces, and may be assessed through visual observation and weight gain, and also by applying fingertip pressure over a bony prominence, e.g. ankle, shin and sacrum. If indentation does not disappear within 30 seconds 'pitting' oedema is present. This indicates increased interstitial volume and is evident when 10% weight gain has occurred (Urden et al 1992).

URINARY SYSTEM

Volume

Urine volume is approximately 1500 ml per day, but can range from 1000 to 2000 ml depending upon intake, other sources of loss and gain, and renal function. As a rule of thumb, normal urine output is about 1 ml per kilogram of body weight, per hour, with parameters of 0.5–2 ml/kg/h (Pestana 1989).

Specific gravity (SG)

Normal range is 1.003–1.035. SG estimates the kidneys' ability to concentrate urine. It measures density or weight of urine compared with 1.000 SG distilled water. As urine contains electrolytes and other substances, its SG is higher than 1.000. SG is elevated in cases of fluid volume deficit, as the kidneys retain fluid, resulting in solutes being excreted in a smaller more concentrated urine volume. A more concentrated urine (increased SG) will occur in solute excess, for example in diabetes mellitus. A decreased SG may indicate the inability of the kidneys to excrete the normal solute load, or increased water loss as a result of diuretics.

Urine osmolality

Renal concentrating capacity declines with age, becoming evident between the ages of 45 and 50. A consequence of this is impaired ability of the kidney.

Normal range is 300–1200 mOsml/l. The urine osmolality accurately reflects the concentrating ability of the kidneys but unlike SG is not significantly altered by the presence of blood, pus or casts in the urine (Colbert 1993). Urine osmolality increases in fluid volume deficit as the kidneys conserve fluid, and decreases in fluid volume excess as fluid is excreted by the kidneys. Simultaneous measurement of serum and urine osmolality provides an accurate measure of fluid status.

BIOCHEMICAL ASSESSMENT

Serum osmolality

Normal values are 280–295 mOsm/kg and reflect the concentration or dilution of vascular fluid. This is determined by the number of particles in solution in relation to the volume of body water. Serum osmolality is mostly determined by serum sodium concentration. Serum osmolality findings increase in dehydration (hypernatraemia) and decrease in overhydration (hyponatraemia).

Serum albumin

Normal values are 3.5–4.8 g/dl. Albumin helps to maintain intravascular volume by maintaining colloid osmotic pressure. If serum albumin is reduced fluid moves from the vascular compartment to the interstitial space, creating peripheral oedema and reducing effective blood volume.

Haemocrit

Normal values are 40–50% in males and 37–47% in females. Changes in the haemocrit can indicate an increase or decrease in intravascular volume. Changes resulting from other processes such as disease, bleeding or haemolysis need to be established. In fluid volume loss the haemocrit can be increased as a result of haemoconcentration: red blood cells are contained in a relatively smaller plasma fluid volume. In fluid volume excess haemocrit can be decreased as a result of haemodilution as red blood cells are contained in a relatively larger plasma fluid volume.

NURSING INTERVENTION IN MAINTAINING

FLUID AND ELECTROLYTE BALANCE

The aim of intervention is to restore and maintain normal fluid and electrolyte balance, thereby enabling homeostatic mechanisms to allow normal cellular function.

Fluid and electrolyte loss

In cases of sudden or continuous fluid and electrolyte loss replacement is necessary, and the intravenous route is invariably utilised for this patient group. In the long term the benefits of tube feeding and parenteral nutrition need to be considered in maintaining fluid and electrolyte balance. The nature and volume of intravenous fluid replacement are decided upon in relation to loss. (See Table 10.7 for examples of intravenous solutions).

Crystalloid electrolyte solutions are named for their potential to form crystals. Once infused into the vein they diffuse through the capillary endothelium, and they are then distributed throughout the ECF compartment as necessary to maintain fluid balance.

Isotonic crystalloid solutions e.g. 0.9% sodium chloride and lactated Ringer's have a sodium concentration similar to ECF. They are distributed throughout the ECF – both plasma and interstitial compartments – very little enters the cells. Isotonic solutions replace deficits of ECF volume. 1 litre of isotonic sodium chloride will expand the ECF by 1 litre; it contributes to both plasma and interstitial compartments but because of their relative size, 1 litre of isotonic saline will theoretically only expand the plasma volume by a quarter of a litre (Smith 1980).

Hypotonic Crystalloid Solutions e.g. 5% dextrose and half strength normal saline have an osmolality of less than serum osmolality, therefore water is distributed equally throughout all fluid compartments – both ICF and ECF. When replacement of total body water is required (in all fluid compartments) 5% dextrose is used as this contributes to all fluid compartments equally. Considering the relative size of the body fluid compartments, 3 litres of dextrose would be needed to expand the ECF by 1 litre (Smith 1980).

> Keeping a meticulous record of fluid and loss gain is essential in building up an hourly picture.

Table 10.7 Intravenous solutions

Solution and contents	Indications/actions	Contraindications/comments
0.9% Sodium chloride (normal saline) (isotonic) • water • sodium 154 mmol/l • chloride 154 mmol/l	• Extracellular Na^+, Cl^-, and H_2O deficits, hypovolaemia • Distributed throughout ECF, does not enter ICF, expands interstitial and plasma compartments without altering normal Na^+ concentration or serum osmolality	• Because of sodium content, potential risk of fluid retention and circulatory overload
4% Dextrose and 0.18%Saline (dextrose saline) • water • glucose 40 g/l • sodium 30 mmol/l • chloride 30 mmol/l	• Used in combined sodium and water depletion • Allows water to enter body cells to correct dehydration, while sodium and small amounts of water remain extracellular to correct sodium depletion	• As for sodium chloride
5% Dextrose (isotonic) • water • dextrose 50 g/l	• Dehydration, in water deficit with no significant electrolyte imbalances • Isotonic only in its container; when in the vascular system dextrose is metabolised leaving water which is distributed evenly throughout the body • Used to replace deficits in total body water, not to expand ECF volume	• Hyperglycaemia • Should not be used in excessive volumes in patients with↑ ADH activity or to replace fluids in hypovolaemic patients (Metheny 1996)
Ringer's solution (isotonic) • water • sodium 146 mmol/l • chloride 152 mmol/l • potassium 4 mmol/l • calcium 2 mmol/l	• Replaces body fluid, provides additional K^+ and Ca^+. More clearly resembles electrolyte composition of blood serum and plasma	• Potential hyperchloraemic metabolic acidosis due to high Cl^- concentration • Potential fluid retention and circulatory overload due to sodium content
Ringer's lactate (Hartman's Solution) (isotonic) • water • sodium 131 mmol/l • chloride 109 mmol/l • potassium 4 mmol/l • calcium 2 mmol/l • lactate 28 mmol/l	• Hypovolaemia, burns and fluid loss in bile or diarrhoea (Metheny 1996) • Treating mild metabolic acidosis • Lactate is converted to bicarbonate (in the liver) which buffers acidosis	• Risk of lactic acidosis particularly with poor tissue perfusion and impaired liver function • Risk of fluid retention and circulatory overload due to sodium content
0.45% Sodium chloride (half strength saline) • water • sodium 77 mmol/500 ml • chloride 77 mmol/500 ml	• Used as maintenance therapy, also in hypovolaemia when hypernatraemia is present	• Potential interstitial and intracellular oedema due to rapid movement of this fluid from the vascular compartment
Albumin preparations Human albumin solution • (HAS) 4.5% • Albuminar-5, • Buminate	• Acute or subacute loss of plasma volume, e.g. burns, haemorrhagic shock pancreatitis, trauma, surgical complications	• Cardiac failure, severe anaemia • Side effects: nausea, fever, chills particularly with rapid infusion

(cont'd...)

(*Table 10.7 cont'd*)

**Plasma substitutes
(colloid solutions)**

• Dextran 70, 110 6% in dextrose or sodium chloride 0.9%	• Volume replacement in shock, burns, septicaemia. • Provide short-term volume expansion, used in place of albumin and blood • Alternative preparations for low blood volume expansion, while waiting for compatible blood	• Cautions: congestive heart failure, renal impairment, x-matching should ideally be done before infusion • Contraindications: severe congestive heart failure, renal failure, bleeding disorders
• Gelofusine • Haemaccel • Hetastarch • Elohes 6% • Hespan	• Low blood volume expansion	• (as for Dextran) • (as for Dextran)

When replacement of total body water is required (pure) water cannot be administered intravenously as it is hypotonic, and would cause haemolysis of red cells – osmosis would pull water into the cells, expanding them until they burst. Adding dextrose renders water isotonic because dextrose is metabolised leaving water without haemolysis ocurring.

Colloid solutions function physiologically like plasma proteins in blood by maintaining colloid osmotic pressure. They are used to replace acute fluid volume losses as they expand the plasma compartment. Once infused they enter the intravascular compartment to maintain fluid volume – the osmotic pressure exerted pulls fluid from the interstitium into the plasma. When the capillary endothelium is functioning normally colloids will remain in the circulation for several days. In conditions that cause the capillary endothelium to leak, e.g. in septic shock, blunt trauma or adult respiratory distress syndrome, colloid will leak into the interstitium pulling fluid with it. Colloids (examples are give in Table 10.7) are given in cases of acute volume depletion, and will maintain intravascular volume in cases of blood loss, until blood transfusion is available.

Assessment findings include:

CASE EXAMPLE 10.1 FLUID LOSS

Mrs Jones is a 72-year-old lady who had an abdominal hernia repair 5 days ago. Over the past 24 hours she has become increasingly unwell with a downward trend in blood pressure. She has a 3-day history of nausea and vomiting and is now unable to tolerate oral fluids. She received crystalloid fluid replacement via a peripheral infusion overnight, but unfortunately her peripheral veins are poor and the infusion tissued several times. On closer examination it appears that her urine output has been gradually tailing off over the past 48 hours. She is also pyrexial. Her medical history includes increasingly debilitating rheumatoid arthritis which has been treated with NSAIDs. Her peripheral infusion is resited but allows infusion of only small amounts of fluid. Despite crystalloid fluid replacement she remains oliguric and hypotensive.

Assessment findings include:

* *BP 90/60 mmHg, P110*
* *Respiratory rate 30/min*
* *Temperature 37.8⁰C. She is perspiring heavily, and is hot and clammy*
* *Perfusional status: generally pale with no evidence of hypoxia*
* *Fluid intake in previous 24 hours Intake: 1000 ml via infusion (infusion issued over-night)*

(Cont'd...)

(Case example 10.1 cont'd)

Fluid loss in previous 24 hours:
- *Urine output: actual volume recorded = 100 ml*
- *Several episodes of incontinence during the night; amount?*
- *Five episodes of diarrhoea; amount?*
- *Vomited 400 ml (approx)*
- *Pressure areas are intact, sacrum and elbows appear red*
- *Oriented to day and time, is distressed and anxious*

Summary of assessment findings

- *The assessment data above indicate fluid volume deficit with both fluid and electrolyte loss exceeding gain. In addition to accountable losses Mrs Jones is also losing fluid through perspiration. A negative fluid balance exists with ongoing fluid loss from several sources and there has been inadequate fluid replacement.*
- *Vital signs reflect reduced circulating volume and hypovolaemia. It is unclear how long Mrs Jones has been hypotensive and oliguric.*
- *Reduced urine output would appear to be as a result of reduced circulating plasma volume (with ADH secretion retaining and conserving water) in response to a poor perfusion state. The most common cause of acute renal failure is a hypovolaemic/ischaemic incident, particularly in patients with an underlying predisposing factor such as long-term use of non-steroidal anti-inflammatory drugs (NSAIDs).*
- *The possibility of ensuing sepsis/capillary leak syndrome needs to be considered.*

Nursing intervention

Mrs Jones has a reduced plasma volume, e.g. hypotension, tachycardia and oliguria, and urgent expansion of the plasma compartment is required to prevent her condition deteriorating any further with resulting organ failure.

Crystalloid fluids are not an efficient means of expanding the plasma volume, which is needed in this instance, as approximately three-quarters of a crystalloid infusion is quickly lost from the plasma (Armstrong et al 1997, p 6). It is decided to perform a fluid challenge, because it is important to ascertain whether oliguria is a result of reduced blood flow secondary to fluid volume loss (pre-renal failure) or acute tubular necrosis because of prolonged hypovolaemia:

- *A CVP line is inserted to monitor pressure in the right atrium which will reflect effectiveness of fluid replacement therapy, with a reading of +1 cm H_2O.*
- *A urethral catheter is inserted – 20 ml of urine are drained. This will enable close monitoring of the hourly urine output in response to replacement fluid, reflecting the health of renal function.*

An algorithm for fluid challenge is suggested by Armstrong et al (1997):

1. *Measure CVP (right atrial pressure).*
2. *Administer 200 ml colloid over 10 minutes.*
3. *Stop after 5 minutes if CVP is increased by 3 mmHg and there is clinical improvement, i.e. improved urine output.*
4. *If there is no increase in CVP repeat steps 2 and 3. Peripheral vasoconstriction may maintain CVP despite hypovolaemia.*

Specific ongoing assessment and intervention
Cardiovascular

Blood pressure, pulse rate and CVP need to be frequently measured to assess response to the increasing ECF volume, observing for signs of stabilising blood pressure, pulse rate and CVP (returning to normal parameters) as fluid volume is replenished.

The following also need to be observed for: continued fluid loss from the vascular compartment, as for example in capillary leak syndrome with persistent hypotension, low

(Cont'd...)

(Case example 10.1 cont'd)
CVP and tachycardia. A steadily rising blood pressure and CVP may result in overloading of the circulation.

Table 10.8 Measurement of urine, and urine and plasma: for the following chemical ratios (Kjellstrand et al (1989)).

	Hypovolaemia (Pre-renal)	Established (ARF)
Urine osmolality	> 400 mOsm/kg	< 350 mOsm/kg
Urine specific gravity	> 1.030	< 1.020
Urine/plasma creatinine ratio	> 30	< 20
Urinary sodium	< 30 mmol/l	> 30 mmol/l

Ongoing fluid losses

Assessment, monitoring and recording all instances and sources of fluid loss and gain is imperative to ascertain an hourly picture of overall fluid balance. These include hourly urine volume measurement, alerting medical staff if this is less than 30 ml/h for 2 consecutive hours. Ensure catheter drainage tubing is carefully 'milked' to account for all urine produced. Urine output should be restored to normal if current decreased output is purely functional and colloid filling has been successful in raising CVP.

Account for all gastrointestinal losses, and monitor fluid loss from respiration and perspiration.

Respiratory

The response to the increasing vascular volume will be reflected in the nature and rate of respiration. Assess for:
- *Ease of breathing and general respiratory effort, which provide an indication of overall patient condition, and should be restored to normal as volume is replaced.*
- *Signs of fluid overload, e.g. dyspnoea, pulmonary oedema and increased production of sputum.*
- *Oxygenation status: general skin colour; and oxygen saturation levels through pulse oximetry and arterial blood gas estimations. Administer prescribed humidified oxygen. Initiate regular physiotherapy, supplementing this as necessary by encouraging deep breathing and leg exercises.*

Biochemistry

Estimation of serum: sodium, potassium, urea, creatinine and haematocrit levels, and serum osmolality.

General

Positioning of the patient is of vital importance, and should be carried out in relation to blood pressure recordings. The aim is for maximum comfort and ease of respiratory effort. Mrs Jones' rheumatoid arthritis will increase her risk of developing pressure areas: risk assessment and scoring are vital in initiating use of the correct pressure relieving aids.

A high standard of oral hygiene will be needed to counteract the effects of fluid volume deficit on delicate muous membranes, thereby reducing the risk of infection.

Replacement of fluid losses should restore blood pressure to within normal range and result in normal volumes of urine production. If this does not occur further circulatory support will be considered, e.g. dopamine, and the use of diuretics such as frusemide and eventually mannitol if oliguria persists. The underlying cause of persisting pyrexia should be further investigated.

(Cont'd...)

- Use intravenous fluid replacement appropriate to loss.
- Frequent estimation of serum electrolytes will guide specific replacement needs. (Table 10.7 outlines content of commonly used solutions and indications for use.)
- In stable patients with normal kidney function: 1000 ml (to cover insensible losses) + previous day's losses e.g. urinary and gastrointestinal.
- Rehydration of previous losses and any ongoing losses must be added.

(Case example 10.1 cont'd)

In simple fluid volume loss immediate restoration of fluid and electrolyte losses with prescribed intravenous fluids such as isotonic crystalloid fluids, e.g. 0.9% sodium chloride will replenish ECF volume and electrolyte losses (Box 10.5). Elderly patients receiving isotonic intravenous fluids are more likely to have a degree of cardiac and renal dysfunction, therefore the kidneys' ability to excrete fluid may well be reduced. Close monitoring and observation are always required. Once a normotensive state is restored hypotonic electrolyte solutions will provide electrolytes and free water for the renal excretion of metabolic wastes (Metheny 1996).

■ **BOX 10.5** Examples of maintenance intravenous fluids (Adapted from Davidson 1987 p 21)

Solution and volume	Providing
• 500 ml 0.9% sodium chloride • 1 L 5% dextrose + 40 mmol K^+ • 1 L 5% dextrose + 40 mmol K^+	Na^+ 75 mmol K^+ 80 mmol H_2O 2500 ml Energy 400 kcal
or	
• 1 L dextrose/saline + 20 mmol K^+ • 1 L dextrose/saline + 20 mmol K^+ • 1 L dextrose/saline + 20 mmol K^+	Na^+ 90 mmol K^+ 60 mmol H_2O 3000 ml Energy 480 kcal

Table 10.9 Diuretics (British National Formulatory 1995)

	Actions/indication	Side effects	Considerations/ nursing actions
Loop diuretics Example: frusemide Oral: 40 mg initially maintenance 20 mg/day resistant oedema 80 mg/day i.v. infusion prescribed for urine output up to 1 g every 24 h	• Inhibits reabsorption in the ascending loop of Henle of the renal tubule • Inhibited reabsorption of sodium and chloride leads to increased water and potassium loss • *Indications*: when potent diuresis needed, oliguria, renal insufficiency, oedema of congestive heart failure	• Hypovolaemia • Hypotension • Electrolyte imbalances: Hypokalaemia Hypomagnesaemia Hypochloraemic Acidosis • Occasional GI disturbances	• Act within 1 hour of oral administration. Diuresis complete within 6 hours • Following i.v. administration have peak effect within 30 minutes • Closely monitor fluid and electrolyte balance • Potassium supplements may be required • Toxicity of digoxin increased with hypokalaemia, observe for toxicity
Thiazide diuretics Example: bendrofluazide Initial 2.5–10 mg 1–3 times	• Inhibit sodium and chloride reabsorption in the distal tubule • *Indications*: hypertension, congestive heart failure,	• Weakness, fatigue • Potassium depletion • Hyponatraemia • Metabolic alkalosis • Hyperglycaemia due	• Act within 1–2 hours of oral administration, mostly have a duration of

(cont'd...)

(Table 10.9 Cont'd)

per week	chronic conditions with sodium and water retention. • Have a moderately potent sustained effect	to reduced glucose tolerance • Gout	action of 24 hours • Usually administered in the morning to avoid night-time diuresis • Monitor fluid and electrolyte balance • Observe for hypotension • Observe potassium levels • Give potassium supplements as prescribed • Check blood sugar levels with impaired glucose intolerance
Potassium sparing Example: amiloride Initial 10 mg daily maximum 20 mg per day Triamterene Initial 150–250 mg daily reducing after 1 week	• Used alone are weak diuretics. Exert effect on the renal tubules – cause a reduction of potassium and hydrogen ion excretion, a mild increase in sodium excretion • *Indications*: oedema, as an alternative to giving potassium supplements with loop diuretics or thiazides	• GI disturbances • Hyperkalaemia • Hyponatraemia • Dry mouth • Rashes • Orthostatic hypotension	• Monitor fluid and electrolyte balance • Do not use potassium supplements • Half-life of digoxin may be increased with potassium sparing diuretics – observe for digoxin toxicity
Spironolactone 100–200 mg daily up to 400 mg if required	• Potassium sparing, that potentiates thiazide or loop diuretics by antagonising aldosterone • *Indications*: oedema of liver cirrhosis, heart failure	• Gynaecomastia • GI disturbances • Hyperkalaemia	
Osmotic diuretics Example: mannitol 10%, 20% and 25% i.v. infusion 50–200 g over 24 hours	• Used in cerebral oedema	• Rarely used in heart failure, may acutely expand the blood volume • Chills, fever	• Extravasation causes inflammation and thrombophlebitis • Monitor fluid balance • Monitor electrolyte balance
Other diuretics Combined diuretics, diuretics with potassium, mercurial diuretics and carbonic anhydrase inhibitors			

See British National Formulary and manufacturer guidelines for complete information

CASE EXAMPLE 10.2 FLUID GAIN

Mr Davies is a 79-year-old man who has been admitted to a medical ward for fluid replacement following a 3-day history of diarrhoea and vomiting. His medical history includes heart failure secondary to hypertension, which has been treated for the past 18 months with diuretics, digoxin and vasodilators. Since admission previous gastrointestinal losses have been replaced with isotonic crystalloids, but the unreliable history provided by Mr Davies made it difficult to approximate fluid loss. Once fluid replacement commenced, he appeared to be improving quickly.

During the early hours of the morning (4 a.m.) Mr Davies's condition deteriorated rapidly and a diagnosis of acute left ventricular failure resulting in pulmonary oedema was made.

Heart failure may be defined as circulatory inefficiency in which the heart fails to supply the metabolic needs of the body (Willats & Winter 1997). Fluid volume excess in heart failure is a result of sodium and water retention. In summary the mechanisms involved include:

- *Low cardiac output which leads to reduced renal blood flow and hence reduced glomerular filtration rate, which result in increased reabsorption of water and sodium by the kidney tubules.*
- *The effective fall in circulating blood volume increases aldosterone and ADH production. Sodium and water retention increase the filling pressure of the myocardium.*
- *Myocardial failure increases venous pressure which increases hydrostatic pressure at the venous end of the capillary. Fluid is forced out into the surrounding tissues resulting in expansion of the interstitial volume in the form of oedema (Fig. 10.6).*

Valuable texts giving specific and detailed rationale include Vander, Sherman & Luciano (1994) and Colbert (1993).

Assessment findings include:

- *Dyspnoea causing distress and great respiratory effort*
- *Rapid respiratory rate – unable to record accurately*
- *Orthopnoea*
- *Production of frothy pink sputum*
- *Perfusional status: warm but developing peripheral cyanosis*
- *Blood pressure 180/110 mmHg*
- *Pulse 120*

(cont'd...)

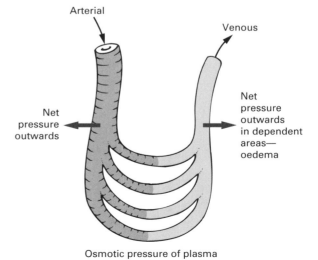

Fig. 10.6 Formation of oedema in heart failure.

Arterial

Venous

Net pressure outwards

Net pressure outwards in dependent areas— oedema

Osmotic pressure of plasma

(Case example 10.2 cont'd)
- Temperature (axilla) 37.2°C
- Agitated and distressed, with increasing disorientation
- Pressure areas intact, extremely red sacral area
- Medication: usual medication prescribed via oral route as no vomiting since admission.
- Fluid intake since admission (13 hours ago):
  — intravenous fluids – 1400 ml
  — oral fluids – difficult to estimate (water jug empty!) but only 300 ml recorded on fluid balance chart
- Fluid loss since admission.
  — Urinary loss: 200 ml
  — x 1 episode of diarrhoea – volume?

Summary of assessment findings

These data indicate a positive fluid balance resulting in fluid volume excess as a result of an overloading of intravenous infusions given too rapidly, combined with unsupervised oral fluid intake in an individual with borderline cardiac function.

The patient's acute respiratory distress, increased blood pressure and pulse rate and reduced urinary output signify the body's compensatory measures to maintain cardiac output:

1. *(Starling mechanism) By increasing the ventricular end diastolic volume (increasing the venous pressure/preload), the end diastolic fibre length is increased and hence so is the stroke volume. However in the failing heart this does not restore the cardiac output adequately and the main effect is to lead to an increase in venous pressure.*
2. *Activation of the sympathetic system leads to an increase in myocardial contractility and heart rate. Increased peripheral vascular resistance improves arterial pressure but at the cost of increased afterload. In addition activation of the renin–angiotensin system increases sodium and water retention and further increases venous pressure (Willats & Winter 1992, p 71).*

The accumulation of fluid in the interstitial spaces of the lungs or in the air spaces themselves impairs gaseous exchange resulting in pulmonary oedema (Fig. 10.7).

Nursing intervention

Management involves promoting oxygenation, improving cardiac output and reducing pulmonary congestion. Interventions include:
- *Sitting the patient upright and administering high flow oxygen.*
- *Reducing cardiac preload by removing excessive salt and water with loop diuretics, e.g. frusemide 80–120 mg or bumetanide 2–3 mg intravenously, causing venodilation as well as diuretic effect.*

(Cont'd...)

Fig. 10.7 Pulmonary oedema.

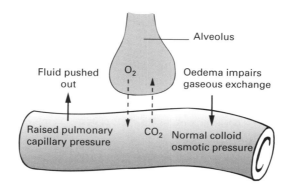

Alveolus

Fluid pushed out

O_2

Oedema impairs gaseous exchange

Raised pulmonary capillary pressure

CO_2

Normal colloid osmotic pressure

(Case example 10.2 cont'd)
- *Administering opiates, e.g. morphine 5–10 mg with an antiemetic. These reduce preload through venodilation and help alleviate distress.*
- *Administer intravenous nitrates, e.g. GTN 1–12 mg/h or isorbide dinitrate 2–10 mg/h via infusion pump. These are powerful venodilators – dose must be adjusted to avoid hypotension.*
- *Vasodilators may be used in conjunction with inotropic agents.*
(Adapted from Guly & Richardson 1996, pp 37–39)

Ongoing assessment and intervention

- *Administration of prescribed drugs.*

Respiration and oxygenation

- *Promote gaseous exchange by positioning the patient in an upright position to help alleviate dyspnoea, aid lung expansion and promote expectoration of excretions.*
- *Administer high flow humidified oxygen.*
- *Monitor and record the depth, rate and nature of respirations.*
- *Observe and monitor oxygenation status – general skin colour, oxygen saturation levels through pulse oximetry and/or arterial blood gas estimations. Blood gases will usually show hypoxia with a low $PaCO_2$. The outcome of successful intervention should be improved oxygenation status indicated by relief of hypoxia and increased $PaCO_2$.*

Cardiovascular

- *Monitor and record heart rate rhythm and BP. Intervention should reduce arterial BP and HR to within normal limits for the patient, but observe for the possibility of hypotension.*
- *A CVP line will enable fluid and drug management as well as evaluation of fluid volume reduction.*
- *Successful intervention should result in heart rate and blood pressure within normal limits, and sinus rhythm and CVP within acceptable parameters indicating a reduced venous pressure.*

Fluid balance

- *Input: all fluid volumes need to be accurately recorded on a fluid balance chart with maintenance of the hourly running total.*
- *Monitor the effects of administered diuretics (Table 10.9 outlines diuretics). Be aware of side effects and take account of outlined nursing considerations.*
- *Output: to accurately monitor urine output a urethral catheter will need to be inserted. Hourly volumes should then be monitored and recorded.*
- *All gastrointestinal losses are measured and recorded.*
- *The outcome of successful intervention should be improved urine output which alleviates general fluid overload.*

General

- *Promotion of skin integrity is vitally important as excess fluid in the tissues can lead to breakdown of the skin, and also a reduction in plasma protein that hinders skin and tissue repair. Mr Davies has an increased risk of developing pressure areas so risk assessment and scoring are vital in initiating use of the correct pressure relieving aids.*
- *Meticulous oral hygiene will counteract the drying effects of oxygen therapy on delicate mucous membranes, and reduce the risk of infection.*
- *Continuously assess the effect of opiates in relieving distress, and effects on respirations.*

Biochemistry

Blood needs to be assessed for estimation of renal function, regular serum potassium levels with diuretic therapy.

ELECTROLYTE IMBALANCES

The acutely ill patient's potential for developing electrolyte imbalances is ever present. The wide variety of presenting clinical features associated with electrolyte imbalance can further complicate the complex clinical scenarios of highly dependent patients. Electrolyte imbalances can occur insidiously without obvious presenting problems. Table 10.10 (p. 267) gives examples of the causes of electrolyte deficits and excess and possible presenting clinical features. Two of the most commonly encountered electrolyte disorders in acutely ill patients are those of potassium and sodium balance and both warrant in-depth exploration.

Potassium

The normal range is 3.5–5.0 mmol/l. Abnormal ranges of K^+ can affect nerve and muscle function, particularly cardiac muscle. Potassium is required for carbohydrate metabolism and is essential for the conversion of glucose to glycogen, and its storage. Serum K^+ levels are maintained through the kidneys' reabsorption and secretion of K^+ ions. This is closely related to reabsorption of Na^+ and H^+ ions. The kidneys adjust the urinary concentration in relation to K^+ intake.

Hypokalaemia

Hypokalaemia (serum K^+ = < 3.5 mmol/l) is a common electrolyte disturbance. Box 10.6 outlines possible causes of potassium loss. It requires prompt treatment because of its potential effect on cardiac muscle. Assessment includes:

- Identification of patients at risk – specifically those receiving digitalis. Hypokalaemia greatly increases its toxicity, and both reduce the excitability of the myocardial membrane (Colbert 1993). Slightly reduced levels can precipitate toxicity resulting in slow irregular pulse, anorexia, diarrhoea and vomiting.
- Estimation of serum K^+ levels.
- Assessment of sources of K^+ intake, e.g. replacement fluids/feeding and sources of loss, e.g. urinary, from the gastrointestinal tract.
- Identification of signs and symptoms of hypokalaemia. These will relate to the level of K^+ deficit, and rarely occur until levels are below 3.0 mmol/l.

Nursing intervention This will depend on prescribed treatment, which will relate to severity of the K^+ deficit. Replacement may be given orally or intravenously. If it is feasible to increase intake orally, a K^+ enriched diet with supplements will suffice. Intravenous replacement needs to be administered cautiously if renal function is compromised as hyperkalaemia can result if there is inadequate excretion. Specific interventions include:

- Administer prescribed K^+ intravenously, in a dilute volume, e.g. 1 l normal saline. In urgent situations a more concentrated solution will need to be given via a central line (concentrated solutions can be irritant)
- Ensure correct rate is calculated and infused via infusion pump
- Observe cardiac rate and rhythm
- Frequently assess serum K^+ levels
- Frequently monitor urine output.

Hyperkalaemia

Hyperkalaemia is characterised by serum K^+ level > 5.0 mmol/l. Possible causes of increased K^+ are outlined in Box 10.6. As with hypokalaemia this affects cardiac muscle and necessitates prompt treatment. Assessment includes:

- Identification of patients at risk, e.g. those with compromised renal function
- Estimation of serum K^+ levels. Haemolysed samples can present artificially increased K^+ levels
- Identification of signs and symptoms of raised K^+, will relate to the level of excess. Most important are those associated with cardiac muscle.

Nursing intervention will depend on the level of serum K+ and resulting cardiac effects. Treatment will be prescribed in relation to these, and possible treatments and effects are shown in Box 10.7.

- Ensure correct rate of administration
- Observe ECG rhythm during and after administration for improvement/deterioration
- Frequently assess serum K^+ levels
- Monitor urine output
- Ensure sources of K^+ e.g. in i.v infusions/feeding do not contain K^+.

Emergency management of hyperkalaemia involves the options given in Box 10.7. Choice will depend on the individual's underlying condition level/cause of raised K^+. In acute emergencies 10 ml 10% calcium gluconate or chloride will protect the heart and allow time for preparation of other measures. Calcium salts potentiate the effects of digitalis, so should be given with caution to patients already receiving cardiac glycocides. Sodium bicarbonate increases the pH and shifts K^+ from the ECF into the cells: overzealous use, particularly in cardiac arrest situations, can lower the K to dangerously low levels (Colbert 1993).

If K^+ levels persist and remain dangerously high, e.g. in renal failure, haemodialysis or haemofiltration would need to be considered.

■ **BOX 10.6** Possible causes of reduced and increased potassium levels

Possible causes of reduced K^+	Presenting signs and symptoms
Reduced K^+ intake • Associated with anorexia, malabsorption and alcoholism **_Excessive loss_** • Excessive diarrhoea and vomiting also in laxative abuse **_Urinary loss_** • In diuretic therapy, diuretic phase of ARF, diabetic ketoacidosis • Increased levels of aldosterone • Associated with Conn's disease. • Found in cardiac and liver failure, and as part of stress response **_Iatrogenic_** • Excessive use of diuretics, prolonged and excessive aspiration of GI tract, i.v. alkali, e.g. sodium bicarbonate in cardiac arrest, nephrotoxic drugs, e.g. aminoglycoside antibiotics (Colbert 1993) **_Rise in blood pH_** (alkalosis) • To correct blood pH imbalance H^+ ions move out of cell into ECF in exchange for K^+, ECF becomes K^+ deplete, although K^+ is not lost from the body.	• Disturbance of cardiac muscle—ECG changes include ST segment depression, T-wave inversion and U waves • Life threatening arrhythmias can potentially occur, leading to cardiac arrest • Disturbed muscle of GI tract – affecting peristalsis – nausea and vomiting, absence of bowel sounds, leading to paralytic ileus • Muscle weakness and loss of muscle tone • Disorientation, confusion and apathy

(cont'd...)

(Box 10.6 cont'd)

Possible causes of increased K⁺

Increased K⁺ intake/iatrogenic causes
K⁺ supplements, excessive infusion of K⁺
Increased supply
- Hypercatabolic states, e.g. MI, cardiac arrest, massive injury/infection, resulting in wide release of K⁺ from the cells into the ECF (Colbert 1993)

Reduced blood pH (acidosis)
- H⁺ ions cross cell membranes into ECF in exchange for K⁺ ions, cells become K⁺ depleted but plasma (ECF) levels increase

Reduced urinary loss
- In chronic renal disease, ARF with inadequate excretion of K⁺ into urine

Endocrine disease
- Aldosterone deficiency, or rarely insulin (Colbert 1993)

- ECG changes as K⁺ levels rise – peaked T waves, widening of QRS complex, cardiac arrythmias and bradycardia, risk of cardiac arrest when levels rise above 7.0 mmol/l
- Neuromuscular weakness
- GI symptoms

Sodium

The normal range is 135–145 mmol/l. Serum sodium levels do not necessarily reflect total body sodium, but the relative content of sodium and water in the ECF.

Hyponatraemia

Hyponatraemia (plasma sodium < 135 mmol/l) is a commonly encountered problem in acutely ill patients. It may result from a loss of sodium or a gain of water,

■ **BOX 10.7** Management options in hyperkalaemia (adopted from Colbert 1993)

Medication	Speed of action	Duration of action	Effect
Calcium gluconate	Minutes	0.25–1 hour	Rapidly, but temporarily reverses adverse effects on the heart
Sodium bicarbonate	Minutes	1–2 hours	By raising pH shifts K⁺ from ECF to ICF
Glucose and insulin	15 minutes	2–4 hours	Drives K⁺ from ECF into cells
Exchange resins, e.g. calcium resonium	1–2 hours	4–6 hours	Exchange calcium ions for K⁺ ions in the bowel
Potassium-losing diuretics	12 hours	24–30 hours	Potassium lost in the urine

In older individuals sodium-conserving capacity declines. The ability of the kidney to reabsorb sodium diminishes with age.

but in either event it is due to a relatively greater concentration of water than sodium (Metheny 1996). Possible causes of sodium loss are shown in Box 10.8. Sodium depletion alone is rare; sodium and water are lost together therefore are isotonic. Acute hyponatraemia can lead to serious neurological disturbances: Colbert (1993) points out that reports indicate there is approximately 50% mortality in patients with serum sodium levels less than 120 mmol/l for 24 hours. Considering the major role sodium plays in the control of ECF volume, it will follow that a reduced level of sodium will affect or be related to fluid balance and volume. When sodium is lost from the body, the osmotic pressure in the ECF is reduced, and water then moves into the ICF leading to overhydration of the cells. Severe hyponatraemia gives rise to neurological disturbances resulting from acute swelling of individual brain cells as water moves from ECF to ICF. A reduced plasma sodium concentration in the ECF results in potassium moving out of the ICF, leading to a potassium imbalance as well as a sodium imbalance. Assessment includes:

- Identification of patients at risk of hyponatraemia, e.g. those predisposed to sodium loss or water gain
- Estimation of serum sodium levels
- Recognition of signs and symptoms of hyponatraemia. These will vary and relate to the level of sodium deficit and underlying cause. A sudden decrease in serum sodium is more likely to produce symptoms than a slow one.

■ BOX 10.8 Hyponatraemia

Possible causes of reduced Na+ levels:

Dietary
- Prolonged restricted dietary Na^+ intake

GI tract loss
- Diarrhoea and vomiting
- GI suction, surgery
- Inappropriate replacement of GI losses, e.g. water without sufficient amounts of sodium

Skin
- Perspiration in fever and in high environmental temperatures, also from the skin surface in burns

Renal
- In salt-losing nephritis: renal tubules do not respond to ADH

Abuse or overuse of diuretics
- **Addison's disease**: ↓ adrenal gland activity → deficient production of aldosterone and ↑ Na^+ loss in urine

Water gain in:
- CCF, liver cirrhosis, nephrotic syndrome. Dilutional hyponatraemia results even though total body Na^+ may be in excess

Syndrome of inappropriate ADH (SIADH). ↑ ADH secretion leads to more water reabsorption, diluting ECF and resulting in hyponatraemia

Presenting signs and symptoms
- Headaches
- Confusion
- Muscle cramps
- Nausea and vomiting
- Coma, convulsions (cell overhydration)
- Disturbance of fluid volume

Nursing intervention This will depend on the prescribed treatment and relate to the cause of hyponatraemia and severity of symptoms, varying from neurological to fluid volume disturbances.

If hyponatraemia is associated with fluid volume deficit, 0.9% sodium chloride will replace sodium and water deficit. In fluid volume excess fluid restriction and occasionally hypertonic 3% or 5% sodium chloride is prescribed. Colbert (1993) urges great caution when replacing sodium in acute hyponatraemia, pointing out that many consider the general objective of raising the blood sodium by 2 mmol/l per hour as excessive, considering that a similar rate of correction in animals damages the brainstem. Specific interventions include:

- Administration of prescribed replacement fluid, careful infusion of hypertonic solutions via an infusion pump
- Observe serum sodium levels in relation to sodium replacement (levels need to increase gradually)
- Institute fluid restriction as necessary
- Monitor intake and output, particularly those that contain sodium
- Observe for signs of improvement and deterioration of neurological and fluid volume status.

Hypernatraemia

Hypernatraemia (serum sodium > 145 mmol/l) is less commonly encountered than hyponatraemia. It is caused by excessive water loss or sodium retention (see Box 10.9). The former is more common, although the latter can occur during intravenous replacement therapy when excessive amounts of sodium are given. If water is not replaced in dehydration, hypernatraemia will develop. In response to increased ECF osmolality, water moves out of the cells, leading to cellular dehydration. The body's response to an increased sodium level – which causes hyperosmolality – is via osmoreceptors in the brain, which stimulate ADH and thirst. The thirst response protects against hypernatraemia and hyperosmolality, as ADH retains water once it has been ingested. Assessment includes:

- Identification of patients at risk (see possible causes) and also patients with renal insufficiency
- Estimation of serum sodium levels
- Identification of signs and symptoms (see Box 10.9).

Nursing intervention Nursing intervention will depend on the underlying cause. If in water loss, hyperosmolality may be corrected with intravenous replacement of water, e.g. 5%, dextrose. If hypernatraemia is associated with fluid excess correction of sodium imbalance may be achieved with restricted intake of sodium and with the use of diuretics. Specific interventions include:

- Administration of prescribed replacement fluids and/or diuretics
- Institute sodium restriction where necessary
- Monitor fluid intake and output
- Observe serum sodium levels
- Observe for signs of improvement or deterioration of neurological, and or fluid volume status.

Other electrolyte imbalances with examples of possible causes and presenting clinical features are outlined in Table 10.10. Clinical features will vary according to the underlying cause and severity of imbalance.

■ **BOX 10.9** Hypernatraemia

Possible causes of increased Na⁺ levels

Dietary
- Increased dietary intake or overinfusion of Na^+ containing fluids. Unlikely to cause hypernatraemia alone but may do in addition to an absent thirst response, e.g. in the elderly, or in debilitated states such as unconsciousness

GI tract
- Severe diarrhoea and vomiting, resulting water loss greater than Na^+

Insensible water loss in excess of Na⁺
- Excessive perspiration in ↑ body or environmental temperatures→ excessive water loss. A dry environment → increased respiratory losses, e.g. in patients with a tracheostomy

Renal
- Insufficiency → retention of Na^+ ions

Renal and CCF failure
- Both involve sodium retention. If water retention is also present pseudohypernatraemia can result

Reduced water intake/inability to respond to fluid deficit
- In deficiency of ADH as a result of diabetes insipidus, pituitary tumours, trauma → brain damage

Presenting signs and symptoms
- Clinical features associated with fluid volume disturbances in excess or deficit
- Disturbance of cerebral cell function due to cell dehydration, e.g. irritability, and in severe hypernatraemia convulsions

Table 10.10 Electrolyte disorders

Electrolyte and normal range	Possible causes of excess and deficit	Clinical features
Calcium (4.5–5.5 mmol/l)		
Hypercalcaemia	Hyperparathyroidism, hypophosphataemia, thyrotoxicosis, bone tumours, prolonged immobilisation, thiazide diuretics	Drowsiness, headache, nausea and vomiting, thirst, polyuria, loss of muscle tone
Hypocalcaemia	Hypoparathyroidism, CRF, Vitamin D deficiency	Irritability, anxiety, tetany (twitching around the mouth, pins and needles in fingers, carpo-pedal spasm, laryngeal spasm and convulsions) ↑ Bleeding tendency ECG changes

(cont'd)

(Table 10.10 cont'd)

Chloride
(95–108 mmol/l)

Hyperchloraemia	↑ Retention or intake Excessive i.v sodium chloride Renal failure Metabolic acidosis	Weakness Lethargy Deep and rapid respirations
Hypochloraemia	Increased loss from GI tract Excessive diuretic use Excessive perspiration Metabolic alkalosis Generally associated with disorders of sodium loss	Those of fluid loss ↓ Respiratory rate Tetany/muscular excitability

Phosphate
(0.8–1.4 mmol/l)

Hyperphosphataemia	Renal failure Hyperparathyroidism	↑ Heart rate Nausea, diarrhoea, muscle weakness
Hypophosphataemia	Hyperparathyroidism Renal failure ↓ Dietery intake (renal failure) Impaired absorption	Lethargy, muscle weakness, nausea, vomiting, ↓WBC function, haemolytic anaemia

Magnesium
(1.5–2.5 mmol/l)

Hypermagnesaemia	Renal failure Excessive magnesium administration e.g. some antacids	Affects cardiac conduction Bradycardia Severe, respiratory and cardiac arrest
Hypomagnesaemia	Large GI losses Excessive use of diuretics Malabsorption Inefficient supplementation with prolonged parenteral nutrition	Muscular weakness, twitching and tremors Cardiac arryhythmias

CONCLUSION

In order to respond rapidly to (and anticipate) the highly dependent patient's fluid and electrolyte needs it is essential that a working knowledge of the underpinning physiological processes is acquired. This chapter has reviewed the fundamental processes; further reading is however recommended in relation to the varying clinical scenarios that face nurses in practice. The aim of rapid assessment and intervention is to prevent a relatively stable patient from becoming a highly dependent patient, and to prevent the patient from requiring intensive care nursing.

Specific causes of fluid and electrolyte imbalances have been reviewed. For the sake of clarity, however, they rarely occur in isolation but are often associated with complex clinical scenarios associated with actual or potential multiorgan deterioration. Examples of patient scenarios have been given to specifically focus on the assessment and intervention required to maintain fluid and electrolyte balance.

ACKNOWLEDGEMENT

Special thanks to Ms Sunita Hansraj for her help with aspects of the chapter.

REFERENCES

Armstrong R F, Bullen C, Cohen S L, Singer M, Webb A R 1997 Critical care algorithms. Oxford Medical Publications, Oxford

British National Formulary March 1995 A joint publication of the British Medical Association and the Royal Pharmaceutical Society of Great Britain

Chandler J 1991 Tabbner's nursing care: theory and practice, 2nd edn. Churchill Livingstone, Edinburgh

Colbert D 1993 Fundamentals of clinical physiology. Prentice Hall, Hemel Hempstead

Davidson T I 1987 Fluid balance. Blackwell Scientific Publications, London

Guly U, Richardson D 1996 Acute medical emergencies. Oxford University Press, Oxford

Kjellstrand C M, Jacobson S, Lins L E 1989 Acute renal failure. In: Maher J (ed.) Replacement of renal function by dialysis, 3rd edn. Kluwer, USA

Marieb E N 1992 Human anatomy and physiology, 2nd edn. Benjamin Cummings, California

Metheny N M 1996 Fluid and electrolyte balance. Lippincott-Raven, Philadelphia

Miller M 1989 Fluid and electrolyte balance in the elderly. Geriatric medicine February: 73–82

Smith K 1980 Fluids and electrolytes: a conceptual approach. Churchill Livingstone, New York

Urden L, Davie J, Thelan L 1992 Essentials of critical care nursing. Mosby Year Book, St Louis

Vander A J, Sherman J H, Luciano D S 1994 Human physiology: the mechanisms of body function, 6th edn. McGraw Hill, New York

Weinstein S M 1993 Plumer's principles and practice of intravenous therapy, 5th edn. Lippincott, Philadelphia

Willats S M, Winter R J 1992 Principles and protocols in intensive care. Farrand Press, London

FURTHER READING

Kassier J P, Hricik D E, Cohen J J 1989 Repairing body fluids: principles and practice. W B Saunders, London

Roberts A 1978 Body water and its control. Nursing Times Vol/pp?

Vanatta J C, Fogleman M J 1988 Moyer's fluid balance: a clinical manual, 4th edn. Year Book. Medical Publishers, London

Pain management

Helena Baxter

Key learning objectives

- To gain an understanding of the physiological and psychological bases of pain generation and modification.
- To discuss the importance of individual assessment, planning and evaluation in pain management.
- To explore nursing issues relating to the pharmacological and non-pharmacological methods of pain relief.
- To gain insight into the nurse's role and responsibilities within the realm of pain management.

Prerequisite knowledge and understanding

- Basic anatomy and physiology of the central nervous system.
- Basic pharmacology of common analgesics.
- Familiarity with patient-controlled analgesia (PCA) devices and epidural analgesia.

INTRODUCTION

The aim of this chapter is to provide a comprehensive, realistic overview of acute pain management. The majority of hospital patients will have presented with a pain-related problem and will require a high degree of nursing skill and care to achieve effective pain control. It is not the intention to give the reader a scientific approach to pain and pain relief; rather it is the intention to discuss the roles and issues related to nursing in the clinical area.

Pain is a unique, unpleasant experience comprising complex sensory, emotional and cognitive components which can be neither seen nor felt by anyone other than the person in pain (Jackson 1995). Pain does not occur as an isolated experience and is more than a sensory perception. According to McCaffery & Beebe pain 'probably disables more people than any single disease entity' (see also Doverty 1994).

Woodforde and Merskey stated that pain is not simply related to tissue damage; it can be positively or negatively influenced by many psychological and social factors, such as fear, anxiety, cultural conditioning and personal experience (O'Connor 1995). With this in mind, it would appear logical that pain management requires a holistic, multidimensional approach in order to be effective.

The lay person might be forgiven for thinking that medical and nursing staff have the skills, ability and technology to alleviate pain. The Royal College of Surgeons and College of Anaesthetists Working Party (1990) and the Audit Commission (1997) however, reported that health professionals working in acute care environments were ineffective when attempting to manage and relieve pain. They also found nurses lacking in knowledge and commitment to achieve satisfactory post-operative pain control (Hunt 1995; Wakefield 1995).

> 'Pain is whatever the patient says it is and occurs whenever the patient says it does' (McCaffrey, as cited in Woodward 1995).

There have been many attempts to define pain, ranging from 'an unpleasant sensory and emotional experience associated with actual or potential tissue damage or described in terms of such damage' (International Association for the Study of Pain, cited in Woodward 1995) to McCaffery's simpler 'pain is whatever the patient says it is and occurs whenever the patient says it does' (Woodward 1995).

In the same way that pain cannot easily be defined there is also no one definitive theory to explain the pain experience. In order to develop an understanding of pain management it is necessary to review some of the basic physiology of pain transmission and current pain theories.

THEORIES OF PAIN

A painful reaction may be considered a protective response. Most pain originates as a result of the stimulation of specific nerve endings which transmit nerve impulses to the brain along pain pathways. The receptors are known as nociceptors (respond to noxious stimuli) and can be divided into two types:

- **A delta fibres** which are found mainly in the skin. These respond to a strong pressure or other stimulus (e.g. heat > 44°C) and warn of potential damage. These fibres form part of the withdrawal reflexes and can transmit impulses rapidly. The result tends to be sharp, bright, localised pain.
- **C fibres** have a smaller diameter than A delta fibres and are widely distributed throughout most tissues. They respond directly to tissue damage, or to chemical mediators formed or released as a result of tissue damage. C fibres transmit impulses more slowly than A delta fibres and tend to result in prolonged, dull, poorly localised pain (Guyton 1986, Park & Fulton 1992).

Pain transmission and interpretation has been the subject of discussion and research for centuries. In the latter half of the nineteenth century, pain was regarded as being a sensory phenomenon in its own right, in a similar fashion to heat and cold. There were thought to be specific receptors for heat, cold, pain or touch with specific routes of transmission through the central nervous system and centres of interpretation in the brain. Further research into this area did not elicit such specificity but did demonstrate that A delta fibres are activated by low intensity stimuli and C fibres by high intensity mechanical, thermal or chemical stimuli (Bond 1979).

Another proposed pain theory is the intensity theory which hypothesises that there are no specific 'pain' fibres and that any stimulus can be interpreted as painful if it is great enough to break through a certain threshold (Bond 1979).

Elements of both theories are now generally accepted, although earlier neurophysiological and biomedical models, such as the specificity theory, reverberating circuit mechanism and input-control theory (Meinhart & McCaffery 1983) have been thrown over in favour of the more comprehensive physiological and psychological approaches of the gate control theory proposed by Melzack and Wall in 1965 (cited in Meinhart & McCaffery 1983).

Gate control theory

The gate control theory is a complex neurophysiological model which takes account of the role of psychological factors in the pain experience.

Put simply, the idea is that a gating mechanism operates in the spinal cord. Depending on circumstances, the gate can either be open, allowing nerve impulses to pass through and reach the brain for interpretation and perception, or it can be closed – blocking impulses at spinal cord level. Alternatively, the gate may be partially open allowing only some of the pain impulses to pass through.

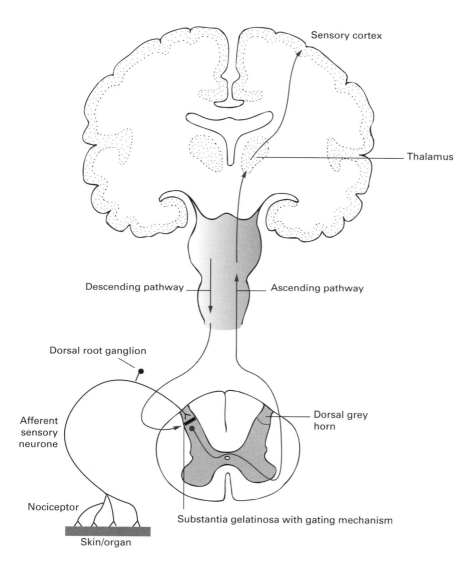

Fig. 11.1 Pain pathway depicting gate control mechanism.

According to this theory, the site of control is in the *substantia gelatinosa* – a group of cells in the grey matter of the dorsal horn. It is here that the afferent sensory neurones from the skin or organs synapse with secondary neurones of the pain pathway and ascend the spinothalamic tract to the brain stem (see Fig. 11.1). Fast pain signals (A delta fibres) pass through the brain stem and thalamus to the cortex where the signals are interpreted. The cortex can accurately localise the area from which the pain signal originates. Slow pain signals (C fibres) are spread over a wide area of the brain stem and thalamus resulting in poor localisation (Bond 1979, Guyton 1986, Davis 1993).

The gate control theory (Box 11.1) suggests two mechanisms for the modification of ascending pain signals:

- Stimulation of large diameter A delta fibres and involvement of the dorsal horn transmission cells of the spinal cord can convey signals of touch or vibration in preference to pain signals.

■ BOX 11.1 Gate control theory (McCaffery & Beebe 1994, p 81)

Structures involved	Gate open/partially closed	Gate open
Spinal cord ? nerve fibres	1. Activity in A delta fibres, e.g. skin stimulation	1. Activity in C fibres, e.g. from tissue damage
Brainstem	2. Inhibiting impulses from brainstem, e.g. adequate stimulation through distraction, guided imagery **or**	2. Facilitatory impulses from brainstem, e.g. insufficient input from monotonous environment or
Cerebral cortex and thalamus	3. Inhibitory impulses from cerebral cortex and thalamus, e.g. through reduced anxiety as a result of information – knowing what pain is and how to relieve it	3. Facilitatory impulses from cerebral cortex and thalamus, e.g. through fear – not knowing what the pain is and when it will end

- Inhibition of the release of chemical transmitters at various synapses in the dorsal horn of the spinal cord and brain through the uptake of naturally occurring endorphins (morphine-like substances) by specialised receptors (Weinman 1987, McCaffery & Beebe 1994).

This second mechanism has its widest use in clinical practice in terms of opioid analgesics which bind to the same receptors as endorphins to reduce pain transmission.

The gate control theory makes no distinction between organic pain (which has a specified origin) and functional pain (which occurs due to a disorder of the mind, without any organic cause (Critchley 1986)). It provides a conceptual framework to incorporate not only the physiological function of pain but also the emotional and cognitive variables which influence the perception and interpretation of pain (Kent & Dalgliesh 1986). This framework is particularly relevant to nursing in that:

- It helps us to appreciate the many factors and individual differences that contribute to the pain experience
- It has implications for developing pain relieving strategies combining physical and psychological therapies (Sofaer 1992, McCaffery & Beebe 1994)

Thus, pain is neither purely physiological nor purely psychological. Its purpose is to aid survival (Green 1990, cited in Hall 1995) and it can be divided into two categories: acute and chronic pain.

ACUTE AND CHRONIC PAIN

Melzack and Wall (1991) characterised acute pain as being a combination of tissue ·damage, pain and anxiety cited in O'Connor 1995, while The World Health Organization (1983) defined chronic pain as being malignant or progressively degenerate (cited in Doverty 1994).

Hanks (1986) identified four factors distinguishing acute from chronic pain (Box 11.2) (cited in Wilkinson 1996).

Acute pain is often associated with anxiety, stress and fear. The autonomic nervous system is stimulated resulting in tachycardia, hypertension, increased

■ **BOX 11.2** Acute and chronic pain (Wilkinson 1996)

Acute	**Chronic**
• An event	• A situation
• Being of predictive and limited duration (usually < 6 months)	• Being of unpredictable duration (lasting > 6 months)
• Tends to diminish	• Tends to increase
• Having meaning or purpose; often localised	• Having no meaning or negative meaning; usually poorly localised

respiratory rate and muscle spasm in the affected area. Conversely, chronic pain rarely results in autonomic stimulation and hence does not give rise to the 'classic' physiological signs of pain. Chronic pain tends to manifest itself in terms of psychological symptoms, such as depression, fatigue, feelings of helplessness and an inability to cope or difficulty in coping. Often it is the perceived threat and loss of control associated with chronic pain which influences coping rather than the actual condition (Walker 1991, Jacques 1994a).

The marked differences between acute and chronic pain necessitate entirely different approaches to effective pain management. It is not within the remit of this chapter to cover both aspects comprehensively, and so it will concentrate more on the acute pain management of the patient with high dependency needs. Acute pain has many causes, including:

- Inflammation
- Ischaemia
- Trauma
- Surgery
- Heat
- Chemicals (e.g. acid, histamine).

The inflammatory response results in the release of prostaglandins, histamine and kinins which sensitise the afferent nerve endings, making them more sensitive. This has the effect of lowering the pain threshold and the pain tolerance level. Pain tolerance varies between individuals and may be reduced by factors such as fatigue and boredom. The character of the pain can also affect tolerance – colicky, intermittent pain is less well tolerated than continuous pain (Gooch 1989, Park & Fulton 1992).

Park and Fulton also noted that surgical patients can be affected not only by the site of the operation, but also by the time of day at which surgery is performed. Morning operations have been associated with less pain than those performed in the afternoon. This may be due to diurnal variations in concentrations of steroid hormones or to changes in the stress response to surgery. While these are interesting facts, what is more important in nursing is to understand the patient's response to pain rather than the pain itself. In order to accomplish this, the patient in pain needs to be fully assessed before any truly effective management can be implemented.

ASSESSING PAIN

Issues of assessing, planning, implementing and evaluating care are indoctrinated into every nurse who has trained in the UK. Although this is referred to as 'the nursing process' it should perhaps be redefined as the nursing purpose, since individual assessment and identification of problems are the crux of holistic patient

■ **BOX 11.3** Pain studies: some facts

- 17 out of 35 nurses felt that patients' self-reports of pain were unreliable (Hunt 1995).
- 52% of qualified nurses did not believe in patients' perceptions of their own pain (Saxey 1986).
- 85% of post-operative patients' pain was not adequately controlled. Nurses felt they had to be able to prove a patient's pain by observing pain behaviours (e.g. grimacing) and checking autonomic signs (pulse and BP) (Seers 1987).
- Nurses underestimated patients' pain in 46% of myocardial infarction situations and overestimated pain in 13% of situations (O'Connor 1995).
- 75% of post-operative patients suffered moderate to severe pain (Cohen 1980).

■ **BOX 11.4** Audit Commission (1998) findings on pain management after surgery

- Effective pain relief is not achieved
- Patients do not tell staff they are in pain
- Nurses underestimate patients' pain
- There is a delay in administering pain relief
- Pain relief is not monitored

care. This shifts the parameters of the biomedical model and understanding illness in terms of subjective experience rather than physiological mishap.

Despite the widespread incidence of pain in clinical practice and the comprehensive framework offered by the gate control theory in assessing and managing pain, nurses still appear to be largely unaware of the emotional and cognitive components of pain. There remains a tendency to concentrate on the pharmacological aspects of pain relief rather than engaging in more complex holistic assessments of the individual pain experience (Haywood 1975; Sofaer 1992; Woodward 1995, Hollinsworth 1995, Willson 1992).

> The nursing process may be redefined as the nursing purpose. Assessing the patient as an individual is the crux of holistic patient care – illness is a subjective experience, not just a physiological mishap.

Nurses may believe that their clinical experience has imparted a certain knowledge of the pain experienced by patients in certain situations and, as such, assessment is not necessary. This is not so; research over the past two decades has consistently shown results of uncontrolled and poorly managed pain by nurses (Cohen 1980, Seers 1987, Sofaer 1992, O'Connor 1995). Equally worrying is that many nurses do not take the patient's self-report of pain seriously (Hunt 1995, Saxey 1986) despite the fact that many nurses can quote McCaffery's 'pain is what the person says it is and occurs whenever the person says it does' verbatim (Box 11.3).

The symptom of pain has been undertreated for the past 20 years, and despite the extensive research and publication in this field, there remains a failure to formally assess and document pain in nursing notes. In some instances, it even fails to be identified as a problem in the care plan (Paice et al 1991, Hollinworth 1995, Audit Commission 1998) (Box 11.4).

Many assessment tools have been devised to measure pain intensity, ranging from simple visual analogue scales to the more complex McGill pain questionnaire.

Visual analogue/numerical scales (VAS)

Both the visual analogue scales and the numerical scales form a quick and easy method for assessing and attempting to quantify pain severity. Essentially a visual

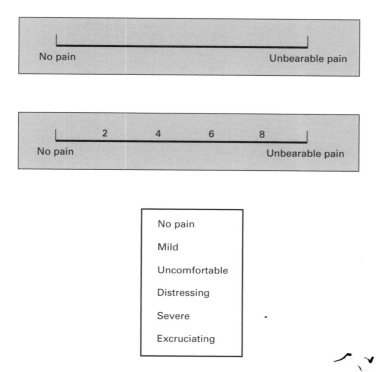

Fig. 11.2 Visual analogue scale.

Fig. 11.3 Visual numerical scale.

Fig. 11.4 Visual description scale.

analogue scale is a 10 cm line with 'no pain' at one end and 'unbearable pain' at the other (see Fig. 11.2). The patient is asked to place a mark on the line which best indicates the severity of his pain.

Numerical scales follow a similar line but are numbered either 0–10 or 0–5; 0 being 'no pain' and 10 (or 5) being 'unbearable pain' (see Fig. 11.3). Generally speaking, the longer 0–10 scale may be a more valuable tool as it allows the patient more points to choose from, and therefore is likely to be more sensitive and reliable. Carpenter and Brockopp (1995) compared a 10 cm visual analogue scale and a 0–5 numerical scale. They found that both patients and nurses did not rate pain in a numerically equivalent way; that is, a score of 3 on the numerical scale did not equate to a 6 cm mark on the visual analogue scale. This shows that while each form has its uses, the scales are not interchangeable.

The main advantages of the visual analogue/numerical scales are that they are quick and relatively easy to use and can be a useful tool in evaluating the effect of analgesia, but their uses are limited. Pain cannot easily be quantified and some patients may not find it easy to understand and score their pain on such a scale.

Visual description scales (VDS)

The visual description assessment tools again follow the same logic as the visual analogue scales, replacing the numbers with adjectives to describe pain intensity (see Fig. 11.4). The patient is asked to choose the word which best describes his pain, ranging from pain free to severe pain.

This form of assessment is also quick and easy to use and may be used to evaluate the effectiveness of analgesia. However, the patient may not be able to choose accurately a word which best describes the pain experienced. As with the VAS method, some pain experiences may not be severe but their constant presence may be annoying or tiring.

Fig. 11.5 Combination scale used in pain assessment chart.

Name: ....   Hospital number: ....

Pain location: ....

Pain character: ....

Patient's goal pain score: ....   Evaluation frequency: ....

| 2   4   6   8 |
No pain   Unbearable pain

      Mild   Moderate   Severe

Pain score

Date/time	At rest	On movement	Comments/action taken	Signature
....	....	....	....	....

■ **BOX 11.5** Examples of descriptors from the McGill Pain Questionnaire

Sensory (temporal)	Affective (punishment)	Evaluative	Miscellaneous
• Flickering	• Punishing	• Annoying	• Tight
• Quivering	• Gruelling	• Troublesome	• Numb
• Pulsing	• Cruel	• Miserable	• Drawing
• Throbbing	• Vicious	• Intense	• Squeezing
• Beating	• Killing	• Unbearable	• Tearing
• Pounding			

Both types of assessment tool may have some bearing on acute pain (e.g. following surgery) which is often finite, with a forseeable end. However, in more chronic or colicky, intermittent pain, words such as 'severe' may have little or no meaning (Scott 1992).

One way to overcome the weaknesses of the VAS and VDS would be to combine the two to make the instrument more valid and more user friendly (see Fig. 11.5).

McGill pain questionnaire (MPQ)

An alternative assessment tool, which is more in tune with the gate control theory, is the McGill pain questionnaire (McCafferey & Beebe 1994). This instrument aims to measure the sensory, emotional and evaluative components of pain separately. The patient is asked to choose the adjectives which best describe his pain from a total of 20 lists. Some lists refer to the sensory components, some the emotional and some the evaluative (see Box 11.5). Acute pain tends to score highly on the sensory components, e.g. throbbing, pounding, whereas chronic pain tends to score highly on the affective, e.g. sickening, tiring (Kent & Dalgliesh 1986).

This is a more holistic approach to pain assessment but may be considered too time consuming for use on a busy ward. Patients with high dependency needs may also find it difficult to use as it is recommended that they read through each category and circle the words describing their pain. This relies heavily on the patient being alert and orientated, motivated to read through 20 lists and not being hampered by too many infusion devices or other equipment. It should also be noted that high dependency care often requires prompt action; a patient suffering sudden onset severe chest pain is likely to require urgent analgesia and investigations to ascertain the cause of the pain. In this case, the patient is unlikely to take too kindly to being asked to complete a pain questionnaire!

The MPQ does take a little time to evaluate but has its benefits in the information it provides. Proper evaluation provides a subjective measure of the pain experience in terms of the number of words chosen, the present pain intensity and the pain rating index. Moreover, its reliability and validity have been ascertained and most patients find that no additional words are needed to describe their pain (Kim et al 1995). This assessment tool can be used to evaluate fully the effect of analgesia and to rate the reduction in pain over time (e.g. post-operatively). In addition, it is much more sensitive in evaluating non-pharmacological interventions in pain management, such as anxiety reduction techniques, the use of guided imagery, etc. However, Kent and Dalgliesh (1986) argue that it could increase the pain experience by focussing the patient's attention on the pain, especially those patients who may be coping by distraction.

It is not the intention of this chapter to advocate the use of one particular assessment tool. When choosing a pain assessment instrument for the clinical area, certain considerations should be taken into account:

- Is it user friendly for both patients and nurses?
- Is it sensitive enough to provide adequate information on pain intensity and evaluate the effect of analgesia?
- Is it appropriate to high dependency care and the conditions likely to be encountered?

It may be that no one form of assessment will be able to encompass all of these all of the time, and there are advantages and disadvantages to each form of assessment. However, it can be argued that any assessment scale is better than none at all. Ideally, they should be used to assess the patient at rest and on movement. It is pointless to have a patient pain free at rest if his pain is only controlled when lying absolutely still. Perhaps more importantly, the reason for using a scale is that each nurse will have the same baseline information and will be utilising the same methodology to assess the patient. In this way, general trends can be monitored, together with the effectiveness of subsequent interventions.

> Assess the patient's pain status at rest and in activity. A patient is not pain free if that means pain free only when immobile.

Assessment tools can be extremely useful for helping patients in pain but should also be used in the wider context of pain management. The instruments are there to improve pain assessment and form only part of the assessment process, particularly the VAS and VDS types. Their main use is to investigate pain severity and to evaluate the effectiveness of medical/nursing interventions. Thus they form part of the assess–evaluate–reassess cycle.

Once the assessment is completed, a holistic care plan can be developed encompassing the physiological and psychosocial components of pain as suggested by the gate control theory. Implicit in this assumption is that nurses are aware of, and able to incorporate, the more cognitive techniques in patient care.

Most pain studies have tended to concentrate on post-operative pain in order to gain a sample of patients undergoing similar procedures as a means of identifying similarities and differences within the sample population (Saxey 1986, Seers 1987, Lovett et al 1994, Knapp-Spooner et al 1995). It is accepted that post-operative pain is predominantly due to the trauma induced by surgery and this generally diminishes as inflammation is reduced and healing takes place. By contrast, obtaining a full description of the pain experienced by medical patients can provide valuable diagnostic clues. As nurses spend much of their time engaged in patient care and building relationships with their patients, they are in a unique position to fully assess the pain experience. For example, a patient presenting with central chest pain may have pain resulting from:

- Myocardial infarction
- Angina
- Pulmonary embolism
- Chest infection
- Musculo-skeletal pain
- Oesophageal reflux.

Often the cause may be determined by ECGs and blood results, but often the diagnosis is not clear for a couple of days. Detailed assessment of the pain experience should include the patient's description of:

- Location
- Radiation (e.g. to back, left arm, jaw)
- Character (tight, gripping, burning, crushing, heavy, catching). Use MPQ at this point
- Intensity (use VAS, VDS, MPQ)
- Duration (constant, intermittent)
- Relieving factors (e.g. rest, sitting forward, heat)
- Associated factors (e.g. breathlessness, exertion, lying down, after eating)
- Impact on lifestyle (e.g. in recurrent problems, such as sickle-cell anaemia or unstable angina).

Scott (1992) identifies three reasons for the failure of adequate pain assessment:

- Poor communication of pain levels by patients to nurses.
- Poor perception by nurses of the patient's pain.
- Poor understanding by nurses of their role in pain management.

The use of open questions and active listening, prompting and empathy can elicit valuable information about the pain itself, its impact on quality of life, anxiety that may be generated, and fears about the future. The nurse and patient can then enter a collaborative relationship. The nurse imparts knowledge of the condition and pain relieving measures available to help alleviate anxiety through information giving (Hayward 1975, Sofaer 1992); the patient communicates any personal coping strategies, such as distraction or the use of heat/massage. Together a plan of care can be devised that incorporates nursing and patient strategies to manage pain.

This may sound idealistic but it is possible. Assessment should be an ongoing process and not all information has to be gathered within the first few hours of admission. It may be that the patient feels too unwell, or is in too much pain to be able to participate in care and would much rather leave this to the nursing and medical professions to sort out. A day or so later, the patient may feel that he wants to become involved in his own care, and this should be encouraged. After all, the nurse may consider herself an expert on matters of health and illness, but the patient *is* an expert on his individual health and the circumstances of his life (Leddy & Pepper 1989, p 320).

The most important aspect of care is that the patient feels 'believed' when reporting pain, and that he is encouraged to report pain when it arises, rather than waiting to be asked by the nurse. There can be few things more frustrating, however, than being asked to report pain when it occurs, only to be told that pain relief cannot be given for another 2 hours. If this is the case, the nurse should be prepared either to liaise with medical staff for further pain relief to be made available,

> In encouraging patients to communicate openly about pain, the real hospital environment must be considered. If you know pain relief is not scheduled for another 2 hours, do not ask your patient how he is – be prepared to seek flexibility in the system to accommodate the patient's pain *now*.

or to explore alternative pain relieving measures with the patient (these will be discussed later).

Evaluation and reassessment are the next key stages in effective pain management. It is pointless to plan and implement care or to administer analgesia if the effectiveness of that care is not being evaluated. At the planning stage, times for evaluation should be noted: for example, pain levels will be formally assessed every hour, and then additionally if the patient complains of pain, and 20 minutes after any analgesia is given. The use of a pain scale before and after analgesia enables the nurse and patient to make a more informed judgement as to whether pain relief is adequate, or whether it needs to be reviewed by the medical team.

PLANNING FOR SHORT-TERM PAIN RELIEF

It is easy to be reminded about the pain management of a patient following surgery or of a patient who has been admitted with pain as the main problem. One problem often encountered in clinical practice, however, is the lack of assessment and planning for *short-term* episodes of pain, or potential pain, such as that encountered during dressing changes or drain removal. Chest drains, for example, tend to cause much discomfort in the first 48 hours following insertion. After this time the inflammation around the insertion site declines, the traumatised area begins to heal and the patient may require only minimal analgesia for the rest of the time the drain is in situ. Pleural drains, conversely, can remain extremely painful for the whole duration of treatment.

Whatever type of drain is used – be it a pleural drain or a simple surgical drain at the wound site – removal of the drain can be a very painful experience, particularly if it has been in for several days, as the tissues may have adhered to the drain itself. Strong analgesics, such as the opioids, or short-acting powerful painkillers such as Entonox, should be given before attempting to remove it.

Similarly, wound dressings, especially those requiring packing or the removal of packing, may cause the patient pain and distress. Although drain removal and wound dressings may be considered a common nursing procedure in high dependency care, it is not a common procedure for the patient. A patient who experiences pain and discomfort during a dressing change is likely to feel apprehensive and anxious for the next one. All too often patients are given analgesia after the event, or they are given analgesics immediately prior to the procedure without giving the drugs time to work before the drain is removed or the dressing changed. It is in this area that nurses can, and should, assess and plan in advance to prevent pain occurring.

Strong analgesics, such as dextromoramide or buprenorphine, have minimal side effects in terms of sedation or respiratory depression and can be very effective for drain removal or dressing changes. They are oral preparations and therefore need to be given approximately 20 minutes before the procedure to achieve their maximum effect. Diamorphine and pethidine can also be used and these have the advantage of being given immediately prior to the procedure if given intravenously.

Entonox (nitrous oxide) is a very effective analgesic for short-term pain but its use and advantages are often forgotten. It is an inhaled drug and so its pain relieving properties are rapid. The patient also has control over the analgesia and can therefore take as much or as little as required. Because the patient has to hold the mask to the face, there is little fear that too much will be taken rendering the patient unconscious.

Although Entonox contains oxygen, oxygen saturation levels may fall if the patient is dependent on high concentrations of oxygen. However, this is rarely a problem if only used for 10–15 minutes.

Some consideration should be given to the period following a drain removal or dressing change as discomfort may persist for several hours. Mild or moderate strength analgesics are normally adequate, but again, this should be included in the plan of care.

Hollinworth (1995) found that neither assessment nor management of pain at dressing changes was documented. She suggests this lack of planning and documentation might compromise the future management of pain during dressing changes as the communication between healthcare professionals is impaired.

NURSING ISSUES CONCERNING THE PHARMACOLOGY OF PAIN RELIEF

The aim of this section is to explore the nursing issues of analgesic agents. Several different groups of analgesics and delivery systems will be discussed in order to gain more understanding of effective, individual pain management. It is not intended to discuss the true pharmacological aspects of analgesia, such as sites and mechanisms of action or routes and duration of action. The interested reader should refer to any standard pharmacology text such as the British National Formulary for this information.

Analgesia for severe pain

Patients with severe pain tend to have high dependency needs for its effective management. Opioid analgesics, such as diamorphine, morphine and pethidine are often the drugs of choice. They work by depressing the appreciation of pain and effects may be euphoric and anxiety reducing. The hypnotic effects may result in sedation and the cough reflex and respiration may also be depressed (Jackson 1995). Their pain relieving properties are invaluable to patients, but the side effects of sedation and respiratory depression appear to cause far more concern to nurses than to the patient.

Respiratory depression   True respiratory depression can be life threatening, although clinically significant opioid-induced respiratory depression rarely occurs (Pasero & McCaffery 1994). Respiratory depression tends to be associated with a decline in the number of breaths per minute, although depth and quality of respiration should be taken into account and the patient assessed on the basis of his normal pattern of breathing.

Each patient will react differently to narcotic analgesics and so there is no 'safe' maximum dose. The first dose carries the greatest risk and the patient should be monitored closely to ascertain the respiratory rate, depth and pattern – particularly if the patient still has anaesthetic agents on board – as these will further increase the risk of respiratory depression until their effects wear off.

Elderly patients may be more sensitive to the opioid effects of sedation and respiratory depression because of a reduced ability to excrete the drug. Similarly, heavy smokers or those patients with pre-existing chronic breathing problems may also be at higher risk of respiratory depression (Pasero & McCaffery 1994). This should not exclude the use of such analgesics for these patients – each should be assessed individually and monitored accordingly.

Respiratory depression is a risk but it is a small one. To some extent, the respiratory rate, tidal volume and minute volume will be affected by the use of narcotics, but this does not necessarily cause adverse effects (Rang & Dale 1987). Pulse oximetry may be helpful in monitoring the respiratory effects, but generally deep sedation will precede the onset of respiratory depression and should alert the nurse to the potential risks.

■ **BOX 11.6** Sedation score (adapted from Pasero & McCaffery 1994, Ferguson, 1995)

1 – Awake and alert.
2 – Occasionally drowsy but easy to arouse **or** sleeping but easily aroused.
3 – Frequently drowsy – can be aroused but falls asleep during a conversation.
4 – Somnolent – minimal/no response to stimuli.

Pasero and McCaffery (1994) recommend close monitoring of respiration and sedation levels (1–2 hourly) for the first 24 hours while an effective dose and frequency regime is being established. If no problems occur during that period, the frequency of monitoring can be reduced to 2–4 hourly.

Sedation High levels of sedation will usually precede any adverse respiratory effects of opioids, and so the amount of sedation effected should be assessed. Many sedation scores have been published (O' Hara 1994, Pasero & McCaffery 1994, Ferguson 1995;), all of which follow similar lines (Box 11.6). Sedation levels of 1 or 2 are perfectly reasonable, but a score of 3 should alert the nurse to potential problems. The opioid dose may need to be reduced or the infusion discontinued until the patient is more rousable. A score of 4 may necessitate the use of naloxone (opioid antagonist) to reverse the unwanted side effects. Used carefully, naloxone can reverse the effects of sedation and respiratory depression without completely eradicating the analgesic benefits (Pasero & McCaffery 1994).

The potential threats of respiratory depression and sedation have resulted in cautious prescribing of opioid drugs on the grounds of safety (Hunter 1991). While this may be attributed to caution on behalf of the medical staff, nurses tend to be more cautious still in their administration of opiates but for different reasons. Despite the research, many nurses believe that patients can easily become addicted to opioids.

Addiction The incidence of addiction to narcotics given for pain relief is low. The Report of the Working Party on Pain after Surgery (Royal College of Surgeons and College of Anaesthetists 1990) suggested that the incidence of addiction to narcotics is probably 1 : 3000 and is not, therefore, a significant reason for nurses to withhold analgesia (Hunt 1995). Ferrell et al (1992) proposed the likelihood of addiction occurring as a result of opioid analgesia for pain control to be less than 1% or non-existent. However, nurses continue to have an exaggerated fear of causing addiction in spite of the need for analgesia. Willson (1992) reported that nearly half of nurses (43%) would only give opioid analgesia for a maximum of 3 days following major surgery or trauma for fear of causing addiction. Some facts relating to opioid analgesia are given in Box 11.7.

Frequency of doses The prescribing of analgesia does not fall under the jurisdiction of nursing, but promoting pain relief and comfort for patients is central to the nurse's role. If the prescribed dose is inadequate or the frequency of doses too small to adequately control pain then the nurse should be prepared to advocate on behalf of the patient. The nurse should have knowledge of the analgesics being administered, and implicit in this assumption is that the nurse is aware of the effects and duration of action. For example, opioids given intravenously tend to have a more profound effect but a shorter half-life than those given intramuscularly. Pethidine loses much of its effectiveness after $1\frac{1}{2}$–2 hours, therefore a prescription for 4-hourly administration is unlikely to result in adequate pain management.

> ### ■ BOX 11.7 Opioid analgesia: some facts
>
> - In a sample of 2459 nurses:
>   24.8% knew the incidence of addiction was less than 1%.
>   21.6% thought addiction would occur in 25% or more of patients. (Ferrell, et al 1992).
> - In a survey of 456 nurses, between 46% and 67% failed to increase the dose of analgesia when the previous dose had been ineffective but had caused no side effects (Ferrell et al 1992).
> - 78% of nurses consider reducing opioid analgesia after 3 days;
>   16% would cut back after the first day
>   43% would be reluctant to give opioids after 3 days (Willson 1992).
> - Only 19% of nurses felt that pain could be relieved completely following surgery (Willson 1992).
> - 33% of nurses believed post-operative pain can only be reduced, not controlled (Kuhn et al 1990).
> - 19 out of 35 nurses agreed with the statement that 'care should be taken when using narcotic drugs as patients easily become addicted' (Hunt 1995).

Do not withhold pain relief through fear of unwanted side effects such as addiction. In effective pain management, the pain and the side effects can be managed together.

Opioid analgesia should not be withheld on the grounds of fear of addiction, respiratory depression or sedation. Although these fears are present in clinical practice they are not founded in medical and nursing research. Careful assessment, initial monitoring and evaluation of analgesia use can result in effective pain management without the unwanted side effects. In addition, it is important not to discontinue an analgesic where a potentially reversible side effect exists: for example, treating the nausea and vomiting with antiemetics as opposed to stopping the analgesia.

Reducing the risk of respiratory depression and sedation can also be achieved by employing different methods of analgesia delivery, such as patient-controlled analgesia pumps and epidural analgesia infusions.

Patient-controlled analgesia (PCA) devices

Patient-controlled analgesia devices have become increasingly popular over the last decade. Initial fears that the patient may accidentally overdose on analgesics have largely been eradicated, and the advantages in terms of effective pain control, patient satisfaction and a reduced workload for nurses have been widely reported (Gooch 1989, Hunter 1991, Scott 1994, Knapp-Spooner et al 1995, Thomas 1995). The infusions usually comprise a diluted dose of opioid analgesia with an antiemetic such as cyclizine which acts on the same receptors as the opioids.

Traditional methods of intramuscular (i.m.) injections of opioids are generally unsatisfactory for several reasons. Firstly, the rigidity of the doses and frequency do not allow for individual differences in pain management. The patient often has to ask for pain relief and as two nurses are required to administer it, the patient may have to wait a while before receiving analgesia. Secondly, bolus i.m. injections result in sharp peaks of narcotic levels causing sedation followed by troughs resulting in pain (Hunter 1991, Thomas 1995).

The value of a PCA pump lies in its ability to provide a constant minimum level of analgesia to maintain comfort with additional bolus doses for use by the patient for breakthrough pain experienced on movement and during dressing changes or physiotherapy. An adequate loading dose should be given when the PCA is first set up to alleviate pain as the background and bolus doses take a while to reach therapeutic levels.

Knapp-Spooner et al's (1995) study of female cholecystectomy patients showed that those patients using the PCA system experienced less pain on their first post-operative day and less fatigue on the second day than their counterparts who received 'traditional' i.m. injections. Similar results were shown in studies by Hunter (1991) and Gooch (1989).

Early fears that patients administering their own opioids may lead to addiction have also been disproven. Studies by Hunter (1991) and Gooch (1989) indicated that while initial analgesic use was high in PCA patients, overall analgesic use was significantly less than in those patients receiving i.m. injections.

Patient assessment

Not all patients will respond well to PCA pumps. For those wishing to gain some control over their illness and care they are extremely beneficial. Some patients, however, will not feel comfortable about the self-administration of drugs and would prefer the nurse to retain control over analgesia. PCA pumps should not, therefore, be seen as the panacea of pain control; their use should be discussed with the patient. The decision to use PCA devices is usually made before surgery when the system can be explained and the patient given instructions on its use, although PCAs have been successfully introduced post-surgery and with trauma and medical patients. However, in order to achieve maximum benefit, the patient should be educated in the use of a PCA, preferably before it is used.

Patients should be assessed not only on their willingness to use PCA devices but also on their suitability. Hiscock (1993) suggests that certain exclusion criteria should apply. These are:

- Allergy to opioids used
- Pregnancy/breastfeeding
- Neurological disease
- Disabilities affecting dexterity
- History of drug abuse
- Language/communication barriers which may prevent full understanding of PCA device.

Nursing care of patients using PCA

It is very easy to assume that a patient using a PCA device will be pain free as the patient can administer bolus doses as required. Most PCAs have a small background infusion rate with a fixed bolus dose, a set lock-out time and a maximum cumulative dose limit during which no further bolus doses can be delivered. Again, close monitoring of the level of sedation and respiratory effect, together with formal assessment using pain scores should be undertaken at regular intervals (at least hourly initially) to evaluate the effectiveness of the analgesia (see Box 11.8).

■ **BOX 11.8** Monitoring of the patient using a PCA pump

- Respiratory rate, depth, oxygen saturation
- Pulse   } 1–2 hourly for first 24 hours, then 2–4
- Blood pressure ∫   hourly during infusion
- Level of sedation
- Pain score at rest and on movement
- Number of tries and successes of bolus doses
- Monitoring checklist/maximum dose (cumulative) been programmed
- Venous access site for signs of extravasation/infection
- Pressure areas and position changes
- Nausea scoring

Fig. 11.6 PCA assessment chart.

Name: ....   Hospital number: ....

Patient's goal pain score: ....

PCA prescription: ....

Background infusion: ....

Bolus dose: ....   mg.

Lock-out time: ....

| Date/time | Pain score | | bolus doses | | total |
	at rest	on movement	No. tries	No. successes	analgesia
....	....	....	....	....	....

The PCA device can elicit a great deal of information, as many systems will keep a record of how many 'tries' and how many 'successes' the patient has had in delivering bolus doses. Thus, if the patient tries to administer bolus doses more often than the system will deliver, and the patient still reports pain, then the analgesia delivery setup should be reviewed. The background infusion may be inadequate, the bolus dose too small or the lock-out time too long. Small adjustments can be made to allow for individual differences in pain control (see Fig. 11.6).

Advantages of PCA

Thomas (1995) cites several advantages of patient-controlled analgesia:

- Nurse-administered analgesics are not necessary.
- Patient satisfaction is increased as patients are more comfortable and able to do more for themselves.
- Patients are more active and therefore less likely to develop complications, such as DVT, chest infection or skin damage.
- More nursing time can be spent in direct patient care rather than in drawing up analgesia – estimated to take up 42 minutes per patient per 24 hours.

EPIDURAL ANALGESIA

Epidural infusion analgesia is becoming increasingly popular and is a greatly under-used resource. Its peri-operative uses are discussed in Chapter 8.

A catheter is inserted into the epidural space, usually between vertebrae T1 and L3 depending on where the blockade is needed. Opioid analgesics (usually diamorphine or fentanyl) and local anaesthetic (usually bupivacaine) are continuously infused, with or without additional 'top-up' doses. The effect is a high degree of pain relief with minimised risks of respiratory depression or sedation associated with the parenteral administration of opioids (Greenland 1995). The combined use of opioids and local anaesthetic agents means that less of each drug needs to be used to achieve the desired effect.

Patient assessment

Epidural analgesia is not without its complications. It is generally set up prior to surgery and so full patient co-operation is needed. The patient should be assessed for suitability for epidural infusion and should be fully informed of the advantages and possible complications of this form of analgesia so that he can make an informed decision. Complete understanding is needed as areas of numbness caused by the blockade may cause unnecessary anxiety and distress to the patient if he is not aware of how epidural analgesia works.

Additionally, most signs of complications with the epidural will be noted first by the patient *before* any changes occur in the vital signs. These will be discussed later. Greenland (1995) suggests that epidural analgesia should not be used in patients with:

- Raised intracranial pressure
- Local skin infections
- Clotting disorders, or those receiving anticoagulation therapy
- Gross obesity
- Arthritis of the spine where the patient has an unyielding back
- Spinal fracture
- An uncooperative attitude.

Nursing care of patients with epidural analgesia

Patients with epidurals may need reassurance from nursing staff as they may worry if their legs feel numb or heavy. Also, the patient may be reluctant to mobilise or change position in bed for fear of dislodging the epidural catheter.

Respiratory/cardiac As with PCAs, close monitoring of the patient's respiration, blood pressure and heart rate is required every five minutes initially, and then at least hourly (Box 11.9).

Unlike parenteral administration of opioids, this frequent monitoring should continue as long as the epidural is in situ, and for 24 hours after it is removed. This is because opiate/anaesthetic levels may accumulate or may rise above the desired level of blockade. If the solution reaches the mid-cervical level respiratory and cardiac innervation may be affected, resulting in severe respiratory depression and/or cardiac insufficiency, with bradycardia and hypotension. The onset is

---

■ BOX 11.9 Monitoring of the patient with epidural analgesia

- Respiration rate, depth and oxygen saturation
- Heart rate and ECG } Every 5 minutes for 1 hour, then hourly
- BP   } during infusion and for 24 hours after
- Conscious level
- Patient positioning – avoid head-down position
- Catheter insertion site for signs of leaking/infection
- Pain scores at rest and on movement
- Level of blockade
- Fluid balance
- Pressure areas and position changes
- Monitoring checklist/maximum dose (cumulative) been programmed

unpredictable and may be delayed, although 30–60 minutes after injection and 6–12 hours post-injection carry the greatest risk. The first period is due to systemic absorption and the latter to spread of the analgesia throughout the cerebrospinal fluid (CSF) to the medulla (Greenland 1995). If this occurs, the infusion should be stopped and the anaesthetist called.

Full resuscitation equipment should be close at hand and naloxone prescribed and available whenever epidural opiates are used.

When the epidural is set up, the patient should be encouraged to tell nursing staff if any altered sensation or numbness is experienced above the level of blockade specified by the anaesthetist. This can be tested by using ice to assess the level of sensation. If decreased sensation to cold is experienced, the infusion should be discontinued until the anaesthetist has reviewed the patient (Greenland 1995).

Patient positioning Two schools of thought exist concerning patient positioning during epidural infusion. After initial injection or 'top-up' dose it is recommended that patients lie supine for 20–30 minutes to reduce the risks of hypotension (Jacques 1994b). Epidural opioids do not affect the sympathetic vasoconstrictor fibres in the cardiovascular system, but local anaesthetics can block these fibres causing decreased peripheral resistance, venous pooling and hypotension. It is worth remembering these effects when attempting to sit patients upright or to mobilise patients with epidurals (Jacques 1994b).

Conversely, Greenland (1995) suggests that respiratory depression may be minimised if the patient is nursed upright, or at an angle of 45°, although posture and gravity may be of limited value in controlling the spread of analgesia in the epidural space. Patients *should not be nursed in the head down position at any time*. This is because bupivacaine is denser than CSF and both this and the opiates will travel towards the head in a short space of time.

Pain scores Again, pain levels should be formally assessed to ensure the analgesia is effective. Epidurals are generally excellent at providing complete pain control, but it is possible to achieve effective blockade on one side of the body and only partial blockade on the other. This does not necessarily mean that the catheter is in the wrong place, but it is due to the positioning of the catheter within the epidural space. There is no easy solution to this, and sometimes it may only be rectified by reinserting the catheter, although there is still no guarantee that it will work.

If a patient suddenly complains of pain when he had previously experienced effective blockade it may indicate that the catheter is blocked or kinked, or has fallen out and should be checked. Any leaking from the catheter site should be reported.

The catheter site should be checked regularly for any signs of inflammation and/or infection. The closed circuit should not be broken unnecessarily and strict asepsis should be observed whenever handling the site, the epidural or breaking the circuit for top-up injections or to change the syringe, to prevent the introduction of infection.

Nausea and vomiting Opioid-induced nausea and vomiting may occur with epidural analgesia, but unlike PCA devices, antiemetics cannot be included in the infusion. The nurse should be aware of this problem as regular antiemetics may be required to prevent further distress and discomfort.

Fluid balance Fluid balance should be monitored carefully as urinary retention may result from epidural analgesia as the blockade can affect bladder tone.

The patient should have a good intake of fluids as dehydration may aggravate systemic hypotension.

Pressure area care As the legs and buttocks will have decreased sensation from the anaesthetic effect of the epidural, patients may not notice discomfort or soreness from sitting or lying in bed. Pressure areas should be checked regularly and the patient encouraged and assisted to change position regularly to prevent tissue damage.

Itching Many patients complain of itching over the legs, face and trunk. This is a fairly common side effect of opioid analgesics, particularly diamorphine, but is generally well controlled with antihistamines such as chlorpheniramine, or with small doses of naloxone.

Complications of epidural analgesia

Despite careful monitoring of the patient, some potentially serious complications can occur. The most common problem is a headache, which often occurs following any dural puncture (including lumbar puncture procedures) and is caused by loss of CSF.

The headache usually resolves after 24 hours, is relieved by lying flat and worse on sitting or standing. Simple analgesia and reassurance will often suffice. However, if the headache increases in severity and is accompanied by visual disturbances, nausea, vomiting and tinnitus, it may be an indication that the epidural catheter has become dislodged and has entered the large epidural veins or perforated the dura (Jacques 1994b). If in doubt, discontinue the infusion and seek help from the anaesthetist.

A more serious neurological complication is a persistent paraplegia known as anterior spinal artery syndrome. This may be due to lack of perfusion to the spinal cord from persistent systemic hypotension (Greenland 1995). Some degree of temporary paraesthesia may exist after the removal of the catheter, but will usually resolve after a few days or weeks.

A misplaced catheter is a serious problem. If the catheter becomes misplaced intrathecally, the analgesic solution could reach the cranial subarachnoid space. This will result in total spinal block paralysing the respiratory muscles and cranial nerves. The patient will become apnoeic, profoundly hypotensive and unconscious, requiring resuscitation and ventilatory support until the effects of analgesia and anaesthetic agents wear off (Greenland 1995). This is unlikely to occur unless the patient's head has been tipped steeply, or the dura has been punctured and gone unnoticed (Jacques 1994b).

Intravascular displacement will result in the drugs being absorbed in the circulatory system. The analgesics are dilute but may still cause respiratory depression. The most serious consequence is the circulation of bupivacaine which can result in cardiac arrhythmias, hypotension and CNS depression (Grahame-Smith & Aronson 1992).

Abcesses or haematomas can form at the catheter site. The patient is likely to complain of severe pain and motor and sensory impairment owing to compression of the spinal nerves. Surgical decompression may be required to prevent permanent damage (Greenland 1995).

Catheter removal

The catheter should be removed with the patient in the fetal position. The site should be observed for any leakage of CSF and covered with an occlusive dressing.

Patient monitoring should continue for 24 hours afterwards, until the analgesic solution is no longer effective.

It should be remembered that the incidence of serious complications is rare, and most patients benefit from epidural analgesia.

Advantages of epidurals

- Continuous, and often complete, pain relief
- Long duration of action
- Early mobilisation, resulting in decreased risk of DVT and chest infection
- Less risk of sedation and respiratory depression (when managed carefully)
- Increased independence and activity
- Less breakthrough pain, and so less fatigue.

Undoubtedly, epidural analgesia and PCA pumps can be extremely beneficial to patients. However, to ensure maximum pain control and maximum patient safety, both delivery systems require high dependency nursing care in order to promote independence and prevent complications.

ANALGESIA FOR MODERATE PAIN

These include oral preparations such as non-steroidal anti-inflammatory drugs (NSAIDs), and opiates like dihydrocodeine, codeine phosphate and oramorph. The injectable preparations of codeine phosphate and dihydrocodeine are more suitable for severe pain.

NSAIDs have recently become fashionable for use in the immediate post-operative period. They are often initially given rectally as this avoids the problem of gastric erosion if taken on an empty stomach. Given regularly, NSAIDs can reduce inflammation and pain following surgery, trauma and in some disease processes. They are particularly useful in pain associated with inflammatory processes, especially those due to bursitis, arthritis and pain of muscular or vascular origin (Rang & Dale 1987).

Lovett et al (1994) advocate early use of NSAIDs in the post-operative period. Their study showed a 20% reduction in narcotic analgesia requirement with combined NSAID use when compared to a control group of narcotic use only. They suggest that NSAIDs should be used in conjunction with opioids in the peri-operative stage rather than being used simply as a step down from opioids. This can then help in the successful weaning off opiates.

ANALGESIA FOR MILD PAIN

Paracetamol, coproxamol and codydramol are among those drugs which are particularly effective for mild pain such as headaches, flu-like symptoms, muscle and joint aches and pains, and generalised discomfort resulting from surgery or trauma. They can be very useful when used as part of a combination of analgesics for moderate to severe pain. There is no rule to say that one pain = one analgesic. Often a combination is needed to achieve the most effective, or complete pain control.

Individuals react differently to different preparations of analgesia and so it is always worth pursuing different approaches and combinations. Some people find coproxamol more effective than paracetamol, others do not; some who gain no relief from either coproxamol or paracetamol may find codydramol effective. The same is true for nearly all drug preparations and there are no hard and fast rules for which preparation to use and when. It should be remembered that the patient is in the best position to evaluate the effectiveness of the analgesia.

Other drugs which may not appear under the title of 'analgesia' can also be effective for different types of pain. For example, nitrates are used for cardiac ischaemic pain, anti-spasmodics such as buscopan are widely used for intestinal colicky/spasm pain, and amitryptiline, primarily used as an antidepressant, has its uses in controlling neuralgia. Diazepam may be used both as an anxiolytic and to relieve pain associated with muscle spasm.

COMMON PROBLEMS WITH CHOOSING
PRESCRIBED ANALGESIA

A nurse will often encounter a blanket prescription for pain relief. These usually range from simple analgesics to diamorphine. The patient complains of pain – which one do you give? There is always a tendency to start with the simplest and work upwards. However, if the pain is more than mild, simple analgesics are unlikely to provide much relief. If the patient really needs diamorphine to achieve comfort, the result will be a patient in pain for several hours while waiting for the more simple analgesics to take effect before moving on to the next one, and so on.

There is nothing wrong with starting at the top, relieving the pain and then preventing its return with milder or more moderate analgesia, but be cautious – diamorphine for a headache is a little overzealous! Formal pain assessments can be very helpful in determining the severity of pain. Again, the patient may be the best judge and should be offered a choice where possible. Generally speaking, if the pain is mild to moderate then an analgesic for moderate pain will probably be effective. If it is moderate to severe then choose an analgesic for severe pain.

Combination therapies have had excellent results in acute pain. It may be useful to have oral preparations, e.g. codydramol or NSAIDs, prescribed and given regularly. Opiates can then be given for immediate pain relief and breakthrough pain, but the combination of opiates and moderate analgesics can reduce or delay the breakthrough resulting in better overall pain control.

'FAST-TRACK' PATIENTS

In the current political climate of the NHS there is a great surge towards day surgery and 'fast-tracking' patients through acute clinical areas. As recently as 1991, coronary artery bypass graft patients would be ventilated at least overnight and spend 24–48 hours in intensive care before being moved to a cardiothoracic ward. They would be expected to remain in hospital for approximately 7–10 days. Current management aims to reduce the amount of acute intervention and includes 'fast-tracking' some patients from theatre to high dependency care, bypassing ICU completely. Ventilation times have been reduced to a couple of hours in some areas, and in others, post-operative ventilation has been eradicated completely. Nowadays, patients can be in and out of hospital within 5 days.

The main problem here is that analgesia can be reduced rapidly – from morphine to coproxamol within 3–4 days. Not surprisingly, moderate to severe pain can persist even after discharge from hospital with inadequate pain relief available to the patient.

Similarly, patients in high dependency care receiving PCA or epidural analgesia may have their devices removed and be transferred to a general ward with a prescription for coproxamol only. The nurse should be aware of these potential

When your patient moves on, ensure that you know where he is going and that satisfactory arrangements have been made for ongoing pain control. The patient's pain does not stop when he leaves the HDU.

Fig. 11.7 Physiological consequences of unrelieved pain.

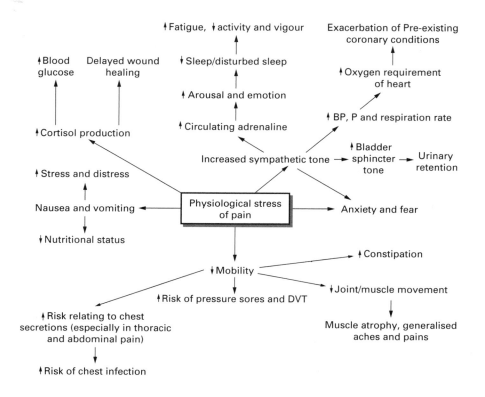

PHYSIOLOGICAL CONSEQUENCES OF UNRELIEVED PAIN

problems and ensure that a reasonable prescription for pain relief is written before discharging the patient from her care.

Many nurses believe that most experiences of acute pain, particularly post-operative pain, cannot be relieved or controlled completely, only reduced (Scott 1992, Hollinworth 1994). This is not true. A study by O'Hara (1994) showed that none of the patients received more than half of the opioid analgesia prescribed to them during the first 48 hours post-operatively, despite the fact that pain was the most common nursing problem among the group.

Leaving a patient in pain when pain relief is available is not only unnecessary and demoralising for the patient, it is morally and ethically unjustifiable. It can also have profound physiological consequences and impede optimal recovery (Ferguson 1995) (Fig. 11.7). Most nurses are taught that the 'classical' signs of acute pain are an increased pulse rate, blood pressure and respiratory rate. These are caused by a rise in sympathetic nervous system activity which, in turn, results in increased hormonal activity (Guyton 1986). The resulting hormonal activity leads to a rise in circulating adrenaline levels which result in increased arousal, consciousness and emotion – typically the 'fight or flight' response. This makes it difficult for the patient to sleep and rest naturally.

> Leaving a patient in pain when pain relief is available is not only unnecessary and demoralising, it is morally and ethically unjustifiable.

Unrelieved pain can cause patients to wake frequently during nocturnal sleep and usually they will not feel rested on waking (McCaffery & Beebe 1994, Knapp-Spooner et al 1995). After a day or two, the patient becomes fatigued which contributes to reduced vigour and physical activity (McCaffery & Beebe 1994, Knapp-Spooner et al 1995).

Severe pain inhibits movement. A patient may try to lie as still as possible in order to minimise pain. Early mobilisation will not be possible and so the patient is further at risk of developing complications of bedrest, such as chest infection, deep vein thrombosis, pressure sores and constipation (Bonica, cited in Hunt 1995). The latter problem may be further exacerbated by the constipating effects of opioid analgesics. Furthermore, lack of movement to minimise pain prevents the natural movement of the joints and muscles resulting in generalised aches and pains, and worsening pre-existing conditions such as arthritis. Muscle atrophy may occur if this is prolonged for more than a day or two.

Pain arising in the abdominal or thoracic regions can cause the patient difficulty with deep breathing and coughing. If unrelieved, secretions may be retained causing chest infection.

Other problems may arise in elderly patients or those with ischaemic heart conditions. The increased demand for oxygen by the heart from stimulation of the cardiovascular system (increased heart rate and blood pressure) may not be met if the coronary arteries cannot accommodate the necessary blood flow. This can lead to angina, ischaemic tissue damage and even infarction (Nursing Times 1995).

The effects of increased sympathetic tone can include reduced intestinal tone and gastric motility. This can further exacerbate the problems of nausea and vomiting which may result as a side effect of opioid drugs or from the pain itself. The patient becomes physically more stressed and emotionally distressed (Jackson 1995). The sphincter tone of the bladder is also affected which contributes to urinary retention (Jackson 1995).

Cortisol levels rise as a result of increased hormonal activity. This has an antagonistic effect on the action of insulin and hence blood sugars rise (Jackson 1995). This is of particular significance in diabetic patients. Insulin dependent diabetics will need an increased dose of insulin to maintain normoglycaemia, and non-insulin dependent diabetics may become insulin dependent during the immediate post-operative phase or during a period of acute illness.

Increased cortisol levels have an anti-inflammatory and catabolic effect and may cause a delay in wound healing (Grahame-Smith & Aronson 1992, Jackson 1995). This is a different mechanism to that encountered with NSAID analgesics which have a more selective effect on the inflammatory process.

Bach et al (cited in O'Hara 1994) suggest that poor peri-operative pain control can lead to sensitisation of the CNS, resulting in long-term pain when normally innocuous stimuli are perceived as painful for many months following surgery.

It should be remembered that a patient does not have to exhibit these physiological signs to be experiencing pain. We are not without our own defence mechanisms to deal with pain. The body has its own opioid analgesics, known as endorphins. It is thought that the release of endorphins is, in part, influenced by the higher centres of the brain, and this is possibly why psychological factors have an important impact on the perception and interpretation of pain (Nursing Times 1995). In fact, the placebo response may be due to the release of endogenous endorphins following the suggestion that pain should be relieved, and not the fact that the pain was imagined and not real in the first place (Gooch 1989, Hollinworth 1994).

> ■ **BOX 11.10** Psychosocial influences on pain perception
>
> • Personality
> • Culture
> • Gender
> • Previous experience
> • Biases

PSYCHOSOCIAL INFLUENCES AND

ALTERNATIVE PAIN RELIEVING STRATEGIES

Certain psychosocial factors can influence the way in which pain is perceived and interpreted both by the patient and by the nurse (Box 11.10).

Gender

Nurses' beliefs about pain and gender affect their clinical decisions. Many nurses believe that female patients more readily exhibit and report pain, have a lower pain tolerance and will exaggerate their pain more than men (Vallerand 1995). Some nurses believe that female patients should be given less narcotic analgesia than men, and decisions based on these beliefs may lead to inadequate treatment of pain in women (Vallerand 1995). Similar problems arise with culture.

> Do women and men feel pain differently? Do you have any personal beliefs about pain which might affect your clinical practice? Do you ever feel that a patient should behave as you feel you would yourself, if his pain were your own?

Culture

A patient's cultural background may influence how pain is perceived and responded to. Some cultures openly express emotions to pain, whereas others believe in the stoical 'stiff upper-lip' approach of emotional suppression.

A study by Madjar showed that Anglo-Australians preferred to be alone, regaining control of their behaviour and emotions, whereas Yugoslavs preferred to have company (Hiscock 1993).

Cultural beliefs should be taken into account when assessing the patient. Nurses should avoid prejudging and labelling a patient's pain on the basis of his nationality or culture as this can lead to misunderstanding and inadequate treatment. Nurses should be aware of how their own cultural biases can affect their nursing care.

Personality

Different personality types respond differently to pain problems, particularly in the healthcare setting. Extroverts tend to be more willing to report pain and request analgesia than introverts. On the other hand, introverts tend to be rewarded for their more stoical approach to pain (Hiscock 1993). Formal pain assessments can therefore be beneficial to introverts as it reduces the necessity of calling a nurse to ask for pain relief.

Personality also involves locus of control. This is the amount of control a person believes he has over certain outcomes. Those with an internal locus believe that their behaviour will influence their outcomes, whereas those with an external locus believe that they have little control. Fate, chance and the influence of powerful others are believed to affect the outcomes of patients with external locus of control (Younger et al 1995). Generally, patients with internal locus of control prefer to be more involved in pain management and respond better to PCA pumps than patients with external locus of control.

Personality can affect pain, but pain can also affect personality. Irritability and frustration can be a symptom of uncontrolled pain and patients may turn their anger on themselves or others (Hiscock 1993).

Previous experience

Inadequate pain relief in the past, or previous experience of poor nursing attitudes, can affect a patient's perception and reaction to pain. Previous experiences of close family members or friends can also influence pain perceptions (Hiscock 1993). This can increase anxiety in the patient which, in turn, can increase the perception and interpretation of pain.

Anxiety

Anxiety may be divided into two types:

- *State anxiety* – a temporary response to a specific situation
- *Trait anxiety* – a characteristic of an individual personality (Hiscock 1993).

Ill-health and admission to hospital are likely to generate anxiety to some degree or another, and this varies from one individual to another. Acute pain is closely associated with anxiety and it is thought that while pain generates anxiety, anxiety can also affect pain perception. The gate control theory postulates that inhibitory signals from the cortex, such as feelings of confidence and control can help close the gate. Unnecessary anxiety and heightened emotions can however lower the pain threshold, open the gate and allow pain impulses to pass (Weinman 1987, Davis 1993).

The gate theory highlights anxiety reduction as a factor inhibiting pain signal transmission. Many researchers (Hayward 1975, Sofaer 1992) have identified pre-operative information as a significant factor in reducing post-operative pain. Preparation for pain may reduce some of its impact by helping patients to increase their feelings of control over the painful stimulus (Weinman 1987). Unfortunately, not all pain can be predicted or prepared for, such as that encountered in trauma or acute illness. However, providing comfort, reassurance and an explanation of what is causing the pain helps remove the uncertainty and therefore reduces anxiety.

The giving of pre-operative information has become quite common practice in nursing, but who can predict the pain a patient may feel? The information given can only be as good as the individual nurse's knowledge and it should be remembered that pain is subjective. Gooch (1989) stated that nurses might rate certain diagnoses or procedures as resulting in a greater degree of pain than more minor ones, and judge pain accordingly. Another problem is what if the patient experiences more pain for much longer than expected from the preop chat? Would this then increase the level of anxiety as the patient may fear there is something amiss? There may be patients who find the best way of coping is not to know. These problems need to be thought through and may be picked up on initial assessment or on later pain assessments. The problems can then be addressed and reassurance and further information can be given as required.

Studies have shown that pre-operative anxiety correlates well with post-operative pain (Scott 1994). The increasing amount of day surgery has resulted in less time being made available for the psychological preparation of patients (Scott 1994). Therefore, there is a great deal of value in providing information regarding post-operative pain control at the 'pre-admission clinic' stage. This should further be seen as a priority for nursing staff working in day surgery units and should not be forgotten when admitting patients for emergency surgery.

■ **BOX 11.11** Pain relieving therapies

- Communication, explanation and education
- Analgesia
- Information and anxiety reduction
- Relaxation
- Distraction and imagery
- TENS
- Heat pads/cold compresses
- Massage
- Changing position and support on movement

The multidisciplinary team (MDT)

Nurses spend a lot of time with patients and are in a unique position to develop an understanding of each patient's pain and involve the MDT accordingly. It may be that the nurse is not the best person to advise the patient. Lyth (1995) found that physiotherapists had the greatest knowledge of phantom limb pain. The consultant did not believe in this syndrome and so the nursing staff became sceptical.

Physiotherapists can assist patients in many ways. They can help promote comfort and independence by teaching them the best way to move around in bed and to mobilise while supporting traumatised areas. Stoma therapy nurses may be the best people to alleviate anxiety in patients who have had stomas formed, and occupational therapists may best advise patients on aids and adaptations available in the home if they have undergone traumatic amputation of a limb.

A list of pain relieving therapies is given in Box 11.11.

Relaxation

As anxiety can reduce the pain threshold, it is thought that relaxation's therapeutic effect is primarily a result of anxiety reduction and may be perceived as increased control by the patient (Weinman 1987). Kent and Dalgliesh (1986) reported that taught relaxation techniques promote activity and reduce analgesia use. However, relaxation programmes are complex and not every nurse has the knowledge, ability or time to teach such programmes. It should be remembered though, that relaxation can be promoted in more simple ways, such as deep breathing exercises or assisting the patient to change into a more comfortable position (Willson 1992).

The importance of effective communication cannot be overstressed. Allowing a patient time to share any worries or fears may in itself relieve some pain (Hayward 1975, Sofaer 1992). This may be because of reduced anxiety, relaxation or perhaps because talking is a form of distraction. Along these lines is another method which aims to encourage the patient to interpret and evaluate information and pain signals in a less distressing way. If the patient can interpret pain in a positive way – for example, as evidence that the tissues are healing–rather than in a negative way (e.g. the tissue damage,) the anxiety surrounding the pain experience tends to be reduced (Kent & Dalgliesh 1986). It should be remembered that patients in acute pain find it extremely hard to relax and tend to tense various muscle groups, often adding to the growing discomfort. In high dependency care, this relaxation technique should be used in conjunction with adequate analgesia.

Distraction and imagery

Distraction therapy and imagery encourage the patient to divert his focus onto something other than the pain. This indicates that attention is limited and attention to one sensory source can reduce or abolish the awareness of another

> Talking about your pain, visualising it, may be a way of diminishing it – attention to one sensory source can reduce or even abolish awareness of another.

(Weinman 1987). This is supported by the gate control theory – adequate sensory stimulation will result in inhibitory impulses from the brain stem (McCaffery & Beebe 1994). Reading, watching television or listening to music have been cited as good distraction techniques, but it may be more difficult to achieve this adequately in hospital than at home. Nurses could encourage distraction in the ward setting but they should also recognise the limitations, particularly at night when distraction techniques to one patient may be disturbance to another. Again, distraction is difficult for a patient with acute pain and it is hard to concentrate on reading or watching television if the pain signals are strong. Although these techniques have some benefits and should not be dismissed, they will not overcome acute pain alone.

Physical therapies

These include the use of heat, cold, transcutaneous electrical nerve stimulation (TENS), massage and support. The gate control theory suggests that pain impulse transmission may be stopped or lessened by activity in the small diameter A nerve fibres, such as that experienced in skin stimulation (McCaffery & Beebe 1994). Many of these physical therapies act by achieving this effect.

Cold compresses are often used in soft tissue injuries (e.g. sprains) to help reduce swelling by reducing the blood flow to the affected area. The blood vessels are constricted by the cold and this helps prevent fluid movement from the vessels into the surrounding tissues. Pain can be relieved possibly as a result of cooling

---

CASE EXAMPLE 11.1

Mandy is a 19-year-old college student with sickle-cell anaemia. She has already had one shoulder replaced due to avascular necrosis, a direct result of her anaemia, and her left hip is now affected.

Mandy has an active social life which she shares with her boyfriend. They live together and plan to get married and start a family when Mandy has completed her studies.

Sickle-cell anaemia is a chronic pain condition with acute exacerbations when a sickle-cell crisis occurs. Crises can be brought on by almost anything – cold, stress, infections and dehydration being the most common causes. When a patient is 'sickling', the red blood cells take on a different shape (sickle shaped) and can become lodged in the capillaries. The resulting pain is ischaemic pain and has been likened to that experienced during a heart attack. This ischaemia can affect any organ or joint; cerebrovascular accidents are common in children and adults, sickle lung can result in devastating respiratory problems and sickling in the coronary arteries can lead to myocardial infarction.

Sickle-cell anaemia used to be regarded as a disease of childhood because so few sufferers lived to be adults. However, modern technology and research have resulted in better understanding of, and ability to treat, this condition.

Mandy copes well. She ensures her flat is kept warm to prevent the precipitation of a crisis through cold. Similarly, on a hot day she takes a coat with her in case the weather turns cold and she ensures she has plenty to drink to prevent dehydration. She has fallen behind in her studies, and although her tutors have tried to be understanding, her missed college time is beginning to cause added strain.

Mandy is a good example of having high dependency needs in pain control. She wants to be as independent as possible and to be discharged as soon as possible. In the past she has been labelled as a pethidine addict by nurses, not because she is, but because the nurses caring for her had very little understanding of her needs and the condition she has. Previously during a crisis, her pain has only been well controlled on 100 mg pethidine at

(Cont'd)

(Case example 11.1 cont'd)

2-hourly intervals. On several earlier admissions, she was prescribed 75 mg pethidine 3–4

hourly. This left her painfully short of analgesia for most of the time and she was left to count the minutes until her next injection was due. As a result she was accused of clock watching and being a pethidine addict.

Stress such as this can worsen and prolong a sickle-cell crisis, but can easily be resolved by proper assessment and understanding by nursing and medical staff. The main treatment for sickle-cell crisis comprises analgesia, i.v. fluids and oxygen. A complete assessment can reveal many factors which, put together, formulate a plan of care to meet Mandy's needs.

CASE EXAMPLE–RESOLUTION

Independence

Mandy wants to be as independent as possible. Her main problem is pain and so to achieve some independence with pain control a PCA pump should be considered.

Previous experience

Pethidine is not the only analgesic available to control sickle-cell pain. Diamorphine has been used effectively in PCA pumps and Entonox can provide relief for some breakthrough pain. Mandy finds pethidine and Entonox the most helpful. She also takes NSAIDs and dihydrocodeine to help control pain at home and would like to continue with these. An effective combination is usually achieved by trial and error, but a combination of analgesics is often more effective than one analgesic alone.

Stress

Mandy's previous admissions have made her wary of health professionals. Offering reassurance and showing an interest in Mandy's needs can help reduce her anxiety. She must always feel that her pain is believed by nurses, and that her interests are at the forefront of nursing care.

Mandy also has stress in her personal life – her college work, her relationship with her partner and the damage to her joints caused by her disease – may all be on her mind. Allowing her time to talk and/or offering to contact a sickle-cell counsellor (if available) may help allay some of her worries.

Cold

Being aware that cold and draughts can precipitate or prolong a crisis is important. Mandy should not be subjected to draughts from open windows, and should have enough bedclothes to keep her warm.

Alternative pain relief

It is always worth exploring alternative methods of pain relief. Like many others, Mandy finds heat pads very useful and she also enjoys listening to music to help her relax. Rubbing the affected joints during moments of pain can also give some relief. **NB** Ice packs should not be used with patients with sickle cell.

Rehydration

Hydration is important and i.v. fluids are often prescribed to help lessen the viscosity of the blood caused by sickling, and therefore reduce pain. Oral fluids should be encouraged, but if the patient finds it hard to drink 2–3 litres per day then alternatives should be explored.

(Case example 11.1 cont'd)

Mandy has poor venous access. To help her maintain her independence she completed her own fluid balance chart. She could not drink 2 litres per day and so subcutaneous fluids were discussed with her to help supplement her oral intake.

Hypoxia

Sickled cells do not carry oxygen properly, and if hypoxia occurs, other cells may begin to sickle, resulting in more pain. Mandy found it hard to tolerate an oxygen mask for long, and her saturations would drop while she was using Entonox. To overcome this, she tried nasal cannulae which she found more comfortable and could continue with oxygen therapy whilst using Entonox.

Partners

Mandy's partner also has needs. If he marries Mandy he marries her condition as well. Conception and childbearing can be a problem for patients with sickle cell and they may require counselling beforehand.

Financial problems exist – many patients find it hard to gain employment and often have problems getting mortgages and life insurance.

Involving partners in care can be very rewarding to the nurse, the patient and the partner. Mandy and her partner will have to continue managing her condition out of hospital, and so the more they are encouraged to participate in care in hospital, the less threatening the illness becomes to the 'outsider' (partner).

down nerve fibres which may reduce their capacity to transmit pain impulses. Cold also stimulates activity in the large diameter A fibres.

Heat pads promote blood flow to a local area and can therefore be beneficial in wound healing. Heat provides warmth and comfort and can help to relax tense muscles. Heat impulses are transmitted by A and C fibres, so may directly block some pain impulse transmission by the C fibres.

TENS has become increasingly popular in recent years as a method of pain control, but its use still appears to be largely confined to chronic pain. It can be used in acute pain and has been beneficial in reducing pain during dressing changes and for women in labour. It works by firing constant, small electrical impulses, mimicking skin stimulation. Other theorists speculate that TENS might act by stimulating the release of endorphins (Davis 1993).

Massage can promote relaxation and comfort, but can also reduce pain impulse transmission in a similar way to TENS. Many people oppose the use of 'true' massage as it can be dangerous or damaging if used by an inexperienced person. However, gentle hand and foot massages given to a patient during the course of conversation or a bedbath can be extremely relaxing and comforting, and aid in promoting pain relief.

Supports such as two towels taped up to make a solid pad are a simple but useful method of helping to control pain on coughing or movement if there is an abdominal or chest wound. The patient holds the pad firmly to the wound area to help support it during movement.

PROFESSIONAL ISSUES

The UKCC Code of Professional Conduct (1992) states that nurses should 'ensure that no action or omission on the nurse's part ... is detrimental to the interests, condition or safety of patients' and that nurses should act in the best interests of their clients.

Although nurses are not yet accountable for prescribing analgesia, they are responsible for the promotion of comfort and administering the analgesia prescribed (Hunt 1995). Lovett et al (1994) suggest that nurses have two specific roles to play in pain management:

- Assisting patients to assess their level of pain
- Providing the means to alleviate the pain.

Adequate pain control can make the difference between a good and bad experience of hospital and nursing care. Nearly all patients requiring high dependency care will experience pain at some time and nurses should be prepared to accept responsibility and accountability to ensure their patients receive proper pain mangement, both in hospital and on discharge.

Increasing awareness of pain management and formally assessing and evaluating nursing care will enhance professional credibility. Nurses have a responsibility to advocate on behalf of their patients if pain is not adequately controlled, involving the multidisciplinary team where necessary. Central to this is that nurses believe patients' reports of pain and that the patients' needs are at the forefront of nursing care. To ignore these needs or to deny pain relief is morally and ethically unjustifiable.

The profession itself has gone some way to addressing the pain management deficit by establishing pain management courses and changing basic nurse education with the advent of Project 2000 (Schofield 1995). However, nurses do not necessarily need to accumulate courses in order to provide effective pain management. They just have to think: 'would this be acceptable to me or a member of my family?'

CONCLUSION

Pause for a moment and reflect on an incident when you have looked after a patient in pain. Did you feel that you had all the information to hand and dealt with the situation with the patient's best interests at heart? Furthermore, if *you* were that patient would you have felt happy with your care? If the answer to this is 'no', then what could you have done to have managed the patient's pain better?

The aim of this chapter was to provide a comprehensive, realistic overview of acute pain management related to high dependency care. Some people may argue that nurses have little authority in pain management, but effective pain management is more than just the prescribing of analgesia. Pain is a noxious experience with complex physiological, psychological and social components. Nurses spend more time with patients on a personal level than any other member of the multidisciplinary team. As such, they are in a unique position to use their skills of communication and assessment to define problems from a patient's perspective, incorporating all the physical and psychosocial elements.

No two people will react to a painful experience or a particular therapy in the same way, or have exactly the same needs. Realistic care plans should be devised which can account for this uniqueness and put the patient's needs at the forefront of nursing care.

It is true that nurses have no accountability for prescribing drugs at present, but they do have responsibility and accountability for prescribing care, and for querying prescriptions and acting as the patient's advocate if the prescription is inadequate or ineffective. Nursing cannot be seen as a profession if it is prepared to sit back and allow poor standards of pain management to continue. As nurses, we can do a great deal to ensure that our patients receive the appropriate level of pain relief and subsequent pain control we would expect for ourselves in a similar situation.

REFERENCES

Audit Commission 1997 Anaesthesia under examination. Audit Commission, London

Audit Commission 1998 Managing pain after surgery. Audit Commission, London

Bond M 1979 Pain – its nature, analysis and treatment. Churchill Livingstone, New York

Carpenter J S, Brockopp D 1995 Comparison of patients' ratings and examination of nurses' responses to pain intensity rating scales. Cancer Nursing 18 (4) : 292–8

Cohen F L 1980 Post-surgical pain relief: patients' status and nurses' medication choices. Pain 9: 265–274

Critchley M (ed) 1986 Butterworth's medical dictionary, 2nd edn. Butterworth, London

Davis P 1993 Opening up the gate control theory. Nursing Standard 7(45): 25–27

Doverty N 1994 Make pain assessment your priority – practitioner led management of pain in trauma injuries. Professional Nurse January: 230–237

Ferguson J 1995 The development of a post-operative pain service (1): an overview. British Journal of Theatre Nursing 5(7): 28–31

Ferrell B R, McCaffery M, Ropchan R 1992 Pain management as a clinical challenge for nursing administration. Nursing Outlook 263–268

Gooch J 1989 Who should manage pain – patient or nurse? Professional Nurse 295–296

Grahame-Smith D G, Aronson J K 1992 Oxford textbook of clinical pharmacology and drug therapy. Oxford University Press, Oxford

Greenland S 1995 A review of the uses of epidural analgesia. Nursing Standard 9(32): 32–35

Guyton A 1986 Textbook of medical physiology, 7th edn. W B Saunders, Philadelphia

Hayward J 1975 Information – a prescription against pain. RCN Series 2, No 5. Royal College of Nursing, London

Hiscock M 1993 Setting up a patient-controlled analgesia service. British Journal of Intensive Care, 149–152

Hollinworth H 1994 No gain? Nursing Times 90(1): 24–27.

Hollinworth H 1995 Nurses' assessment and management of pain at wound dressing changes. Journal of Wound Care 4(2): 77–83

Hunt K 1995 Perceptions of patients' pain: a study assessing nurses' attitudes. Nursing Standard 10(4): 32–35

Hunter D 1991 Relief through teamwork. Nursing Times 87(17): 35–38

Jackson A 1995 Acute pain – its physiology and the pharmacology of analgesia. Nursing Times 91(16): 27–28

Jacques A 1994a Physiology of pain. British Journal of Nursing 3(12): 607–610

Jacques A 1994b Epidural analgesia. British Journal of Nursing 3(14): 734–738

Kent G, Dalgliesh M 1986 Psychology and medical care, 2nd edn. Baillire Tindall, Eastbourne

Kim H S, Schwartz-Barcott D, Holter I M et al 1995 Developing a translation of the McGill pain questionnaire for cross-cultural comparison: an example from Norway. Journal of Advanced Nursing 21: 421–426

Knapp-Spooner C, Karlik B, Pontieri-Lewis V et al 1995 Efficacy of patient-controlled analgesia in women cholecystectomy patients. International Journal of Nursing Studies. 32(5): 434–442

Kuhn S, Cook K, Collins M et al 1990 Perceptions of pain after surgery. British Medical Journal 300: 1687–1690

Leddy S, Pepper J M 1989 Conceptual bases of professional nursing, 2nd edn. J B Lippincott, Philadelphia

Lovett P E, Stanton S L, Hennessy D et al 1994 Pain relief after major gynaecological surgery. British Journal of Nursing 3(4): 159–162

Lyth H 1995 Invisible problem. Nursing Times 91(19): 38–40

McCaffery M, Beebe A 1994 Pain – clinical manual for nursing practice. Mosby/Times Mirror, London

Meinhart N, McCaffery M 1983 Pain – a nursing approach to assessment and analysis. Appleton Century Croft, Connecticut

Nursing Times 1995 Pain – knowledge for practice. Professional Development Series Unit 20 part 1/3. Nursing Times 91(36)

O'Connor L 1995a Pain assessment by patients and nurses, and nurses' notes on it, in early acute myocardial infarction. Part 1. Intensive and Critical Care Nursing 230–237

O'Connor L 1995 Pain assessment by patients and nurses, and nurses' notes on it, in early acute myocardial infarction. Part 2. Intensive and Critical Care Nursing 10: 283–292

O'Hara R 1994 Changing practice in pain management. Nursing Standard 8(39): 25–28

Paice J, Mahon M, Faut-Callaghan M 1991 Factors associated with adequate pain control in hospitalized post-surgical patients diagnosed with cancer. Cancer Nursing 14(6): 298–305

Park G, Fulton B 1992 The management of acute pain. Oxford University Press, Oxford

Pasero C L, McCaffery M 1994 Avoiding opioid-induced respiratory depression. Australian Journal of Nursing 25–30

Rang H P, Dale M M 1987 Pharmacology. Churchill Livingstone, Edinburgh

Royal College of Surgeons and College of Anaesthetists 1990 Pain after surgery. Royal College of Surgeons, London

Saxey S 1986 Nurses' response to post-operative pain. Nursing 3(10): 377–381

Schofield P 1995 Using assessment tools to help patients in pain. Professional Nurse 10(11): 703–706

Scott I 1992 Nurses' attitudes to pain control and the use of pain assessment scales. British Journal of Nursing 2(1): 11–16

Scott I 1994 Effectiveness of documented assessment of post-operative pain. British Journal of Nursing 3(10): 494–501

Seers K 1987 Perceptions of pain. Nursing Times 33(48): 37–39.

Sofaer B 1992 Pain – a handbook for nurses 2nd edn. Chapman & Hall, London

Thomas N 1995 Patient-controlled analgesia. Nursing Standard 9(35): 31–35

United Kingdom Central Council for Nursing, Midwifery and Health Visiting 1992 Code of professional conduct. UKCC, London

Vallerand A H 1995 Gender differences in pain. Image: Journal of Nursing Scholarship 27 (3): 235–237

Wakefield A 1995 Pain – an account of nurses' talk. Journal of Advanced Nursing 21: 905–910.

Walker J 1991 Living with pain. Nursing Times 87(43): 28–32

Weinman J 1987 An outline of psychology as applied to medicine, 2nd edn. Wright, UK

Wilkinson R 1996 A non-pharmacological approach to pain relief. Professional Nurse 11(4): 222–224

Willson H 1992 Painful facts. Nursing Times 88(35): 32–33

Woodward S 1995 Nurse and patient perceptions of pain. Professional Nurse 10(7): 415–416

Younger J, Marsh K J, Grap M J 1995 The relationship of health locus of control and cardiac rehabilitation to mastery of illness-related stress. Journal of Advanced Nursing 22: 294–299

Index

Page number in **bold** indicate figures
and tables.